Current Concepts in the Management of Proximal Interphalangeal Joint Disorders

Editor

KEVIN C. CHUNG

HAND CLINICS

www.hand.theclinics.com

Consulting Editor
KEVIN C. CHUNG

May 2018 • Volume 34 • Number 2

ELSEVIER

1600 John F. Kennedy Boulevard • Suite 1800 • Philadelphia, Pennsylvania, 19103-2899

http://www.theclinics.com

HAND CLINICS Volume 34, Number 2
May 2018 ISSN 0749-0712, ISBN-13: 978-0-323-58356-5

Editor: Lauren Boyle
Developmental Editor: Kristen Helm

Hand Clinics (ISSN 0749-0712) is published quarterly by Elsevier Inc., 360 Park Avenue South, New York, NY 10010-1710. Months of publication are February, May, August, and November. Business and Editorial Offices: 1600 John F. Kennedy Blvd., Ste. 1800, Philadelphia, PA 19103-2899. Customer Service Office: 3251 Riverport Lane, Maryland Heights, MO 63043. Periodicals postage paid at New York, NY and at additional mailing offices. Subscription price is $422.00 per year (domestic individuals), $772.00 per year (domestic institutions), $100.00 per year (domestic students/residents), $481.00 per year (Canadian individuals), $898.00 per year (Canadian institutions), $541.00 per year (international individuals), $898.00 per year (international institutions), and $256.00 per year (international and Canadian students/residents). Foreign air speed delivery is included in all *Clinics* subscription prices. All prices are subject to change without notice. **POSTMASTER:** Send address changes to *Hand Clinics*, Elsevier Health Sciences Division, Subscription Customer Service, 3251 Riverport Lane, Maryland Heights, MO 63043. Customer Service (orders, claims, online, change of address): Elsevier Health Sciences Division, Subscription **Customer Service, 3251 Riverport Lane, Maryland Heights, MO 63043. Tel: 1-800-654-2452 (U.S. and Canada); 314-447-8871 (outside U.S. and Canada). Fax: 314-447-8029. E-mail: journalscustomerservice-usa@elsevier.com (for print support); journalsonlinesupport-usa@elsevier.com (for online support)**.

Reprints. For copies of 100 or more of articles in this publication, please contact the Commercial Reprints Department, Elsevier Inc., 360 Park Avenue South, New York, New York 10010-1710. Tel.: 212-633-3874; Fax: 212-633-3820; E-mail: reprints@elsevier.com.

Hand Clinics is covered in *MEDLINE/PubMed (Index Medicus), Current Contents/Clinical Medicine, EMBASE/Excerpta Medica,* and *ISI/BIOMED.*

Contributors

CONSULTING EDITOR

KEVIN C. CHUNG, MD, MS
Chief of Hand Surgery, University of Michigan
Health System, Charles B.G. de Nancrede
Professor of Plastic Surgery and Orthopaedic
Surgery, Assistant Dean for Faculty Affairs,
Associate Director of Global REACH,
University of Michigan Medical School,
Ann Arbor, Michigan, USA

EDITOR

KEVIN C. CHUNG, MD, MS
Chief of Hand Surgery, University of Michigan
Health System, Charles B.G. de Nancrede
Professor of Plastic Surgery and Orthopaedic
Surgery, Assistant Dean for Faculty Affairs,
Associate Director of Global REACH,
University of Michigan Medical School,
Ann Arbor, Michigan, USA

AUTHORS

EMILY ALTMAN, DPT, CHT
Hospital for Special Surgery, New York,
New York, USA

FRANCIS J. AVERSANO, MD
Department of Orthopedic Surgery,
Washington University School of Medicine
in St. Louis, St Louis, Missouri, USA

NICHOLAS M. CAGGIANO, MD
Hand Surgery Fellow, Department of
Orthopaedic Surgery, Beth Israel Deaconess
Medical Center, Boston, Massachusetts,
USA

RYAN P. CALFEE, MD, MSc
Associate Professor, Department of
Orthopedic Surgery, Washington University
School of Medicine in St. Louis, St Louis,
Missouri, USA

JAMES CHANG, MD
Chief, Division of Plastic and Reconstructive
Surgery, Johnson & Johnson Distinguished
Professor of Surgery (Plastic Surgery) &
Orthopedic Surgery, Hand & Microsurgery,
Stanford University, Palo Alto, California, USA

KEVIN C. CHUNG, MD, MS
Chief of Hand Surgery, University of Michigan
Health System, Charles B.G. de Nancrede
Professor of Plastic Surgery and Orthopaedic
Surgery, Assistant Dean for Faculty Affairs,
Associate Director of Global REACH,
University of Michigan Medical School,
Ann Arbor, Michigan, USA

CASEY M. DEDEUGD, MD
Resident, Department of Orthopedic
Surgery, Mayo Clinic, Rochester, Minnesota,
USA

NATHAN P. DOUGLASS, MD
Hand Fellow, Department of Orthopedic
Surgery, Robert A. Chase Hand & Upper Limb
Center, Stanford University, Redwood City,
California, USA

PAIGE M. FOX, MD, PhD
Assistant Professor, Department of Surgery,
Division of Plastic Surgery, Stanford University,
Palo Alto, California, USA

CHARLES A. GOLDFARB, MD
Professor and Vice Chair, Department of
Orthopedic Surgery, Chief, Pediatric and
Adolescent Orthopedic Surgery, Co-Chief,
Hand and Microsurgery Service, Washington
University School of Medicine in St. Louis,
St Louis, Missouri, USA

RANJAN GUPTA, MD
Professor, Orthopaedic Surgery, University of
California, Irvine, Orange, California, USA

BRANDON HAGHVERDIAN, MD
Resident Physician, Orthopaedic Surgery,
University of Pennsylvania, Philadelphia,
Pennsylvania, USA

CARL M. HARPER, MD
Instructor, Department of Orthopaedic
Surgery, Harvard Medical School, Beth Israel
Deaconess Medical Center, Boston,
Massachusetts, USA

JAMES P. HIGGINS, MD
Chief of Hand Surgery and Attending Surgeon,
The Curtis National Hand Center, MedStar
Union Memorial Hospital, Associate Professor,
Department of Plastic Surgery, Johns Hopkins
University School of Medicine, Baltimore,
Maryland, USA; Associate Professor,
Georgetown University School of Medicine,
Division of Plastic Surgery, Washington, DC,
USA; Adjunct Associate Professor of Surgery,
University of Pennsylvania School of Medicine,
Division of Plastic Surgery, Philadelphia,
Pennsylvania, USA

HELEN E. HUETTEMAN, BS
Research Assistant, Department of Surgery,
Section of Plastic Surgery, University of
Michigan, Ann Arbor, Michigan, USA

ELIZABETH INKELLIS, MD
Hospital for Special Surgery, New York,
New York, USA

JAMES JUNG, MD
Resident Physician, Orthopaedic Surgery,
University of California, Irvine, Orange,
California, USA

SIRICHAI KAMNERDNAKTA, MD
International Research Fellow, Department
of Surgery, Section of Plastic Surgery,
University of Michigan, Ann Arbor, Michigan,
USA; Division of Plastic Surgery, Department
of Surgery, Faculty of Medicine, Siriraj
Hospital, Mahidol University, Bangkok,
Thailand

RYAN D. KATZ, MD
Attending Surgeon, The Curtis National Hand
Center, MedStar Union Memorial Hospital,
Baltimore, Maryland, USA

AMY L. LADD, MD
Professor, Department of Orthopedic Surgery,
Robert A. Chase Hand & Upper Limb Center,
Stanford University, Redwood City, California,
USA

W.P. ANDREW LEE, MD
Milton T. Edgerton, MD Professor and
Chairman, Department of Plastic and
Reconstructive Surgery, Johns Hopkins
University School of Medicine, Baltimore,
Maryland, USA

ERIC QUAN PANG, MD
Department of Orthopaedic Surgery, Stanford
University, Stanford, California, USA

PAYMON RAHGOZAR, MD
Hand Fellow, Department of Surgery,
Section of Plastic Surgery, University of
Michigan, Ann Arbor, Michigan, USA

MARCO RIZZO, MD
Professor of Orthopedics, Department of
Orthopedic Surgery, Mayo Clinic, Rochester,
Minnesota, USA

TAMARA D. ROZENTAL, MD
Chief, Hand and Upper Extremity Surgery,
Associate Professor, Department of
Orthopaedic Surgery, Harvard Medical
School, Beth Israel Deaconess Medical
Center, Boston, Massachusetts,
USA

BRADLEY HART SAITTA, MD
Resident, Department of Orthopaedic Surgery
and Rehabilitation Medicine, University
of Chicago Hospitals, Chicago, Illinois,
USA

SAMI H. TUFFAHA, MD
Resident, Department of Plastic and
Reconstructive Surgery, Johns Hopkins
University School of Medicine, Baltimore,
Maryland, USA

JENNIFER MORIATIS WOLF, MD
Professor, Department of Orthopaedic
Surgery and Rehabilitation Medicine,
University of Chicago Hospitals, Chicago,
Illinois, USA

SCOTT WOLFE, MD
Hospital for Special Surgery, New York,
New York, USA

MICHIRO YAMAMOTO, MD, PhD
International Research Fellow, Department of
Surgery, Section of Plastic Surgery, University of
Michigan Health System, Ann Arbor, Michigan,
USA; Associate Professor, Department of Hand
Surgery, Nagoya University Graduate School of
Medicine, Nagoya, Aichi, Japan

SARAH M. YANNASCOLI, MD
Hand and Microsurgery Fellow, Department of
Orthopedic Surgery, Washington University
School of Medicine in St. Louis, St Louis,
Missouri, USA

JEFFREY YAO, MD
Department of Orthopaedic Surgery, Stanford
University, Stanford, California, USA

ANDY F. ZHU, MD
Orthopaedic Surgery Resident, Department of
Orthopaedic Surgery, University of Michigan,
Ann Arbor, Michigan, USA

Contents

Anatomy and Biomechanics of the Finger Proximal Interphalangeal Joint 121

Eric Quan Pang and Jeffrey Yao

A complete understanding of the normal anatomy and biomechanics of the proximal interphalangeal joint is critical when treating pathology of the joint as well as in the design of new reconstructive treatments. The osseous anatomy dictates the principles of motion at the proximal interphalangeal joint. Subsequently, the joint is stabilized throughout its motion by the surrounding proximal collateral ligament, accessory collateral ligament, and volar plate. The goal of this article is to review the normal anatomy and biomechanics of the proximal interphalangeal joint and its associated structures, most importantly the proper collateral ligament, accessory collateral ligament, and volar plate.

Surgical Exposure of the Proximal Interphalangeal Joint 127

Casey M. DeDeugd and Marco Rizzo

There are 3 main surgical approaches to the proximal interphalangeal (PIP) joint, dorsal, volar, and lateral, and several described modifications to these main approaches. Historically, the dorsal approach has been the standard for the most common procedures of the PIP joint. The volar approach is advantageous for surgical interventions requiring access to the volar plate. It spares the central slip insertion from possible disruption, as does the lateral approach. This article describes the surgical approaches to the PIP joint, explains the rationale for choosing each approach, and discusses some of the most common complications.

Treating Proximal Interphalangeal Joint Dislocations 139

Bradley Hart Saitta and Jennifer Moriatis Wolf

Proximal interphalangeal (PIP) joint dislocation is a common injury. Usually, concentric stable reduction can be achieved with closed reduction. Occasionally, PIP joint dislocations are irreducible and open reduction is necessary. Complications include prolonged splinting and delay in presentation with subluxation or persistent dislocation. Surgery is often recommended for contracture or joint reduction. Surgical techniques focus on contracture release, joint reduction, and range of motion. Techniques have evolved from primary repair to tenodesis and suture anchor reconstruction. Most studies on PIP joint dislocations are retrospective case reports with good outcomes, but chronic mild contracture and deformity are consistent in the literature.

Management of Proximal Interphalangeal Joint Fracture Dislocations 149

Nicholas M. Caggiano, Carl M. Harper, and Tamara D. Rozental

Fracture dislocations of the proximal interphalangeal (PIP) joint of the finger are often caused by axial load applied to a flexed joint. The most common injury pattern is a dorsal fracture dislocation with a volar lip fracture of the middle phalanx. Damage to the soft-tissue stabilizers of the PIP joint contributes to the deformity seen with these fracture patterns. Unfortunately, these injuries are commonly written off and left untreated. A late-presenting PIP joint fracture dislocation has a poor chance of regaining normal range of motion. The provider must be suspicious of these injuries. Treatment options and algorithm are reviewed.

Swan neck and boutonniere deformities of the proximal interphalangeal (PIP) joint are challenging to treat. In a swan neck deformity, the PIP joint is hyperextended with flexion at the distal interphalangeal (DIP) joint. In a boutonniere deformity, there is flexion of the PIP joint with hyperextension of the DIP joint. When the deformities are flexible, treatment begins with splinting. However, when the deformity is fixed, serial casting or surgery is often necessary to restore joint motion before surgical correction. Many surgical techniques have been described to treat both conditions. Unfortunately, incomplete correction and deformity recurrence are common.

This article is an in-depth analysis of proximal interphalangeal joint arthrodesis indications and surgical techniques. There is a wide variety of indications for proximal interphalangeal joint arthrodesis with relatively few contraindications. Moreover, although there is a limited surgical approach, there is a wide breadth of modalities in which to obtain the arthrodesis, of which several are listed here. Proximal interphalangeal joint arthrodesis has been shown to have excellent outcomes and a high success rate.

Proximal interphalangeal (PIP) joint arthritis is a debilitating condition. The complexity of the joint makes management particularly challenging. Treatment of PIP arthritis requires an understanding of the biomechanics of the joint. PIP joint arthroplasty is one treatment option that has evolved over time. Advances in biomaterials have improved and expanded arthroplasty design. This article reviews biomechanics and arthroplasty design of the PIP joint.

This article analyzes various surgical exposures and implant designs for proximal interphalangeal (PIP) joint pathology. A literature review by the authors found that silicone implants using a volar approach had the best arc of motion, least extension lag, and lowest complication rates compared with all the other implant designs and approaches. Surface replacement arthroplasties had more frequent surgical revisions compared with silicone implants. Continued efforts toward the development of improved PIP joint implants are necessary.

Microvascular toe interphalangeal joint transfer can serve as a means of autogenous digit proximal interphalangeal joint (PIPJ) arthroplasty. Among surgical options for treating dysfunctional, absent, or destroyed PIPJs, free toe joint transfer is the most technically challenging and carries the greatest donor site cost to patients. Despite drawbacks, free toe joint transfer is a valuable tool with considerable advantages over conventional arthroplasty in the appropriate clinical setting. Particular advantages include lifelong durability, coronal plane stability, low infection risk, and growth potential in skeletally immature patients. This technique requires a balanced assessment of the risk-to-benefit ratio for each patient.

Salvaging a failed proximal interphalangeal (PIP) joint implant arthroplasty remains a considerable technical and rehabilitation challenge. Experienced arthroplasty surgeons have reported 70% survival of revision PIP implants at 10 years. with 25% of patients requiring subsequent revision surgery. At this time, there is no consensus surgical approach or implant proven superior for revision implant arthroplasty of the PIP joint. Secondary arthrodesis or amputation may be required to salvage the failed PIP implant arthroplasty with compromised bone stock or soft tissue envelopes that are inadequate for implant arthroplasty.

Proximal interphalangeal joint (PIPJ) flexion contracture is a challenging and often frustrating problem. Treatment of PIPJ contracture begins with conservative measures. With good compliance and prolonged use, favorable results can be achieved using these modalities. For contractures that fail to respond to conservative treatment, surgical intervention can be considered. The affected structures that can be released during surgery include the accessory collateral ligaments, volar plate, checkrein ligaments, retinacular ligaments, and flexor and extensor tendons. A stepwise approach to release is typically favored in which active motion is tested after each release to determine the need for subsequent releases.

The management of congenital proximal interphalangeal joint deformity, also known as camptodactyly, is challenging. There are numerous theories on the cause of this abnormal finger posture, leading to variations in classification, definition, and treatment approaches. This article assesses the previous literature and provides clarity and guidance for the practical treatment of camptodactyly.

Flexor pulley ruptures with severe proximal interphalangeal (PIP) joint contracture present a complex challenge for the hand surgeon. Four patients were treated with a delayed presentation of pulley rupture and fixed PIP flexion contracture with a technique of external extension torque application followed by splinting without pulley reconstruction. Using this technique, the PIP joint contractures improved from an average of 66° to an average of 19°, patient satisfaction was high, and the pulley injuries were managed with splinting alone without open pulley reconstruction.

Complications of Proximal Interphalangeal Joint Injuries: Prevention and Treatment

Sirichai Kamnerdnakta, Helen E. Huetteman, and Kevin C. Chung

Proximal interphalangeal joint injuries are one of the most common injuries of the hand. The severity of injury can vary from a minor sprain to a complex intraarticular fracture. Because of the complex anatomy of the joint, complications may occur even after an appropriate treatment. This article provides a comprehensive review on existing techniques to manage complications and imparts practical points to help prevent further complications after proximal interphalangeal joint injury.

Therapy Concepts for the Proximal Interphalangeal Joint

Nathan P. Douglass and Amy L. Ladd

The principles of hand therapy for proximal interphalangeal joint disorders include protecting injured structures, minimizing patient discomfort, and optimizing patient recovery. Comprehension of hand anatomy, the nature of the injury being treated, and the phases of healing are critical when designing a safe and effective hand therapy program. Hand therapists use a combination of orthoses, guided exercises, and modalities to improve edema, sensitivity, range of motion, and function.

HAND CLINICS

THE CLINICS ARE AVAILABLE ONLINE!
Access your subscription at:
www.theclinics.com

HAND CLINICS

Preface

Current Concepts in the Management of Proximal Interphalangeal Joint Disorders

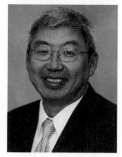

Kevin C. Chung, MD, MS
Editor

The proximal interphalangeal (PIP) joint facilitates the motion of the fingers, first initiated through the arc of the metacarpophalangeal joint in completing the Fibonacci curve through the PIP joint and ending with the terminal distal interphalangeal joint. The PIP joint plays a crucial role in the motion of the hand in rendering precision and strength for functional performance. However, the PIP joint often is subjected to traumatic insult and is afflicted with a number of arthritic conditions. It is one of the most commonly injured joints in sports activities. Furthermore, arthritic conditions, including osteoarthritis and rheumatoid arthritis, destroy the articular surfaces and ligamentous support, causing chronic pain and limited function.

Because of the multitude of injuries and diseases affecting this joint, this issue of *Hand Clinics* provides much needed guidance regarding the latest evidence on prevention and treatment. This issue is dedicated to the Sterling Bunnell Fellowship in honoring the father of hand surgery, who promoted the practice during World War II. Dr Bunnell traveled around the country to teach the principles of this discipline. In the spirit of education and research, the American Foundation for Surgery of the Hand launched the Sterling Bunnell Fellowship in 1981, and, 36 years later, countless Sterling Bunnell Fellows have represented the American Society for Surgery of the Hand as ambassadors of the society to institutions in the United States and around the world. All of the articles in this issue were contributed by past Sterling Bunnell Fellows in collaboration with their trainees or junior faculty members. The Bunnell Fellows represent the ideals of the American Society for Surgery of the Hand to promote innovative care of hand surgery patients through inquiry and discovery.

This issue provides contemporary insight on this critical joint to help you take care of your patients predictably and effectively. I am grateful to my fellow Sterling Bunnell Fellows, who make my editing job so much easier by delivering scholarly contributions that require virtually no revisions. I hope you will enjoy reading these articles as much as I have.

Kevin C. Chung, MD, MS
Michigan Medicine
University of Michigan Medical School
2130 Taubman Center, SPC 5340
1500 East Medical Center Drive
Ann Arbor, MI 48109, USA

E-mail address:
kecchung@med.umich.edu

hand.theclinics.com

Hand Clin 34 (2018) xiii
https://doi.org/10.1016/j.hcl.2018.01.002
0749-0712/18/© 2018 Published by Elsevier Inc.

Anatomy and Biomechanics of the Finger Proximal Interphalangeal Joint

Eric Quan Pang, MD, Jeffrey Yao, MD*

KEYWORDS

- Proximal interphalangeal joint • Proper collateral ligament • Accessory collateral ligament
- Volar plate • Anatomy • Biomechanics

KEY POINTS

- The proximal interphalangeal joint is more than a simple hinge and has motion in the axial, coronal, and sagittal planes.
- The proper collateral ligament is the primary lateral stabilizer of the proximal interphalangeal joint in flexion.
- The accessory collateral ligament and volar plate confer stability in extension.

INTRODUCTION

The proximal interphalangeal joint (PIPJ) is a complex anatomic structure. There are several variations on surgical approaches to the PIPJ via volar, dorsal, or lateral incisions.[1] Regardless of the approach used, a complete understanding of the anatomy is critical. The basic anatomy of the PIPJ is well described, yet there continues to be new research regarding the mechanical properties and subsequent contributions of the various associated structures to the stability and motion of the PIPJ. The purpose of this article is to review the normal anatomy and biomechanics of the PIPJ and its associated ligamentous structures, most importantly the proper collateral ligament (PCL), accessory collateral ligament (ACL), and volar plate.

OSSEOUS ANATOMY

The osseous anatomy of the PIPJ plays an important role in the joint's stability. The PIPJ is composed of the articulation between the head of the proximal phalanx and the base of the middle phalanx.

The head of the proximal phalanx has a trapezoidal configuration in the axial plane divided by the intercondylar groove that increases in depth from dorsal to volar (**Fig 1**).[2–4] In the sagittal plane, the articular surface is tilted palmarly 1° to 29° with the articular surface spanning 160° to 210° without significant difference between the radial and ulnar condyles (**Fig 2**).[2,3,5] On the radial and ulnar surfaces of the proximal phalangeal head, there are concave areas dorsally from which the collateral ligaments arise and there is a subsequent large flat area that extends from the concave area to the joint surface.[2,4] Lastly, in the coronal plane, there is not much difference in condylar width of the radial and ulnar condyles of the proximal phalanx.[6]

The anatomy of the middle phalanx acts as a counterpart to that of the proximal phalanx. In the axial plane, the middle phalangeal base is composed of 2 asymmetric concave ellipses separated by a median ridge that corresponds with the intercondylar groove of the proximal phalanx (see **Fig 1**).[5] The dorsal extent of the median ridge serves as the insertion point of the central slip of the extensor mechanism.[2,4] On the volar side there is a rough, flat area proximally to which the volar plate inserts. Additionally, there are small tubercles radially and ulnarly to which there are

Department of Orthopaedic Surgery, Stanford University, 300 Pasteur Drive, Room R144, Stanford, CA 94305-5341, USA
* Corresponding author.
E-mail address: jyao@stanford.edu

Hand Clin 34 (2018) 121–126
https://doi.org/10.1016/j.hcl.2017.12.002
0749-0712/18/© 2017 Elsevier Inc. All rights reserved.

hand.theclinics.com

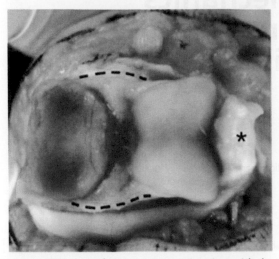

Fig. 1. Axial view of PIPJ. Intraoperative view with the PIPJ shot gunned open. The PCL (*dashed lines*) and volar plate (*asterisks*) are visualized by this approach as well. (*From* Cheah AE, Yao J. Surgical approaches to the proximal interphalangeal joint. J Hand Surg Am 2016;41(2):302; with permission.)

some capsular attachments.[2,4] In the sagittal plane, the middle phalanx is biconcavoconvex to match the bicondylar proximal phalanx with the concave portion separating the convex areas. Overall there is approximately 64° of articular surface in this plane.[3] The depth of the concavities of the middle phalanx depends on the height of the corresponding condyles of the proximal phalanx.[5]

OSSEOUS MECHANICS

The mechanics of the PIPJ were originally described as a hinge model. However, subsequent observations have demonstrated that the articulation is not, in fact, a perfect hinge because of the incongruities at the PIPJ between the proximal and middle phalanx.[2,7] In the coronal plane, there is a mismatch between the radius of curvature of the middle phalanx and the proximal phalanx creating 2 points of contact located centrally to the condyles of the proximal phalanx (**Fig 3**).[3] Thus, the PIPJ has

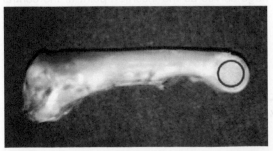

Fig. 2. Lateral view of proximal phalanx. Flat area circled (*red*).

potential for motion in abduction/adduction, axial rotation, and sagittal rotation around the center of rotation of the condyles of the proximal phalanx as well as the center of rotation of the concavity of the middle phalanx. Rotation about the center of rotation of the condyles of the proximal phalanx allows for motion without translation of the point of contact or line of force between the two articulations. Rotation around the center of rotation of the middle phalanx, however, results in dorsal migration of the point of contact and axial force on the middle phalanx and results in joint space widening. In reality, rotation occurs simultaneously around both centers of rotation resulting in rotation around the "instantaneous rotational axis"[3] which lies on the line between the two centers of rotation. More complex motion than a simple hinge is further supported by the work of Hess and colleagues[8] who used a combination of computed tomography (CT) imaging and motion capture to create a 3-dimensional (3D) model of the PIPJ demonstrating motion in the axial, coronal, and sagittal planes.

COLLATERAL LIGAMENT ANATOMY

The collateral ligament complex is composed of the proper and accessory collateral ligaments (**Fig 4**). The collateral ligaments are primarily composed of type I and III collagen with type I collagen being the dominant type based on recent messenger RNA (mRNA) analysis.[9] These laterally based ligaments span the PIPJ and serve to support against varus and valgus motion in different degrees of flexion. The details of the anatomy and function are discussed next.

PROPER COLLATERAL LIGAMENTS

The PCL was previously described in anatomic studies as a cordlike structure arising eccentrically from the concavities on the radial and ulnar proximal phalangeal head.[2,4] Recent microscopic analysis suggests that the origin of the PCL extends more proximal and dorsal to the radial and ulnar concavities of the proximal phalangeal heads than previously described. In regard to the orientation of the fibers, Allison[6] used histologic analysis to describe differential orientation of the dorsal and volar fibers of the PCL. His work demonstrates the dorsal fibers are more parallel to the middle phalanx and the volar fibers are oriented more obliquely to the joint line. The insertion has been classically described as a long broad insertion that blends with the volar plate and periosteum.[2,10] Allison[6] did not observe a confluence between the PCL and volar plate in his dissection but did acknowledge that subtle confluence may be difficult to

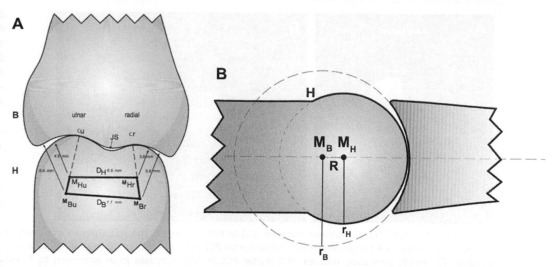

Fig. 3. Osseous biomechanics. (*A*) In the coronal plane, the concavities of the proximal phalanx (H) each have a contact point (contact point radial [Cr], contact point ulnar [Cu]) with the base of the middle phalanx (B). Note that there is a small joint cavity between the heads of the distal proximal phalanx (JS). Notably, there are differential centers of rotation of the concavities of the distal phalanx (M_{Br} and M_{Bu}) and the convexities of the proximal phalanx (M_{Hr} and M_{Hu}). The distance between the different centers of rotation are noted as D_H and D_B. (*B*) In the sagittal plane, rotation about the center of rotation of the condyles of the proximal phalanx (M_B) allows for motion without translation compared with rotation around the center of rotation of the middle phalanx (M_H), which results in translation of the articulation point. (*From* Dumont C, Albus G, Kubein-Meesenburg D, et al. Morphology of the interphalangeal joint surface and its functional relevance. J Hand Surg Am 2008;33(1):9–18; with permission.)

identify consistently. Regardless, recognizing the broad origin and insertion can be beneficial during the various exposures, as the PCL can be recessed from its origin and/or insertion to increase exposure rather than fully releasing the ligament.[1]

ACCESSORY COLLATERAL LIGAMENTS

The ACL is not as well defined as the PCL but arises from the volar portion of the PCL and inserts on the volar plate. The ACL is deep to and

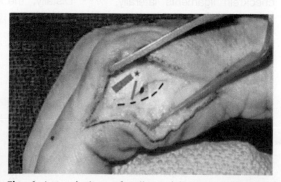

Fig. 4. Lateral view of collateral ligament complex. Lateral exposure of the PIPJ exposing the proper collateral ligament (*thick blue line*), accessory collateral ligament (*thin blue line*), and volar plate (*dashed black line*). The *asterisk* represents the P1 head. (*From* Cheah AE, Yao J. Surgical approaches to the proximal interphalangeal joint. J Hand Surg Am 2016;41(2):299; with permission.)

contiguous with the transverse retinacular ligament. Although not as substantial as the PCL, the ACL serves to suspend the volar plate as well as complete the capsule. The inner portion is lined by synovial tissue.[2,6] The ligament has a more oblique orientation in extension with the palmar fibers shorter than the dorsal fibers. In flexion, the ACL becomes more triangular reorienting the fibers in a more dorsal to palmar arrangement.[11]

COLLATERAL LIGAMENT BIOMECHANICS

The collateral ligaments serve as the primary stabilizer to varus and valgus stress.[2,12,13] Leibovic and Bowers[2] demonstrated that the PCL is the primary lateral stabilizer of the PIPJ in flexion, whereas the ACL and volar plate confer stability from 0° to 15° of flexion. More recently, Chen and colleagues[14] used 3D reconstructions of CT scans to model the behavior of the ACL and PCL during flexion and extension. In their model, they found the dorsal PCL increased in length from 0° to 90° (2.0 mm) and decreased from 90° to full flexion (0.5 mm). Meanwhile, the volar PCL decreased in length 2.6 mm from full extension to full flexion. Lastly, the distally inserting fibers of the ACL decrease their length from full extension to full flexion by 2.9 to 3.0 mm and the more proximally inserting fibers of the ACL do not significantly change their length (**Fig 5**). Subsequently, other biomechanical

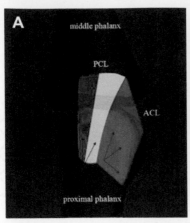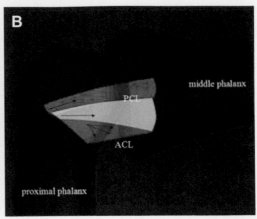

Fig. 5. Sagittal orientation of collateral ligament complex. (*A*) In PIPJ extension, the ACL (*green*) and volar PCL (*yellow*) are in their most elongated position, whereas the dorsal PCL (*blue*) length is decreased. (*B*) In flexion, the ACL and volar PCL length decreases, whereas the dorsal PCL length increases from extension to flexion. The *arrows* represent the orientation of the fibers of the ACL and PCL. (*From* Chen J, Tan J, Zhang AX. In vivo length changes of the proximal interphalangeal joint proper and accessory collateral ligaments during flexion. J Hand Surg Am 2015;40(6):1132; with permission.)

studies have supported the importance of the PCL with additional findings that up to half of the ligament can be sectioned without significant alteration in stability.[12] However, it should be noted that a partial tear may predispose to a complete injury at that site with continued stress.[15] Together, these findings further support the function of the collateral ligaments as lateral stabilizing structures of the PIPJ.

Different mechanisms of failure of the collateral ligament complex have been demonstrated including midsubstance tears, proximal or distal failures, or avulsion fractures.[13,15,16] Rhee and colleagues[15] reported a greater incidence of failure through distal fractures of the insertion of the PCL when force was applied at higher speeds (ie, 10 mm/s) and conversely higher incidence of midsubstance tears at lower applied speeds (ie, 1 mm/s). They did not find any correlation of the failure mechanism to the overall force applied with an average of 176.9 ±5.9 N applied to create ligament failure. Similarly, Kiefhaber and colleagues[13] stressed cadaveric PIPJs, performed postfailure dissections, and proposed a sequential failure of

the palmar PCL fibers progressing dorsally, followed by failure at the PCL-ACL junction, and finally failure at the distal palmar plate.

VOLAR PLATE

The volar plate is a stout fibrous structure that spans the volar PIPJ (**Fig 6**). Similar to the collateral ligaments, mRNA analysis demonstrates that the volar plate is composed primarily of type I collagen but does contain a small proportion of type III collagen as well.[9] Proximally, the volar plate has a much larger surface area of attachment compared with its distal attachment. This proximal portion includes the membranous portion of the volar plate centrally made up of disorganized connective tissue and the checkrein ligaments laterally.[11,17,18] Distally, the volar plate is more stout and fibrocartilaginous, which lends to its resistance of hyperextension. The lateral insertions extend more distally than the central attachments. The existence and significance of any connection of the distal volar plate and the ACL and A3 pulley remain unclear.[6,11,18] Proximally, the checkrein ligaments blend into the periosteum

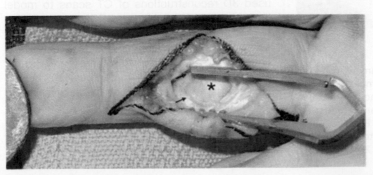

Fig. 6. Volar plate (VP). The VP spans the volar PIPJ. Arrows indicate the 2 slips of the flexor digitorum superficialis. The *asterisk* represents the volar plate. (*From* Cheah AE, Yao J. Surgical approaches to the proximal interphalangeal joint. J Hand Surg Am 2016;41(2):296; with permission.)

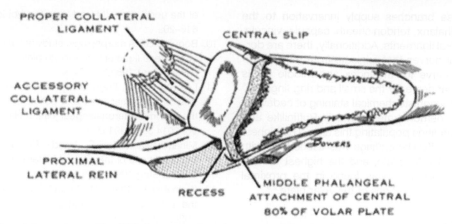

Fig. 7. Volar plate anatomy. The PIPJ demonstrating the recess at the distal volar insertion of the volar plate. (*From* Saito S, Suzuki Y. Biomechanics of the volar plate of the proximal interphalangeal joint: a dynamic ultrasonographic study. J Hand Surg Am 2011;36(2):266; with permission.)

over the length of their attachment in contrast to the distal lateral attachments that insert directly onto bone via Sharpey fibers laterally.[11,18,19] The volar plate also serves as the volar extent of the capsule lined with synovial tissue dorsally and conversely acts as a gliding surface for the overlying flexor tendons lined with teno-synovium volarly.[2,18–20]

VOLAR PLATE BIOMECHANICS

The function of the volar plate is primarily to resist hyperextension at the PIPJ.[2,4,20–22] Bowers and colleagues[20] loaded cadaveric specimens in extension at the PIPJ and found the radial digits to be more resistant to hyperextension compared with the ulnar digits suggesting that the strength of the volar ligamentous complex differs between fingers. Subsequently, Komurcu and colleagues[23] demonstrated the thickness of the volar plate differing between fingers with the fifth finger having the thinnest central and lateral thickness corresponding with the findings of Bowers and colleagues.[20]

The volar plate distal insertion was previously described as a uniform insertion into the middle phalanx but has since been revised to include a recess in the volar plate originally described by Bowers and colleagues[20] (**Fig 7**).[18] Dynamic ultrasound suggest that, through an arc of flexion, the volar plate slides proximally and is elevated by the A3 pulley, allowing the middle phalanx to roll into the recess without impinging (**Fig 8**).[21] This recess allows for the volar plate to fall away from the joint in flexion to avoid impingement. Additionally, the recess creates a foldlike protrusion of the volar plate into the PIPJ. This protrusion has been likened to a meniscus serving as a cushion between the two articulations.[18,20] Proximally, the membranous portion of the volar plate folds onto itself during flexion.[11]

INNERVATION

The PIPJ is innervated by both dorsal and volar nerve branches.[2,24,25] Gross dissection demonstrates both distal and proximal articular branches from the palmar digital nerves that supply the volar

1ˢᵗ phase: sliding

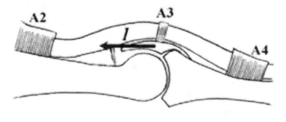

2ⁿᵈ phase: elevating

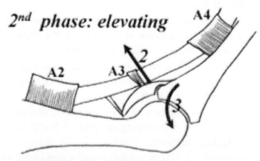

3ʳᵈ phase: rolling in the recess

Fig. 8. Volar plate mechanics. Saito and Suzuki[21] describe 3 phases of volar plate motion: sliding, elevation, and rolling. The A3 pulley elevates the volar plate during the elevation phase and leads to the rolling phase. A2 and A4 represent the annular ligaments. (*From* Saito S, Suzuki Y. Biomechanics of the volar plate of the proximal interphalangeal joint: a dynamic ultrasonographic study. J Hand Surg Am 2011;36(2):270; with permission.)

PIPJ. These branches supply innervation to the proximal phalanx, tendon sheath, capsule, vincula, and collateral ligaments. Additionally, there are dorsal articular nerves that originate from the superficial radial nerve for the index and middle PIPJs and the ulnar nerve for the small and ring fingers.[24] Further immunohistochemical staining of cadaveric specimens demonstrates primarily Ruffinilike and Pacinilike endings populating this area. The highest density of Ruffinilike endings was associated with the proximal volar plate, and the highest density of Pacinilike endings was found in the proximal radial and ulnar insertions of the volar plate.[25]

SUMMARY

Despite the wealth of knowledge we have regarding the anatomy of the PIPJ, it remains a subject of ongoing investigation. As our understanding of the anatomy and biomechanical properties contributing to normal motion and stability evolves, we will continue to improve our treatment and reconstructive designs in those situations when motion and stability are no longer normal.

REFERENCES

1. Cheah AE, Yao J. Surgical approaches to the proximal interphalangeal joint. J Hand Surg 2016;41(2):294–305.

2. Leibovic S, Bowers W. Anatomy of the proximal interphalangeal joint. Hand Clin 1994;10(2):169–78.

3. Dumont C, Albus G, Kubein-Meesenburg D, et al. Morphology of the interphalangeal joint surface and its functional relevance. J Hand Surg 2008;33(1):9–18.

4. Kuczynski K. The proximal interphalangeal joint. Anatomy and causes of stiffness in the fingers. J Bone Joint Surg Br 1968;50(3):656–63.

5. Lawrence T, Trail IA, Noble J. Morphological measurements of the proximal interphalangeal joint. J Hand Surg 2004;29(3):242–7.

6. Allison DM. Anatomy of the collateral ligaments of the proximal interphalangeal joint. J Hand Surg 2005;30(5):1026–31.

7. Bullough PG. The geometry of diarthrodial joints, its physiologic maintenance, and the possible significance of age-related changes in geometry-to-load distribution and the development of osteoarthritis. Clin Orthop 1981;156:61–6.

8. Hess F, Farshad M, Sutter R, et al. A novel technique for detecting instability of the distal radioulnar joint in complete triangular fibrocartilage complex lesions. J Wrist Surg 2012;01(02):153–8.

9. Cheah A, Harris A, Le W, et al. Relative ratios of collagen composition of periarticular tissue of joints of the upper limb. J Hand Surg Eur Vol 2017;42(6):616–20.

10. Bogumill GP. A morphologic study of the relationship of collateral ligaments to growth plates in the digits. J Hand Surg 1983;8(1):74–9.

11. Lee SW, Ng ZY, Fogg QA. Three-dimensional analysis of the palmar plate and collateral ligaments at the proximal interphalangeal joint. J Hand Surg Eur Vol 2014;39(4):391–7.

12. Minamikawa Y, Horii E, Amadio PC, et al. Stability and constraint of the proximal interphalangeal joint. J Hand Surg 1993;18(2):198–204.

13. Kiefhaber TR, Stern PJ, Grood ES. Lateral stability of the proximal interphalangeal joint. J Hand Surg 1986;11(5):661–9.

14. Chen J, Tan J, Zhang AX. In vivo length changes of the proximal interphalangeal joint proper and accessory collateral ligaments during flexion. J Hand Surg 2015;40(6):1130–7.

15. Rhee R, Reading G, Wray C. A biomechanical study of collateral ligaments of the proximal interphalangeal joint. J Hand Surg 1992;17(1):157–63.

16. Ali MS. Complete disruption of collateral mechanism of proximal interphalangeal joint of fingers. J Hand Surg Br 1984;9(2):191–3.

17. Watson HK, Light TR, Johnson TR. Checkrein resection for flexion contracture of the middle joint. J Hand Surg 1979;4(1):67–71.

18. Watanabe H, Hashizume H, Inoue H, et al. Collagen framework of the volar plate of human proximal interphalangeal joint.pdf. Acta Med Okayama 1994;48(2):101–8.

19. Williams EH, McCarthy E, Bickel KD. The histologic anatomy of the volar plate. J Hand Surg 1998;23(5):805–10.

20. Bowers W, Wolf J, Nehil J, et al. The proximal interphalangeal joint volar plate. I. An anatomical and biomechanical study. J Hand Surg Am 1980;5(1):79–88.

21. Saito S, Suzuki Y. Biomechanics of the volar plate of the proximal interphalangeal joint: a dynamic ultrasonographic study. J Hand Surg 2011;36(2):265–71.

22. Gad P. The anatomy of the volar part of the capsules of the finger joints. J Bone Joint Surg Br 1967;49:362–7.

23. Kömürcü M, Kirici Y, Korkmaz C, et al. Morphometric analysis of metacarpophalangeal and proximal interphalangeal palmar plates. Clin Anat 2008;21(5):433–8.

24. Chen Y, McClinton M, DaSilva M, et al. Innervation of the metacarpophalangeal and interphalangeal joints-a microanatomic and histologic study of the nerve endings.pdf. J Hand Surg Am 2000;25(1):128–33.

25. Chikenji T, Suzuki D, Fujimiya M, et al. Distribution of nerve endings in the human proximal interphalangeal joint and surrounding structures. J Hand Surg 2010;35(8):1286–93.

Surgical Exposure of the Proximal Interphalangeal Joint

Casey M. DeDeugd, MD, Marco Rizzo, MD*

KEYWORDS

- Surgical approaches • Proximal interphalangeal joint • Dorsal approach • Volar approach
- Lateral approach • Chamay approach

KEY POINTS

- The primary approaches are dorsal, volar, lateral, chamay.
- Indications for approach to proximal interphalangeal (PIP) joint include arthroplasty, open reduction internal fixation, and osteotomy.
- Approach is determined by indication for surgery.
- Given the nature of the PIP joint, motion is notoriously difficult to improve.
- Dedicated postoperative therapy is customized to the patient.

INTRODUCTION

Surgical access to the proximal interphalangeal (PIP) joint is necessary for a variety of procedures, including PIP implant and surface arthroplasty, open reduction internal fixation (ORIF) of dorsal fracture-dislocations and condylar fractures, contracture treatments, deformity corrections and intra-articular corrective osteotomies. There are several different approaches, including variations of dorsal, volar, and lateral. In the context of implant arthroplasty, Swanson first described a dorsal approach to the PIP joint in the 1960s, and this remains the preferred technique for access to the joint. This approach provides essentially safe access and wide exposure of the entire joint surface. Over the last 20 to 30 years, there has been interest in use of a volar approach for these procedures.[1–7] Although technically more challenging, the volar approach offers the advantage of preserving the extensor mechanism and avoids any issues with adhesions, extensor lag, or loss of motion in the extension arc. Although

many consider the lateral approach to be more recently advocated, years ago Carroll and colleagues[8] described a lateral approach for PIP arthroplasty. Since this early report, there have been only a few reports of outcomes of PIP procedures using this approach.[9–11] Of the 3 approaches, the lateral remains the most infrequently utilized.

The main determining factor for the method of accessing the PIP joint is the surgical indication. For example, the dorsal approach is typically used in surface replacement arthroplasty (SRA) because of the reliability of generous exposure of the joint surface and the preservation of the collateral ligaments for anatomic stability.[12,13] In addition, the technique, alignment, and cutting guides used with these implants were designed for use though a dorsal exposure. Thus for modular implants, a volar approach may prove too challenging. Despite demonstrating that successful implant placement was achievable via a volar approach, Stoecklein and colleagues admitted challenges associated with this technique,

Disclosure Statement: No disclosures (C.M. DeDeugd). Consultant Zimmer-Biomet (M. Rizzo).
Department of Orthopedic Surgery, Mayo Clinic, 200 First Street Southwest, Rochester, MN 55905, USA
* Corresponding author.
E-mail address: rizzo.marco@mayo.edu

Hand Clin 34 (2018) 127–138
https://doi.org/10.1016/j.hcl.2017.12.003

hand.theclinics.com

highlighting the need for instrumentation to be refined to help surgeons choosing this approach. Most of the published series with the volar approach have been in patients who underwent silicone arthroplasty. Several reasons may be proposed for this. First, because the hinged silicone implant functions more like a spacer than an anatomic joint replacement, its placement is less technically demanding than the modular metal/plastic or pyrocarbon implants. In addition, the volar approach offers the surgeon exposure to address and treat volar plate problems such as seen in swan neck deformities.

Similarly, the complication profile of the surgery is predicated upon the approach used. According to Murray and colleagues,[14] the surface replacing PIP arthroplasty in their series failed more often when implanted via a volar approach versus a dorsal approach. Moreover, Yamamoto and colleagues[15] showed in their systematic review that the silicone implants performed using a volar approach have lower revision rates, less incidence of extension lag, and improved gains in arc of motion compared with dorsal and lateral approaches. Underscoring the difficulties in general of improving motion regardless of approach, most studies examining motion following arthroplasty show no significant improvement compared with preoperative measures. This article will highlight the various surgical approaches to the PIP joint, explain rationale for choosing 1 approach over another, and discuss some of the most common complications and how to avoid them (**Table 1**).

Table 1
Indications of the dorsal, volar and lateral approaches

Indication	Possible Approach
PIP silicone implant arthroplasty	Volar, dorsal, or lateral
PIP surface replacement arthroplasty	Volar or dorsal
PIP hemi-hamate arthroplasty	Volar
Open reduction internal fixation	Volar, dorsal, or lateral
PIP arthrodesis	Dorsal
Volar plate arthroplasty	Volar
Corrective osteotomy	Volar or dorsal
Deformity correction (swan neck)	Volar
Deformity correction (boutonniere)	Dorsal
Contracture treatment	Volar, dorsal

SURGICAL TECHNIQUE/PROCEDURE
Preoperative Planning

Thorough history should include: previous trauma, infection, inflammatory arthritis, previous surgeries (affected digit or others), and instability.

Preoperative imaging should include AP and true lateral radiographs of affected and contralateral digit and magnified views of the PIP joint. Additionally, patients should be evaluated for medullary canal sclerosis, deformity, and dorsal joint widening ("V-sign"). In cases of severe bone loss or complex fractures, computed tomography may be helpful. MRI helps to delineate the soft tissues, degree of synovitis, mass effects, and soft tissue and bony lesions.

Preoperative clinical evaluation should be determined based on the pathology. All patients are tested for active and passive range of motion, crepitus versus smooth, concentric gliding of the joint, with range of motion. Varus and valgus joint stability is assessed via stressing of the radial and ulnar collaterals. Dorsal-volar stability is ascertained by shucking the middle phalanx manually dorsally and volarly. Coronal plane and rotational deformity are also important to assess.

PREPARATION AND PATIENT POSITIONING

Anesthesia should include general, regional, or local anesthesia with digital block; alternatively the patient may be wide awake with local anesthesia. Type of anesthesia will depend on which procedure is to be performed.

Antibiotics are patient dependent (allergies, intolerances, previous infections), although surgeon preference also plays a role. The decision to use antibiotics also depends on the procedure to be performed, as certain procedures may not require intravenous antibiotics.

Positioning is determined by surgeon preference and is usually supine with a hand table versus using the base of the fluoroscopy image intensifier as a table. The lead hand is used for retraction of other digits.

Sterile tourniquet, draped in tourniquet, or tourni-cot may be used. A tourni-cot is often too close to the exposure to be sufficient, depending upon procedure to be performed.

SURGICAL APPROACH
Volar

Approach
Step one Skin incision is based on the indication for surgery. The possible incisions for a volar approach are Bruner type (**Fig. 1**), Bruner-midlateral hybrid or zig-zag incision with apices

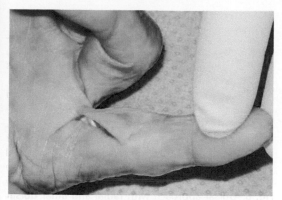

Fig. 1. Bruner incision for the volar approach.

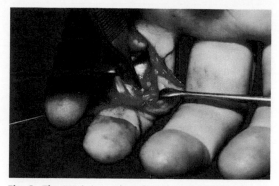

Fig. 3. The PIP joint volar plate is exposed by retracting the flexor tendons (radially/ulnarly). *Green dot* is volar plate.

at the flexion creases. For more exposure, use the Bruner midlateral hybrid or zig-zag.[5] The base of the flap is best positioned on the more involved side of the fracture dislocation.[5]

Step two Identify and protect the flexor tendon sheath centrally and neurovascular bundles on radial and ulnar sides (**Fig. 2**).

Step three Next, the approach to the volar plate must be performed. Either a radially based flap can be raised by incising the flexor sheath from the A2 to the A4 pulley or the entire FDP can be retracted 1 side, and the volar plate can be accessed between the 2 slips of the flexor digitorum superficialis (FDS) or to the side of the retracted FDS (**Fig. 3**). If the access between the slips of the FDS is chosen, the FDS split can be taken more proximally to increase exposure.[16] If the FDS and FDP are retracted to the same side, a single FDS slip release can be done to increase the exposure of the joint.[16]

Step four The volar plate must then be released from the collateral ligaments by incising the attachment of the collateral ligament from the

proximal or distal aspect. The extent of this release is determined by the amount of access required for the procedure being performed.

Closure
Step five Involves repairing the volar plate and collateral ligaments as needed.

Step six Involves skin closure with nonabsorbable nylon or prolene sutures.

Step seven Involves postoperative dressing, and splinting (if at all) is individualized depending on the indication and satisfaction with the surgery. If single digit, the authors typically recommend the use of tube-gauze compressive dressings reinforced with plaster molded splint. If multiple digits, they recommend using a volar-dorsal compressive dressing and plaster splint. Obtain intraoperative radiographs following splint application to customize the amount of flexion and extension as needed.

Dorsal

Approach
Step one Skin incision is based on surgical indication. The incisions from this approach include

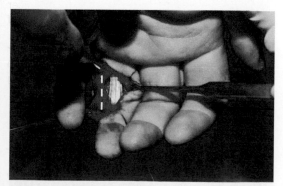

Fig. 2. Exposed flexor tendon sheath with ulnar neurovascular structure marked by dashed white line and radial neurovascular structures protected by retractor.

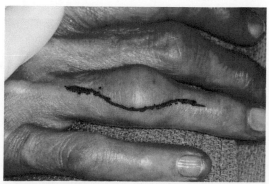

Fig. 4. Curvilinear incision for dorsally based approaches.

midline longitudinal, curvilinear (**Fig. 4**), or lazy S (**Fig. 5**). This is typically 2 to 3 cm in length. A straight incision is a utilitarian approach, while a curved (C-shaped or last S) can be utilized to avoid the extensor tendon and theoretically prevent adhesions and scar formation. Use a sharp knife through skin vertically all the way to the extensor tendon and then Jones scissors to dissect down to the level of dorsal veins.

Step two Identify and protect dorsal veins; elevate them with your skin flaps (**Fig. 6**).

Step three Elevate lateral skin flaps to visualize the extensor mechanism both proximal and distal to the PIP joint.

Step four Exposure can be obtained by detaching the central slip or splitting the extensor tendon longitudinally (**Fig. 7**) while maintaining the central slip insertion.[16] Additional exposure if necessary can be facilitated with release of the collateral ligaments. If the extensor mechanism is incised, it must be done sharply, and detached from the base of the middle phalanx. If this step is taken, the extensor mechanism must be repaired following the surgical procedure. This approach with extensor mechanism splitting, favors extension, and thus the patient is more likely to have a flexion lag.

Closure
Step five Close the longitudinal incision in the extensor mechanism, if present (**Fig. 8**). When closing a tendon-splitting approach, the digit should be extended at the PIP and flexed at the distal interphalangeal (DIP) joint to ensure the appropriate tension on the dorsal tendon to avoid overtightening, which invites risk of swan neck deformity postoperatively. Use of nonabsorbable sutures may cause prominence underneath the skin, which can be avoided with an inverted figure 8 repair with the knots buried deep to the extensor mechanism.

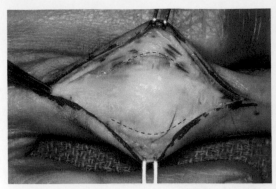

Fig. 6. Dorsal approach with radial and ulnar dorsal veins marked with dashed blue lines.

Step six This involves skin closure with nonabsorbable nylon or prolene sutures.

Step seven If single digit, the authors recommend the use of tube-gauze compressive dressings reinforced with plaster molded splint. If multiple digits, they recommend using a volar-dorsal compressive dressing and plaster splint. Obtain intraoperative radiographs following splint application to customize the amount of flexion and extension as needed.

Lateral

Approach
Step one A midaxial lateral incision from the midpoint of P1 to the midpoint of P2 (**Fig. 9**) is used. A dorsal skin incision can also be utilized. The radial or ulnar side may be utilized. The decision for this is based on surgeon preference as well as the presence of clinical instability or deformity. Classically, the incision is preferentially placed on the ulnar side of the finger in the index finger and on the radial side of the finger in the small finger. However, the lateral approach to the

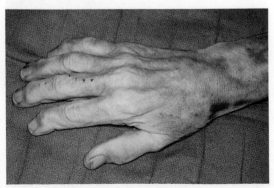

Fig. 5. Lazy S incision for dorsally based approaches.

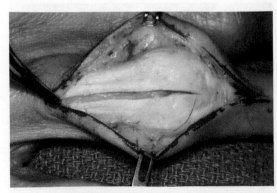

Fig. 7. Longitudinal split of the extensor tendon, maintaining central slip insertion.

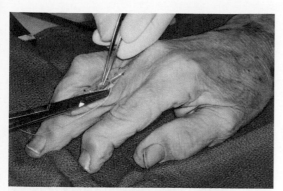

Fig. 8. Interrupted inverted figure of 8 repair of the extensor mechanism.

joint may also be performed via a dorsal skin incision.

Step two Elevate lateral skin flaps dorsally and volarly to maintain the transverse retinacular ligament in the center of the operative field (**Fig. 10**).

Step three Use retractors to keep the extensor tendons dorsal and the neurovascular bundle volar. The proper digital nerves are protected by the volar skin flap.

Step four Make a longitudinal incision on the transverse retinacular ligament (**Fig. 11**) to expose the insertion of the collateral ligamentous complex. There are options for dividing the collateral ligament. One option is done by reflecting the upper half of the collateral ligament dorsally beneath the extensor mechanism and leaving it attached to the proximal phalanx neck (**Fig. 12**), leaving a proximally based dorsal flap of the collateral ligament (**Fig. 13**). Volarly, leave the attachment of the collateral ligament distally and dissect proximally to the Checkrein ligaments, which can be

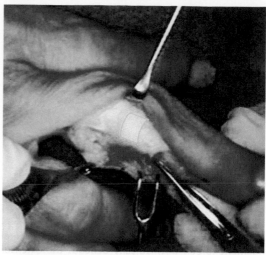

Fig. 10. Elevation of skin flaps dorsally and volarly to expose the transverse retinacular ligament, marked by blue line.

released on the operative side (radial/ulnar) as long as they remain intact on the nonoperative side to prevent hyperextension. Alternatively, one can release the accessory collateral ligament from its proximal insertion on the volar plate and release the proper collateral ligament from its origin. Further release of the volar plate can be performed if additional access to the joint is needed. The joint capsule is then incised in line with the incision. Gentle but deliberate manipulation will facilitate exposure of the joint up to and including shot-gunning the PIP to facilitate full exposure (**Fig. 14**).

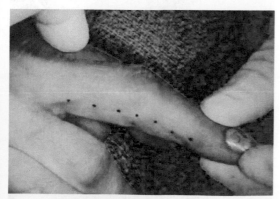

Fig. 9. Midlateral incision of the lateral approach, which can vary in length but usually extends from at least the midpoint of P1 to the midpoint of P2.

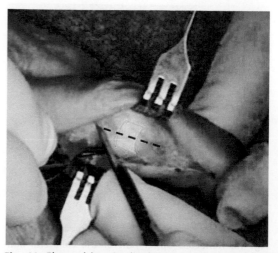

Fig. 11. Planned longitudinal incision (seen as *black dashed line*) of transverse retinacular ligament marked by blue line.

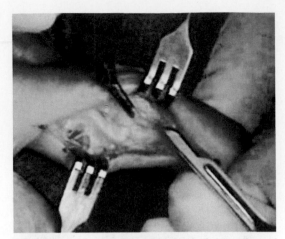

Fig. 12. Reflection of the upper half of the collateral ligament (*green dot*) dorsally beneath the extensor mechanism and leaving it attached to the proximal phalanx neck (*blue dot*).

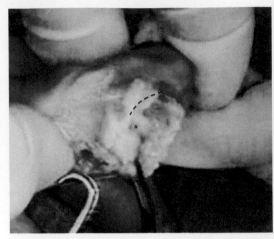

Fig. 14. Shot-gunned proximal interphalangeal joint with P1 head marked with red dot and lateral bands shown by dashed black line as seen from the lateral approach.

Closure

Step five Repair the volar plate if violated. Repair the edges of the collateral ligaments (**Fig. 15**) or repair the accessory collateral ligament to its proximal insertion or to the proper collateral, depending on approach used. This will allow for appropriate tensioning. Repair the transverse retinacular ligament. These repairs will provide stability to the joint.

Step six This involves skin closure with nonabsorbable nylon or prolene sutures (**Fig. 16**).

Step seven If single digit, the authors recommend the use of tube-gauze compressive dressings

reinforced with plaster molded splint (**Fig. 17**). Upon initiation of motion, the finger can be buddy taped to the adjacent digit to protect the ligament repair. If multiple digits, the authors recommend using a volar-dorsal compressive dressing and plaster splint. Obtain intraoperative radiographs following splint application to customize the amount of flexion and extension as needed.

Chamay

Approach
Step one This is an alternative dorsal approach to the standard dorsal approach described previously. Again, the skin incision is based on the surgical indication. The incisions from this approach

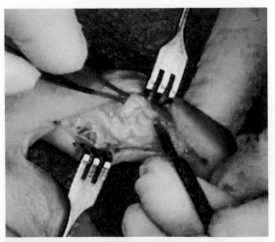

Fig. 13. Reflected upper half of the collateral ligament (*green dot*) dorsally beneath the extensor mechanism still attached to the proximal phalanx neck (*blue dot*).

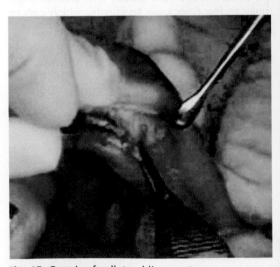

Fig. 15. Repair of collateral ligaments.

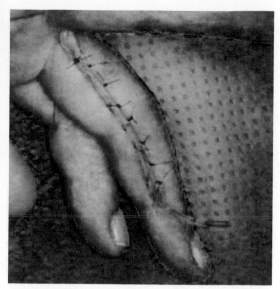

Fig. 16. Skin closure using interrupted nonabsorbable suture.

include midline longitudinal, curvilinear (see **Fig. 4**), or lazy S (see **Fig. 5**). This is typically 2 to 3 cm in length. A straight incision is a utilitarian approach, while a curved (C-shaped or last S) can be utilized to avoid the extensor tendon and theoretically prevent adhesions and scar

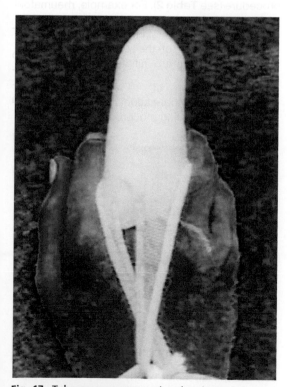

Fig. 17. Tube gauze compressive dressing.

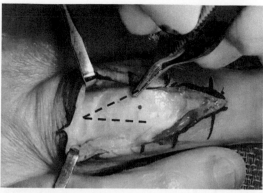

Fig. 18. The planned isosceles triangle incision of the distally based extensor tendon flap for the Chamay approach (*dashed lines*). The red dot shows the insertion of the central slip, which will be preserved.

formation. Use a sharp knife through the skin vertically all the way to extensor tendon and then Jones scissors to dissect down to the level of dorsal veins.

Step two Identify and protect dorsal veins; elevate them with skin flaps (see **Fig. 6**).

Step three Elevate lateral skin flaps to visualize the extensor mechanism both proximal and distal to the PIP joint.

Step four This is where the Chamay approach deviates from a standard dorsal approach. Exposure can be obtained by a v- or u-shaped elevation of the extensor tendon over the proximal phalanx. Typically, a distally based extensor tendon flap is made based on a v-shaped isosceles triangle (**Fig. 18**). This flap is incised sharply while leaving the central slip insertion intact (**Figs. 19–22**). The lateral bands are not included in this flap and will

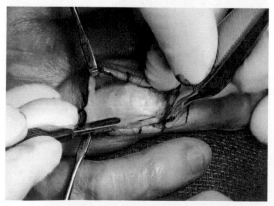

Fig. 19. Ulnar extensor limb of the Chamay extensor flap approach.

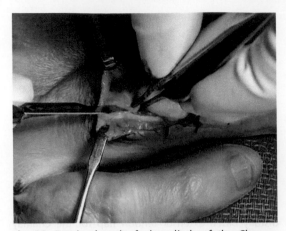

Fig. 20. Proximal end of ulnar limb of the Chamay extensor flap approach.

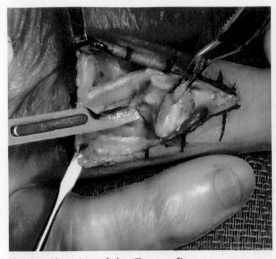

Fig. 22. Elevation of the Chamay flap.

fall volarly to help with the exposure of the joint (**Fig. 23**).

Closure

Step five Careful repair of the triangular flap is then performed using interrupted absorbable suture (**Fig. 24**). This repair is performed with the PIP in extension.

Step six This involves skin closure with nonabsorbable nylon or prolene sutures.

Step seven If single digit, the authors recommend the use of tube-gauze compressive dressings reinforced with plaster molded splint. If multiple digits, they recommend using a volar-dorsal compressive dressing and plaster splint. Obtain intraoperative radiographs following splint application to

customize the amount of flexion and extension as needed.

COMPLICATIONS AND MANAGEMENT

Complications and management are described in **Table 2**.

POSTOPERATIVE CARE

Postoperative care is specific to the patient and procedure (see **Table 2**). For example, rheumatoid patients with largely preoperative deformity may require longer periods of immobilization to ensure stability. Depending on the surgery performed, the following protocols are initiated for variable time periods:

- Immediate mobilization of DIP joint to encourage gliding motion of lateral bands

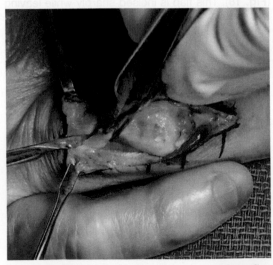

Fig. 21. Radial limb of the Chamay extensor flap approach.

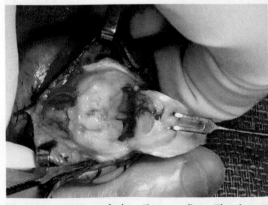

Fig. 23. Elevation of the Chamay flap. The lateral bands (*green dots*) are not included in this flap (*red dot*) and will fall sublux volarly to help with the exposure of the joint.

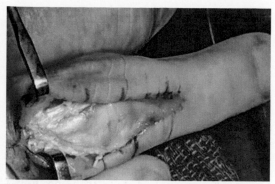

Fig. 24. Careful repair of the triangular flap is then performed using interrupted absorbable suture.

- Period of immobilization of the PIP joint
- Nighttime static forearm- or hand-based resting splints
- Avoid hyperextension for the longitudinal splitting dorsal approach to protect the extensor mechanism

- Initiation of mobilization using orthoses and/or protected motion via dynamic splinting
  - Usually aggressive ROM
  - Multiple repetitions per day (hourly/10 x per day)
  - Extension blocks for hyperextension
  - Night time static flexion blocks
- Buddy taping to the adjacent digits once active extension is maintained

REHABILITATION PROTOCOLS

Specific protocols are designed based on the surgeon and institution. The following are examples of approach-specific protocols. The supervision of a hand therapist is recommended to provide guidance and encouragement.

General postoperative care recommendations will be detailed as follows (approach-specific instructions are given subsequently in this article and instructions may vary because of a patient's individual limitations):

Table 2
Complications and management of approaches to the proximal interphalangeal joint

Approach	Complication	Management
Volar	Damage to neurovascular bundle	• Repair under loupe magnification or microscopy
	Damage to flexor tendons	• Repair under loupe magnification or microscopy
	Bowstringing of flexor tendons (aggressive release of sheath)	• Pulley reconstruction
	Swan neck deformity (VP disruption)	• VP repair, superficialis hemitenodesis
Dorsal	Damage to central slip	• Reattachment to P2 base or repair
	Boutonniere deformity (dorsal slip detachment)	• Reattachment of dorsal slip Boutonniere reconstruction • Arthrodesis
	Swan neck deformity (overtightening the closure)	• Close extensor mechanism with the DIP joint in flexion to minimize the amount of hyperextension through the PIP • Swan neck reconstruction • Extensor plication
Chamay	Inadequate repair/failure to restore tension of extensor apparatus	• Revision of repair • Tenolysis and early ROM
Lateral	Damage to neurovascular bundle	• Repair under loupe magnification or microscopy
	Coronal plane instability (collateral ligament damage)	• Collateral ligament reconstruction/revision repair • Arthrodesis
All approaches	PIP extensor lag	• Avoid by not overtightening dorsal closure (dorsal) • Custom splinting/hand therapy • Tenolysis for adhesions
	Decreased range of motion	• Custom splinting/hand therapy • Tenolysis for adhesions
	Instability/dislocation	• Revision surgery (depending on original procedure)

- The finger will typically be immobilized in compressive dressing for 1 to 7 days based on surgeon's discretion and preoperative and intraoperative assessments.
- Motion exercises may begin cautiously with isolated flexion of the DIP on the first postoperative day.
- Progressive PIP flexion may begin slowly but with return to full extension during each cycle, blocking hyperextension.
- If extension cannot be obtained after each flexion, a dynamic extension exercise splint is applied during exercise periods. A static extension splint for rest periods and nighttime can be used for a period of time in order to obtain satisfactory extension.
- Elevation during both daytime and nighttime is important to control swelling and avoid postoperative stiffness. Elastic wrapping for edema control, especially for nighttime wear, may also helpful.

After Dorsal Approach

The DIP joint may be flexed independently as soon as the patient is capable, usually in the first 24 to 48 hours, with an initial range of motion of 30° to 40° to protect the extensor tendon repair.

Begin PIP exercise gradually, at 2 to 7 days. Start with a limited arc of motion of the PP, 30° to 40°. This will provide tendon excursion of 3 to 5 mm. Exercise periods should last 5 to 10 minutes, and performed 5 to 6 times per day. It is important to return the finger to neutral after each flexion exercise and to avoid a flexion deformity at the PIP joint. The exercise period should gradually increase depending on patient tolerance.

Dynamic extension splinting with active flexion is recommended. One should also prescribe a nighttime static splint in order to hold the finger in full extension.

If the finger is swollen, try placing elastic wraps during rest periods.

A static extension block should provide extension of the PIP joint and prevent extensor lag. Once active extension is achieved, usually after 4 to 5 weeks, discontinue the dynamic splint. The static nighttime splint should be used for 7 to 10 weeks.

An ideal range of motion to achieve is 0° to 80°. However, if a stable, pain-free 60° arc of motion is achieved, this will also be considered a success.

If an extension lag increases, use a static splint in extension for an additional 2 to 4 weeks. Also, passive motion (stretching into flexion) should be discouraged for the first 6 weeks postoperatively.

If the preoperative deformity was a swan neck, holding the finger in flexion of 10° to 15° is recommended to prevent recurrence of the swan neck deformity. A volar sublimis tenodesis or similar procedure may be indicated. The therapy is modified to protect the volar repair with limited finger extension at the same time that there is active finger flexion.

After Volar Approach

If dorsal extension insertion integrity is satisfactory, the finger may be held in 15° to 20° flexion for the first 2to 3 days with a dorsal support splint.

Depending on patient comfort and degree of swelling, motion exercises can begin on the first postoperative day with isolated flexion of the DIP joint. More palmer flexion is possible initially with the palmar approach, up to 45° as tolerated by the patient. Protect against hyperextension.

On the second to third day, active PIP flexion begins with return to full extension after each cycle of flexion and extension. Avoid hyperextension.

During rest periods, the joint should be held by a static extension splint, in 10° to 15° flexion. This splint should also be worn at night for a period up to 6 weeks.

The goal is to maintain close to full extension but not allow hyperextension, which is a risk with the volar approach and release of the volar plate.

Elevation during the day and at night is important to control swelling and avoid postoperative stiffness. Elastic wrapping for edema control is also helpful. The finger will be somewhat swollen for a few weeks following surgery. In addition, skin sutures should be removed once healing is completed, generally at 10 to 14 days after surgery and up to 3 weeks for rheumatoid disease.

If the preoperative deformity was a swan neck deformity, the DIP is supported in neutral with a volar splint at absolute 0°, and the PIP joint is splinted in flexion of 20° to 25°. This is recommended so that the lateral bands stay lateral and do not migrate dorsally. Range of motion should be 10° to 15° short of full extension with flexion to 75° to 80°. The patient can have controlled motion with a protective splint under therapist supervision but not alone. The PIP should be held at 10° to 15° flexion with splinting to prevent dorsal displacement of the lateral bands.

For boutonniere injuries with extensor tendon repair techniques, motion can be started as soon as 3 days postoperatively, as inflammation subsides but with limited flexion. The goal is a limited arc of motion to maintain tendon gliding without disruption of the reconstructed extensor tendon central slip attachment. For the first 3 weeks, the range of motion should be between 30° to 45° of flexion with a limited arc, gradually having the motion progress under supervision of a hand therapist.

The affected finger will be somewhat swollen for several weeks postoperatively. Furthermore, the finger may remain somewhat enlarged at the joint level for several months and up to 1 year. Postoperative medications should be started or continued in accordance with the surgeon's standard protocol and discretion.

Hand therapy, including finger mobility exercises, should begin approximately 1 to 7 days postoperatively, subject to the physician's assessment of the patient's healing, and should continue until patient reaches maximum medical improvement. Skin sutures can be removed when healing is completed, usually between 10 to 14 days.

OUTCOMES

Although many studies report outcomes of various surgical interventions to the PIP joint, there are few studies reporting outcomes specifically approach related. Although it is difficult to compare approach related complications specifically, there are reasonable conclusions that can be drawn when comparing 1 approach to the other. There are risks to every surgical approach, and structures at risk can be generalized. For example, the volar approach puts the digital neurovascular bundle, volar plate, and the collateral ligaments at risk; the dorsal approach puts the central slip at risk, and the Chamay approach intentionally incises the extensor mechanism. The risk is inadequacy of the repair and extensive bed of scar tissue that may limit range of motion. Finally, the lateral approach puts the neurovascular bundle and collateral ligaments at risk. These are generalizations however, and most common complications such as volar plate disruption and collateral ligament damage of dorsal slip detachment can occur with any approach leading to poor clinical outcomes.[16]

In an article Herren and Simmen,[17] outcomes after flexible implant arthroplasty via the palmar and dorsal approach to the PIP joint were compared. This retrospective review compared results of 59 PIP arthroplasties, 39 via the palmar approach and 21 via the dorsal approach utilizing well-matched cohorts. They found no significant difference in range of motion or postoperative stability. Moreover, in an early study of the volar approach, Lin and colleagues[3] found no significant difference between their cohort of exclusively volar approach PIP arthroplasties when comparing with comparable studies using the dorsal approach such as the

historical dorsal approach only data from Swanson, Dryer,[18] and Pelligrini.[19] The aforementioned study by Lin and colleagues[3] included 69 PIP joint arthroplasties in 36 patients using an exclusively volar approach.

Additionally, a recent retrospective review of reoperations following PIP joint nonconstrained arthroplasties.[20] In this study, various approaches were used including extensor tendon-splitting dorsal, central slip reflection approach, Chamay, lateral, and volar approaches. They found the average number of reoperations to the PIP joint was 1.6 (range from 1 to 4), and extensor mechanism dysfunction was the primary reason for reoperation. Interestingly, extensor mechanism dysfunction was found to be related to the surgical approach used, as it was more significantly common in the Chamay (90%) and central slip reflection (84%) approaches. This study also found that the lateral approach had the lowest rate of reoperation (33%).

A recent systematic review of the various surgical approaches to the PIP joint looked to clarify the importance of surgical approach on range of motion, complications, and clinical outcomes.[15] According to Yamamoto and colleagues,[15] the incidence of extension lag was variable depending on the procedure performed. They found that the extension lag from least to greatest was seen in silicone arthroplasty with a volar approach, silicone arthroplasty with a dorsal approach, silicone arthroplasty with a lateral approach, SRA with a dorsal approach, and finally SRA with a volar approach.[15] This complication can be treated by pulling the digit to full extension and converting to a Stack boutonniere splint for day and nighttime use followed by slowly reinitiating of flexion.

Similarly, there are known benefits from each approach. For example, the volar approach does not violate the extensor mechanism in any way and provides the advantage of immediate range of motion. However, there are certain patient such as those with swan neck deformities, boutonniere deformities, and PIP instability in whom the volar approach would be contraindicated despite its proposed benefits. The dorsal approach provides excellent access to joint, the P1 head, the central slip, and oblique retinacular ligament in the event that the patient has concomitant pathology of those structures.

SUMMARY

With its constrained bony congruity and adjacent soft tissues, maintaining motion and function following trauma and/or surgery of the PIP joint remains very challenging. A proper understanding of the various surgical approaches and their indications, technique, and pitfalls will help optimize patient outcomes. Comfort with each approach will help the surgeon minimize complications, improve function, and individualize treatment for conditions affecting the PIP joint. Improved instrumentation accommodating alternative approaches will help diversify approaches for surgeons. Postoperative therapy is also individualized depending on the condition and surgery and is helpful in minimizing stiffness and maximizing functional outcomes.

REFERENCES

1. Proubasta IR, Lamas CG, Natera L, et al. Silicone proximal interphalangeal joint arthroplasty for primary osteoarthritis using a volar approach. J Hand Surg Am 2014;39(6):1075–81.
2. Lautenbach M, Kim S, Berndsen M, et al. The palmar approach for PIP-arthroplasty according to Simmen: results after 8 years follow-up. J Orthop Sci 2014;19(5):722–8.
3. Lin HH, Wyrick JD, Stern PJ. Proximal interphalangeal joint silicone replacement arthroplasty: clinical results using an anterior approach. J Hand Surg Am 1995;20(1):123–32.
4. Bouacida S, Lazerges C, Coulet B, et al. Proximal interphalangeal joint arthroplasty with Neuflex(R) implants: relevance of the volar approach and early rehabilitation. Chir Main 2014;33(5):350–5.
5. Cheah AE, Tan DM, Chong AK, et al. Volar plating for unstable proximal interphalangeal joint dorsal fracture-dislocations. J Hand Surg Am 2012;37(1):28–33.
6. Duncan SF, Merritt MV, Kakinoki R. The volar approach to proximal interphalangeal joint arthroplasty. Tech Hand Up Extrem Surg 2009;13(1):47–53.
7. Stoecklein HH, Garg R, Wolfe SW. Surface replacement arthroplasty of the proximal interphalangeal joint using a volar approach: case series. J Hand Surg Am 2011;36(6):1015–21.
8. Carroll RE, Taber TH. Digital arthroplasty of the proximal interphlangeal joint. J Bone Joint Surg Am 1954;36-A(5):912–20.
9. Merle M, Villani F, Lallemand B, et al. Proximal interphalangeal joint arthroplasty with silicone implants (NeuFlex) by a lateral approach: a series of 51 cases. J Hand Surg Eur Vol 2012;37(1):50–5.
10. Stahlenbrecher A, Hoch J. Proximal interphalangeal joint silicone arthroplasty–comparison of Swanson and NeuFlex implants using a new evaluation score. Handchir Mikrochir Plast Chir 2009;41(3):156–65 [in German].
11. Hage JJ, Yoe EP, Zevering JP, et al. Proximal interphalangeal joint silicone arthroplasty for posttraumatic arthritis. J Hand Surg Am 1999;24(1):73–7.
12. Dickson DR, Nuttall D, Watts AC, et al. Pyrocarbon proximal interphalangeal joint arthroplasty: minimum five-year follow-up. J Hand Surg Am 2015;40(11):2142–8.e4.
13. Storey PA, Goddard M, Clegg C, et al. Pyrocarbon proximal interphalangeal joint arthroplasty: a medium to long term follow-up of a single surgeon series. J Hand Surg Eur Vol 2015;40(9):952–6.
14. Murray PM, Linscheid RL, Cooney WP 3rd, et al. Long-term outcomes of proximal interphalangeal joint surface replacement arthroplasty. J Bone Joint Surg Am 2012;94(12):1120–8.
15. Yamamoto M, Malay S, Fujihara Y, et al. A systematic review of different implants and approaches for proximal interphalangeal joint arthroplasty. Plast Reconstr Surg 2017;139(5):1139e–51e.
16. Cheah AE, Yao J. Surgical approaches to the proximal interphalangeal joint. J Hand Surg Am 2016;41(2):294–305.
17. Herren DB, Simmen BR. Palmar approach in flexible implant arthroplasty of the proximal interphalangeal joint. Clin Orthop Relat Res 2000;(371):131–5.
18. Dryer RF, Blair WF, Shurr DG, et al. Proximal interphalangeal joint arthroplasty. Clin Orthop Relat Res 1984;(185):187–94.
19. Pellegrini VD Jr, Burton RI. Osteoarthritis of the proximal interphalangeal joint of the hand: arthroplasty or fusion? J Hand Surg Am 1990;15(2):194–209.
20. Pritsch T, Rizzo M. Reoperations following proximal interphalangeal joint nonconstrained arthroplasties. J Hand Surg Am 2011;36(9):1460–6.

Treating Proximal Interphalangeal Joint Dislocations

Bradley Hart Saitta, MD[a], Jennifer Moriatis Wolf, MD[b],*

KEYWORDS

- PIP joint • Dislocation • Volar plate • Irreducible

KEY POINTS

- Proximal interphalangeal (PIP) joint dislocations are a common hand injury, especially in the athlete, and have good outcomes if treated properly.
- Soft tissue interposition can prevent concentric reduction and is an indication for acute surgical intervention.
- Prolonged splinting or self-immobilization can lead to PIP joint contracture.
- Subluxation or neglected dislocations typically require open reduction and stabilization.

INTRODUCTION

Dislocations of the proximal interphalangeal (PIP) joint are among the most common injuries of the hand, particularly in athletes.[1] In a study of hand injuries in the National Football League, the incidence of PIP joint dislocations was second only to metacarpal fractures.[2] These finger dislocations are often treated by onlookers, athletic trainers, and emergency department personnel, often without oversight or intervention by a hand surgeon.[3,4] Outcomes can vary from minimal disability to contracture, deformity, or chronic subluxation. This article defines the epidemiology, etiologic factors, and nonoperative and operative management of these injuries, stratified by dislocation type.

Epidemiology

Though PIP joint dislocations are common,[4] there are very little data about their prevalence. According to Chinchalkar and Gan,[3] the lack of hard data

is explained by a tendency for bystanders to perform reduction before radiographic evaluation and diagnosis, with another subset being reduced in the primary care or emergency room setting. Many PIP joint dislocations are known as coach's finger because they are commonly reduced on the field of play.[4]

Hindle and colleagues[5] evaluated all dislocations presenting to the Royal Infirmary of Edinburgh between November 2008 and October 2009. Dislocations involving the small joints of the hand were found to have a bimodal distribution, occurring most frequently in

- A younger cohort between 40 to 44 years of age
- An older cohort averaging 90 years of age
- Men more commonly than women (2.9:1 male to female ratio)
- At the PIP joint (10% of all dislocations).

In this study, PIP joint dislocation by joint occurred in a distribution as follows:

Disclosure Statement: None.
[a] Department of Orthopaedic Surgery and Rehabilitation Medicine, University of Chicago Hospitals, 5841 South Maryland Avenue, Chicago, IL 60637, USA; [b] Department of Orthopaedic Surgery and Rehabilitation Medicine, University of Chicago Hospitals, 5841 South Maryland Avenue, Room P-211, MC 3079, Chicago, IL 60637, USA
* Corresponding author.
E-mail address: jwolf@bsd.uchicago.edu

Hand Clin 34 (2018) 139–148
https://doi.org/10.1016/j.hcl.2017.12.004
0749-0712/18/© 2018 Elsevier Inc. All rights reserved.

- 5% at the index finger
- 10% at the middle finger
- 14% at the ring finger
- 24% at the small finger.

The frequency and distribution of PIP joint dislocations was similar to the findings of Joyce and colleagues.[6] The investigators reported that 69% of dislocations were reduced in the emergency room, with 19% treated in the community, and 8% in the operating room.

Etiologic factors

PIP joint dislocations are defined by the position of the middle phalanx in relation to the proximal phalanx.[1] These are classified as

- Dorsal
- Volar
- Lateral.

Each has a specific mechanism, findings, associated soft tissue injury, management, and complications.

Dorsal dislocations represent almost all PIP joint dislocations. They are characterized by the following:

- Mechanism: forced hyperextension, axial load,[7] and radial or ulnar deviation[8]
- Volar plate rupture at its distal attachment
- A split between the accessory collateral ligament and proper collateral ligament with detachment of the proper collateral ligament from its proximal attachment[9]
- The volar plate is maintained beneath the condyle, held by intact attachment to the accessory collateral ligament[1]
- When a torsional mechanism is involved, soft tissue interposition can block reduction.[10]

Lateral dislocations (**Fig. 1**) are less common and characterized by

- Mechanism: direct radial or ulnar stress on the PIP joint with axial load
- The collateral ligament on the side of the force fails under tension, avulsing from its proximal attachment
- Continued force causes disruption of the volar plate on the side of the force.[1,7]

The least common is dislocation in the volar direction, with or without a rotatory component (**Fig. 2**). This was described in 1970 by Spinner and Choi[11] in a series of 5 cases. Their cadaveric study demonstrated that volar dislocation required force in 2 vectors:

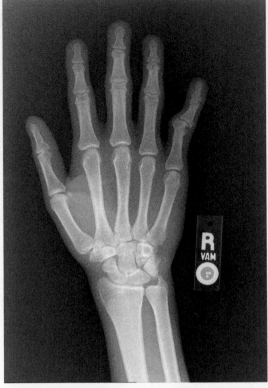

Fig. 1. Lateral dislocation of the small finger PIP joint. Failure of the collateral ligament and volar plate on the side of force results in lateral angulation and translation of the middle phalanx.

- Ulnar or radial deviation causing rupture of the collateral ligament and volar plate
- A second vector with volar force against the middle phalanx.

Volar PIP joint dislocation can result in 1 of 2 patterns of soft tissue injury:

- Volar dislocation without torsion
  - Direct volar translation of middle phalanx, resulting in central slip rupture
  - Accompanied by rupture of volar plate and 1 collateral ligament
- Volar dislocation with torsion
  - 1 condyle of the proximal phalanx slides past the central slip
  - Longitudinal tear forms between intact central slip and intact lateral band
  - Attenuation of triangular ligament[12]
  - The proximal phalanx subluxates between central slip and lateral band
  - The middle phalanx dislocates volarly and rotates around the intact collateral ligament.

Both mechanisms result in extensor lag at the PIP joint.

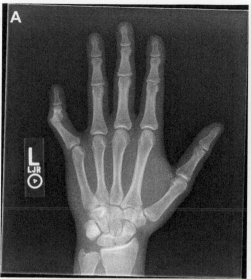
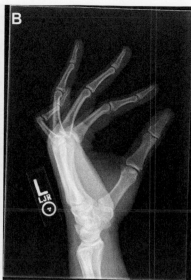

Fig. 2. Two varieties of volar PIP joint dislocation. (*A*) When a torsional component is involved, 1 condyle of the proximal phalanx slides past an intact central slip. (*B*) Without a torsional component, direct volar force results in rupture of the central slip, volar plate, and 1 collateral ligament.

TECHNIQUE: CLOSED REDUCTION OF THE PROXIMAL INTERPHALANGEAL JOINT

Each of the 3 dislocation types has a distinct reduction maneuver due to the differential soft tissue injury and mechanism. Digital block is usually sufficient to anesthetize the affected digit and allows relatively easy and painless reduction:

- Dorsal
  - Longitudinal traction, gentle PIP joint flexion[7]
  - Gentle volar force along dorsal side of the middle phalanx can aid reduction[7,13]
- Lateral
  - Longitudinal traction with ulnar or radial directed force, based on direction of dislocation
  - The joint will often reduce with longitudinal traction alone
- Volar
  - Longitudinal traction, dorsal directed force, and extension[7]
  - Performing reduction with the metacarpophalangeal (MCP) joint in flexion relaxes the lateral band through which the proximal phalanx is buttonholed[1]
  - If there is a rotatory component to the mechanism, a reciprocal rotatory maneuver is required for reduction.[1]

As with all dislocations, it is important to assess the stability after reduction both clinically and fluoroscopically by taking the finger through active and passive range of motion (ROM) and testing the collateral ligaments. In general, dorsal and lateral

dislocations reduce easily without a soft tissue block to reduction,[7] whereas reducibility of volar dislocations depends on the status of the central slip and the presence or absence of soft tissue interposition.

IRREDUCIBLE DISLOCATIONS OR BLOCK TO REDUCTION

A small subset of PIP joint dislocations is irreducible by closed means. Soft tissue interposition is usually the cause of irreducible dislocation and the exact identity of the interposed tissue depends on the type of dislocation.

Dorsal dislocations are at the lowest risk for irreducibility, so much so that many of the major texts on hand surgery fail to mention it.[4] The risk, however, is not zero because irreducible dorsal dislocations (**Fig. 3**) have been described in several case reports[4,14–17] (**Table 1**). The most common block to reduction is the volar plate, which falls into the joint when rupture occurs at its proximal membranous attachment and is no longer supported by the accessory collateral ligaments.[1] Successful reduction is achieved after retrieval of the plate from the joint. Reduction can also be blocked by the intact flexor digitorum profundus (FDP) and flexor digitorum superficialis (FDS),[15] buttonholing of the proximal phalanx between the FDS slips,[18] or buttonholing of the proximal phalanx through the volar plate[16] (see **Table 1**).

Volar dislocations of the PIP joint, which are less common, can be difficult to reduce. Paradoxically, it is the less severe volar dislocations that are commonly irreducible.[3] One of the earliest reports

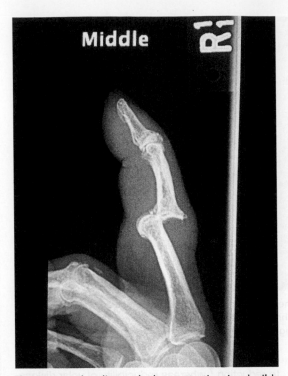

Fig. 3. Lateral radiograph demonstrating irreducible dorsal dislocation of the long finger PIP joint. An incarcerated volar plate was responsible; however, FDS, FDP, and buttonholing of the volar plate have been implicated in irreducible dorsal dislocations.

of an irreducible volar dislocation was in 1966 by Johnson and Greene,[19] who described an intact central slip, ulnar collateral ligament rupture, and buttonholing of the proximal phalanx head between the central slip and lateral band. Reduction of the central slip and lateral band allowed for reduction and a stable joint. Several investigators have described similar findings.[20–23] Reduction can also be blocked by an isolated lateral band with a ruptured central slip[11,24,25] or an isolated lateral band with an intact central slip[26] (see **Table 1**).

Irreducible lateral dislocations are rare and reports in the literature are scarce (see **Table 1**). In 2004 Isshiki and colleagues[27] reported a case in which a collateral ligament and joint capsule had detached in a sleeve-like fashion and become interposed in the joint. Blocks to reduction also include the collateral ligament alone[28] and an intact extensor tendon.[29]

REHABILITATION FOR CLOSED OR REDUCIBLE DISLOCATIONS

General postreduction management of PIP joint dislocations consists of

- Minimal immobilization for soft tissue rest (2–3 days)
- Rapid mobilization to support cartilage health
- Supportive taping to decrease edema.

Table 1		
Summary of cases describing soft tissue block to reduction of the proximal interphalangeal joint		
Type	**Authors, Year**	**Findings: Blocks to Closed Reduction**
Dorsal	Green & Posner,[4] 1985	• 4 cases: 3 primary, 1 delayed
		• Avulsed proximal volar plate in joint
	Oni,[17] 1985	• Avulsed proximal volar plate in joint
	Takami et al,[15] 2001	• Intact FDP and FDS in joint
	Kung et al,[18] 1998	• Proximal phalanx buttonholed in FDS slip
	Kjeldal,[16] 1986	• 1 case of buttonholing through volar plate
		• 2 cases with flexor tendons in joint
Lateral	Isshiki et al,[27] 2004	• Collateral ligament and capsule subluxated into joint
	Redler & Williams,[28] 1967	• Collateral ligament in joint
	Neviaser & Wilson,[29] 1972	• Intact extensor tendon in joint
Volar	Johnson & Greene,[19] 1966	• Intact central slip, UCL rupture
		• Proximal phalanx between central slip and lateral band
	Murakami,[21] 1974	• Intact central slip, UCL rupture
		• Proximal phalanx between central slip and lateral band
	Posner & Kapila,[22] 1986	• Intact central slip, UCL rupture
		• Proximal phalanx between central slip and lateral band
	Ostrowski & Neimkin,[23] 1985	• Intact central slip, UCL rupture
		• Proximal phalanx between central slip and lateral band
	Inoue & Maeda,[20] 1990	• Central slip and lateral band subluxated into joint
	Nanno et al,[24] 2004	• Ruptured central slip, lateral band in joint
	Peimer et al,[25] 1984	• Ruptured central slip, lateral band in joint
	Spinner & Choi,[11] 1970	• Ruptured central slip, lateral band in joint
	Chamseddine et al,[26] 2009	• Lateral band in joint with central slip intact.

Dorsal dislocation typically results in rupture of the volar plate and 1 collateral ligament. If reduction is achieved and congruity of the joint surfaces is confirmed, these PIP joint dislocations are amenable to nonoperative treatment. Often, a small volar avulsion fragment is visualized after reduction, consistent with a volar plate injury. Eaton and Littler[1] described splinting in full extension to prevent flexion contracture, with unstable joints splinted in a position of stability; however, this led to hyperextension contracture. Chinchalkar and Gan[3] recommended either dorsal block splinting or pinning to block extension while maintaining flexion for 4 to 6 weeks, making sure to continue flexion and extension exercises:

- Rehabilitation for stable dorsal dislocation
  - Buddy taping for 2 weeks to prevent hyperextension[30]
  - Progressive active ROM, preventing passive hyperextension
- Rehabilitation for unstable dorsal dislocation
  - Extension block splinting at point of stability using a figure-of-8 splint[6]
    - Active flexion allowed
    - The distal interphalangeal (DIP) joint is not included in splint
  - Obligatory extension decreased 25% weekly over 4 weeks
    - Weekly radiographs to evaluate stability.

Modifications include use of buddy taping in stable dislocations and figure-of-8 splinting in unstable dislocations. Joyce and colleagues[6] evaluated the effect of splint style on patient outcomes, finding figure-of-8 splinting superior to dorsal blocking, buddy taping, and immobilization. The superiority of figure-of-8 splinting is due to

- Rigid protection of the collateral ligaments
- Prevention of hyperextension
- Simultaneously allowing full flexion at the PIP and DIP joints.

This splint supports

- Smooth flexor tendon gliding
- Decreased swelling
- Prevention of arthrofibrosis.

Simple buddy taping of stable dislocations is supported by a randomized trial by Paschos and colleagues[30] that demonstrated faster resolution of edema and earlier return to baseline ROM in subjects treated with buddy taping than those treated with aluminum extension block splinting.

Most lateral dislocations with good articular congruence and minimal lateral instability are amenable to nonoperative management as long as lateral instability is less than 20°.[7] Intact flexion and extension mechanisms provide significant joint stability despite ligamentous injury. In 1976, Eaton and Littler[1] recommended immobilization in approximately 25° to 30° of flexion for 2 to 3 weeks. Since then, there has been a paradigm shift to dynamic splinting. Chinchalkar and Gan[3] recommended

- Extension block splinting (between 10° and 15°), leaving the DIP joint free
- Progression to full active extension over 2 to 3 weeks
- Buddy taping on the side of the injured collateral ligament for an additional 3 to 4 weeks.

Suboptimal management of volar dislocations can lead to pain, stiffness, and a boutonniere deformity.[11,22,25,31] It is of the utmost importance to evaluate the patient's ROM because an extensor lag of greater than 30° suggests a significant disruption of the extensor mechanism and surgical intervention is indicated. If extensor lag is less than 30° and the joint is stable through ROM, nonoperative management is acceptable.[1] The recommended regimen is

- The PIP joint splinted in full extension, the DIP joint left free
  - This position approximates central slip to anatomic insertion
  - DIP joint flexion and extension in the splint is encouraged
  - This promotes gliding of the lateral bands and decreases tension on the central slip
- Immobilization for 3 to 4 weeks
- Dynamic extension splinting for 2 weeks
- Progressive passive flexion and strengthening
- Active extension.

SEQUELAE

The long-term sequelae of PIP joint dislocations depend on which structures around the PIP joint are injured, as well as the adequacy of splinting and rehabilitation course.

Dorsal dislocations have good outcomes when hyperextension is limited because it allows the volar plate to heal back to its distal attachment. However, splinting the patient in too much flexion or for an extended period puts the patient at risk for flexion contracture and pseudo-boutonniere deformity.[8]

Daily flexion and extension exercises in the splint and aggressive ROM rehabilitation after the patient comes out of the splint help prevent contracture. For a stable dorsal dislocation, immobilization should be limited to 3 to 7 days. The other extreme occurs when the finger is splinted in hyperextension. The volar plate becomes attenuated and the lateral bands subluxate dorsal to the PIP joint with resultant DIP joint extensor lag, resulting in a swan neck deformity.[8]

Lateral dislocations occur when 1 collateral ligament is completely disrupted. If improperly immobilized, the collateral ligament will fail to heal or will heal in an attenuated fashion. This results in persistent instability, which can cause pain, swelling, dysfunction of the digit, and susceptibility to recurrent trauma.[32]

The most common complication of a volar dislocation is a boutonniere deformity. Most volar dislocations are accompanied by rupture of the central slip. With the loss of extensor tendon continuity, the imbalance of forces results in flexion at the PIP joint. Stretching of the triangular ligament then leads to dorsal subluxation of the lateral bands at the level of the DIP joint and obligatory hyperextension at the DIP joint. This is initially correctable with passive extension exercises at the PIP joint, resulting in a flexible boutonniere. If left untreated, this can develop into a permanent contracture and a fixed boutonniere deformity. Correction with splinting is possible until approximately 6 weeks after injury. After that time, surgical intervention is recommended, highlighting the importance of a thorough clinical examination and evaluation of the extensor lag as close to the time of injury as possible.[25]

CHRONIC DISLOCATION AND INSTABILITY

Although most patients do well following concentric reduction of a simple PIP joint dislocation, chronic dislocation or instability can occur with delay in treatment or nonconcentric reduction. Chronic instability is

- Greatest in volar dislocation because both ligamentous and tendinous restraints are compromised
- Dorsal and lateral dislocation are at lower risk because only ligamentous structures are affected.

If the PIP joint is not immobilized in extension after volar dislocation, the central slip will heal in a retracted location due to the pull of extensor digitorum communis. This differs from the volar plate, which in most cases will heal in an acceptable location.

Chronic dislocation is defined as persistent dislocation or subluxation of the joint, often seen when a patient presents for treatment after delay or neglect of a finger injury. At 6 weeks after injury, closed management is unlikely to result in favorable outcomes.[25] If chronic subluxation is present,

there is uneven wear on the cartilage surfaces of the proximal and middle phalanges, which can quickly lead to stiffness, arthritis, pain, swelling, deformity, and poor function.[1,12,22,33–35] As a result, chronic subluxation is an indication for surgery, with the goal of reducing the articular surfaces to prevent further damage.

SURGICAL TECHNIQUE: OPEN REDUCTION OF THE PROXIMAL INTERPHALANGEAL JOINT

Indications for surgery include

- Acute irreducible dislocation
- Chronic dislocation or subluxation
- Lateral instability greater than 20°.

Preoperative Planning

It is critical to analyze the direction of the original dislocation because this helps the surgeon to identify which structures have been compromised and need repair or reconstruction.

Patient Positioning

The patient is positioned supine with the arm on a hand table. A tourniquet, if used, is placed high on the arm to allow the arm to be supinated or pronated for surgical approaches without the bulk of the tourniquet.

Surgical Approach

This differs depending on the type of dislocation. Each type of approach is detailed in the following sections.

Open reduction for dorsal dislocation of the proximal interphalangeal joint: acute

Surgical intervention for both acute and chronic dorsal dislocations is focused at repairing or reconstructing the volar plate (**Table 2**). If the volar plate is blocking reduction, it must be removed from the joint surgically:

- Using a lead hand, the arm is supinated to expose the volar side of the hand
- The PIP joint is approached from a volar Bruner-type extensile approach, or a midlateral approach
- Care is taken to protect the digital arteries and nerves, which can be tented or prominent volarly
- If the flexor tendons have subluxated behind the proximal phalanx, they must first be reduced
- If the volar plate is interposed within the joint, this is then directly visualized and extracted from the joint.

Table 2
Published outcomes for open reduction of acute irreducible dorsal dislocations

Authors, Year	Technique Notes	Outcomes

Green & Posner,[4] 1985	• No repair of volar plate
	  ○ K-wire fixation or extension block splint
		• 2/3 subjects near full ROM
		  ○ 1/3 subjects 65° flexion contracture, full flexion

Kjeldal,[16] 1986	Primary repair of volar plate	• ½ subjects regained full painless ROM • ½ subjects ROM 20°–100° of flexion
Takami et al,[15] 2001	• No repair of volar plate ○ K-wire fixation in slight flexion	10° shy of full extension, full flexion
Muraoka et al,[14] 2010	• No repair of volar plate • Immobilized in aluminum splint	• Full painless ROM • Persistent swelling

Postoperative care

- The digit is immobilized via splinting or Kirschner wire (K-wire) fixation for 1 to 2 weeks
- Rehabilitation with graded increases in ROM and dynamic extension splinting is then initiated.

Technique: reduction of chronic dorsal dislocation

With chronic dislocation, the volar plate and collateral ligaments retract and scar down and are, therefore, no longer able to heal to their original insertion. Several techniques have been described that use local or remote tendon autograft to reconstruct the volar plate (**Table 3**). The earliest technique was described by Bate[36] in 1945, involving primary repair of the volar plate and collateral ligament. Currently, the most common technique involves

tenodesis using 1 slip of the FDS. It was initially described by Littler[37]; however it was popularized by Catalano and colleagues,[38] who described it more thoroughly and published promising results:

- The PIP joint is approached via a volar Bruner incision, with the apex at the radial midaxial line
- Full-thickness flaps are used
- The flexor tendon sheath is incised in an L-shaped fashion, with the transverse leg at the proximal end of the A1 pulley and the longitudinal limb on the radial side of the sheath
- The ulnar FDS slip is transected at its most proximal end without damaging the main tendon
  ○ The length of the slip is maximized by extending the wrist at the time of transection
  ○ The slip is mobilized proximal to distal

Table 3
Published outcomes following reconstruction for chronic dorsal proximal interphalangeal dislocation

Authors, Year	Technique Notes	Outcomes
Bate,[36] 1945	• Volar plate and collateral ligaments repaired primarily	• Full flexion, 20° flexion contracture
Adams,[35] 1959	• Palmaris longus autograft criss-cross through bone tunnels	• 2/3 subjects full ROM • 1/3 subjects full flexion, 25° flexion contracture
Wiley,[34] 1965	• Intact FDS slip tacked to volar plate base of middle phalanx with pullout suture	• 1/3 lacked full extension • 1/3 ROM 35°–90° • 1/3 ROM 20°–75°, pain with ADLs
Catalano et al,[38] 2003	• FDS tenodesis to proximal phalanx with bone tunnel or suture anchor	• 12 subjects, average ROM 12°–100° • 10/12 with excellent function • 2/12 with fair function and flexion contracture (60°–90°) • 12/12 subjects returned to preoperative employment
Onishi et al,[39] 2007	• FDS tenodesis using suture anchor without crossing FDS under FDS or FDP, VP repair	• 1 subject, full flexion, 20° flexion contracture. • Lateral stability
Swanstrom et al,[40] 2016	• FDS tenodesis at mid-diaphysis of proximal phalanx	• 5/5 with without recurrent deformity, apprehension, or deformity • Mean ROM -1-96°, achieved by 3 mo

- The FDS slip is passed deep to the FDP and radial FDS slip
- A transverse tunnel is made in the head of the proximal phalanx
- The transected slip is passed through the tunnel from radial to ulnar and tensioned with the PIP joint at 5° to 8° of flexion
- The tendon slip is sutured to the periosteum at the entry and exit from the tunnel, or can be stabilized using a suture anchor.

Postoperative care
- The hand is immobilized in a short arm cast incorporating the adjacent digits for 7 to 10 days
- At that point, flexion and extension is begun with a dorsal blocking splint that limits terminal 10° to 15° of extension
- Full motion is allowed 4 weeks postoperative, avoiding hyperextension.

SURGICAL TECHNIQUE: VOLAR PROXIMAL INTERPHALANGEAL JOINT DISLOCATIONS

Volar dislocations become irreducible when

- The proximal phalanx buttonholes between an intact central slip and lateral band[3]
- Most of the soft tissue restraint is intact.

Open reduction of irreducible volar dislocation can be accomplished via the following technique:

- The PIP joint is approached by a curved incision over the dorsum of the joint
- Thick flaps are raised, with care taken to protect the neurovascular bundles
- Structures that lie within the joint are bluntly removed and replaced in the native positions:
  o Central slip[19–21,23]
  o Lateral band[20,24–26,41]
  o Ruptured collateral ligaments[28]
- The joint usually reduces easily by the maneuver previously described
- If the central slip is ruptured, it is repaired to its insertion, typically using 1 or 2 small or miniature suture anchors
- The longitudinal split between the central slip and the lateral band is repaired primarily with resorbable suture (eg, 2-0 Vicryl or similar)
- The joint is splinted in extension, either for 5 to 7 days in the absence of central slip rupture, or for 3 weeks if the injury required repair of the central slip.

Untreated volar PIP joint dislocation can go on to develop chronic instability, subluxation, and boutonnière deformity as the result of an attenuated central slip, dorsally subluxated lateral bands, and volar plate contracture. Reconstruction is complicated because of the complex balance of the extensor mechanism. It includes reconstruction of the central slip at its native insertion while releasing the contracted lateral bands, collateral ligaments, and volar plate.

Outcomes

There has been little written specifically on surgical treatment of chronic volar PIP joint dislocation due to its relative scarcity. Peimer and colleagues[25] published a series on 15 subjects with volar PIP joint dislocations, with a reported delay to presentation averaging 11 weeks after injury. Twelve of 15 required open reduction with ligament and tendon repair, and none recovered full motion, with a reported PIP joint arc of motion between 50° to 100°. Posner and Kapila[22] reported on 7 subjects with chronic volar PIP joint dislocations treated with advancement of the central slip and mobilization of the lateral bands, combined with pinning, and noted an average arc of motion was 57° with minimal pain.

SURGICAL TECHNIQUE: LATERAL PROXIMAL INTERPHALANGEAL JOINT DISLOCATIONS

There is controversy regarding surgical intervention for lateral dislocation because the injured collateral ligament has good potential to heal with immobilization (Table 4). Redler and Williams[28] advocated for repair of complete collateral ligament injuries, as opposed to partial tears, because of the risk of prolonged swelling and stiffness. Bindra and Foster[7] recommended surgical intervention with

- Instability greater than 20°
- Involvement of the small or index finger PIP joints
- High functional demand based on patient activity.

Technique: Lateral Approach

- The PIP joint is approached from a midlateral incision on the injured side.
- The collateral ligament is identified; if interposed into the joint, it is extracted and replaced in an anatomic position.
- The ligament is typically torn from its proximal attachment, as shown by Kiefhaber and colleagues.[42]
- The collateral ligament is repaired, typically using a microsuture anchor.[43,44]
- If detached, the volar plate is repaired back to its insertion at the base of the middle phalanx using resorbable sutures.
- The PIP joint is immobilized in 10° to 15° of flexion for 2 to 3 weeks in a dorsal splint, which

Table 4
Published outcomes following repair of the lateral collateral ligaments

Authors, Year	Technique Notes	Outcomes
Redler & Williams,[28] 1967	• 14 subjects • Primary repair of proximal rupture	• Joint stability achieved in 14/14 subjects • None lost >10° flexion or extension
McCue et al,[32] 1970	• 30 acute, 5 chronic • Repair with Bunnell suture over button on opposite side • Volar plate repaired with dissolvable suture	• Acute: 30/30 with lateral stability, 5/30 lost 5°–10° ROM • Chronic: 2 stable, 3 with lateral laxity, flexion contractures 0°–20°
Ali,[45] 1984	• RCT, 14 treated with surgery, 14 without • Ligament repaired with stainless suture through 2 bone tunnels	• Operated: stable, painless on lateral stress, 14/14 reached preoperative function • Unoperated: 14/14 had pain and laxity, 64% with functional disability • ROM equal between groups, 79% ROM >0°–90°

pairs the digit with the adjacent digit on the side of the collateral ligament injury. Protected motion is permitted with buddy taping.

SUMMARY

Pure dislocations of the PIP joint are common and are often reduced before the patient presents for care. These injuries should be treated and mobilized promptly due to the debilitating sequelae that can result from delayed management. Dorsal, volar, and lateral dislocations all have distinct tissue injuries and require different closed and open treatment. Chronic or neglected dislocations require operative reduction and possible tendon and ligament reconstruction, generally resulting in stiffness and loss of function.

REFERENCES

1. Eaton RG, Littler JW. Joint injuries and their sequelae. Clin Plast Surg 1976;3(1):85–98.
2. Mall NA, Carlisle JC, Matava MJ, et al. Upper extremity injuries in the national football league: part I: hand and digital injuries. Am J Sports Med 2008;36(10):1938–44.
3. Chinchalkar SJ, Gan BS. Management of proximal interphalangeal joint fractures and dislocations. J Hand Ther 2003;16(2):117–28.
4. Green SM, Posner MA. Irreducible dorsal dislocations of the proximal interphalangeal joint. J Hand Surg Am 1985;10(1):85–7.
5. Hindle P, Davidson EK, Biant LC, et al. Appendicular joint dislocations. Injury 2013;44(8):1022–7.
6. Joyce KM, Joyce CW, Conroy F, et al. Proximal interphalangeal joint dislocations and treatment: an evolutionary process. Arch Plast Surg 2014;41(4):394–7.
7. Bindra RR, Foster BJ. Management of proximal interphalangeal joint dislocations in athletes. Hand Clin 2009;25(3):423–35.
8. Prucz RB, Friedrich JB. Finger joint injuries. Clin Sports Med 2015;34(1):99–116.
9. Arora R, Lutz M, Fritz D, et al. Dorsolateral dislocation of the proximal interphalangeal joint: closed reduction and early active motion or static splinting; a retrospective study. Arch Orthop Trauma Surg 2004;124(7):486–8.
10. Freiberg A. Management of proximal interphalangeal joint injuries. Can J Plast Surg 2007;15(4):199–203.
11. Spinner M, Choi BY. Anterior dislocation of the proximal interphalangeal joint. A cause of rupture of the central slip of the extensor mechanism. J Bone Joint Surg Am 1970;52(7):1329–36.
12. Freeman BH, Haskin JS Jr, Hay EL. Chronic anterior dislocation of the proximal interphalangeal joint. Orthopedics 1985;8(3):385–8.
13. Bielak KM, Kafka J, Terrell T. Treatment of hand and wrist injuries. Prim Care 2013;40(2):431–51.
14. Muraoka S, Furue Y, Kawashima M. Irreducible open dorsal dislocation of the proximal interphalangeal joint: a case report. Hand Surg 2010;15(1):61–4.
15. Takami H, Takahashi S, Ando M. Irreducible open dorsal dislocation of the proximal interphalangeal joint. Arch Orthop Trauma Surg 2001;121(4):232–3.
16. Kjeldal I. Irreducible compound dorsal dislocations of the proximal interphalangeal joint of the finger. J Hand Surg Br 1986;11(1):49–50.
17. Oni OO. Irreducible buttonhole dislocation of the proximal interphalangeal joint of the finger (a case report). J Hand Surg Br 1985;10(1):100.

18. Kung J, Touliopolis S, Caligiuri D. Irreducible dislocation of the proximal interphalangeal joint of a finger. J Hand Surg Br 1998;23(2):252.

19. Johnson FG, Greene MH. Another cause of irreducible dislocation of the proximal interphalangeal joint of a finger. J Bone Joint Surg Am 1966;48(3):542–4.

20. Inoue G, Maeda N. Irreducible palmar dislocation of the proximal interphalangeal joint of the finger. J Hand Surg Am 1990;15(2):301–4.

21. Murakami Y. Irreducible volar dislocation of the proximal interphalangeal joint of the finger. Hand 1974; 6(1):87–90.

22. Posner MA, Kapila D. Chronic palmar dislocation of proximal interphalangeal joints. J Hand Surg Am 1986;11(2):253–8.

23. Ostrowski DM, Neimkin RJ. Irreducible palmar dislocation of the proximal interphalangeal joint. A case report. Orthopedics 1985;8(1):84–6.

24. Nanno M, Sawaizumi T, Ito H. Irreducible palmar dislocation of the proximal interphalangeal joint of a finger evaluated by magnetic resonance imaging: a case report. Hand Surg 2004;9(2):253–6.

25. Peimer CA, Sullivan DJ, Wild DR. Palmar dislocation of the proximal interphalangeal joint. J Hand Surg Am 1984;9A(1):39–48.

26. Chamseddine AH, Jawish R, Zein H. Irreducible volar dislocation of the proximal interphalangeal finger joint. Chir Main 2009;28(4):255–9.

27. Isshiki H, Yamanaka K, Sasaki T. Irreducible lateral dislocation of the proximal interphalangeal joint–a case report. Hand Surg 2004;9(1):131–5.

28. Redler I, Williams JT. Rupture of a collateral ligament of the proximal interphalangeal joint of the fingers. Analysis of eighteen cases. J Bone Joint Surg Am 1967;49(2):322–6.

29. Neviaser RJ, Wilson JN. Interposition of the extensor tendon resulting in persistent subluxation of the proximal interphalangeal joint of the finger. Clin Orthop 1972;83:118–21.

30. Paschos NK, Abuhemoud K, Gantsos A, et al. Management of proximal interphalangeal joint hyperextension injuries: a randomized controlled trial. J Hand Surg 2014;39(3):449–54.

31. Bot AG, Bekkers S, Herndon JH, et al. Determinants of disability after proximal interphalangeal joint sprain or dislocation. Psychosomatics 2014;55(6):595–601.

32. McCue FC, Honner R, Johnson MC, et al. Athletic injuries of the proximal interphalangeal joint requiring surgical treatment. J Bone Joint Surg Am 1970; 52(5):937–56.

33. Hussin P, Mahendran S, Ng ES. Chronic dislocation of proximal interphalangeal joint with mallet finger: a case report. Cases J 2008;1(1):201.

34. Wiley AM. Chronic dislocation of the proximal interphalangeal joint: a method of surgical repair. Can J Surg 1965;8(4):435–9.

35. Adams JP. Correction of chronic dorsal subluxation of the proximal interphalangeal joint by means of a criss-cross volar graft. J Bone Joint Surg Am 1959; 41-A(1):111–5.

36. Bate JT. An operation for the correction of locking of the proximal interphalangeal joint of finger in hyperextension. J Bone Joint Surg 1945;27(1): 142–4.

37. Littler J. The hand and wrist. In: Howorth MB, editor. A textbook of orthopedics. Stamford (CT): Dorman; 1959. p. 284–5.

38. Catalano LW, Skarparis AC, Glickel SZ, et al. Treatment of chronic, traumatic hyperextension deformities of the proximal interphalangeal joint with flexor digitorum superficialis tenodesis. J Hand Surg 2003;28(3):448–52.

39. Onishi Y, Fujioka H, Doita M. Treatment of chronic post-traumatic hyperextension deformity of proximal interphalangeal joint using the suture anchor: a case report. Hand Surg 2007;12(01):47–9.

40. Swanstrom MM, Henn CM, Hearns KA, et al. Modified sublimis tenodesis: surgical technique for treating chronic traumatic proximal interphalangeal joint hyperextension instability. Tech Hand Up Extrem Surg 2016;20(1):48–51.

41. Posner MA, Wilenski M. Irreducible volar dislocation of the proximal interphalangeal joint of a finger caused by interposition of the intact central slip: a case report. J Bone Joint Surg Am 1978;60(1): 133–4.

42. Kiefhaber TR, Stern PJ, Grood ES. Lateral stability of the proximal interphalangeal joint. J Hand Surg 1986;11(5):661–9.

43. Morris SF, Yang D, Milne AD, et al. Reconstruction of the proximal interphalangeal joint collateral ligaments using the mitek micro arc anchor: an in vitro biomechanical assessment. Ann Plast Surg 1999; 42(2):124–8.

44. Kato H, Minami A, Takahara M, et al. Surgical repair of acute collateral ligament injuries in digits with the Mitek bone suture anchor. J Hand Surg 1999;24(1): 70–5.

45. Ali M. Complete disruption of collateral mechanism of proximal interphalangeal joint of fingers. J Hand Surg Br 1984;9(2):191–3.

Management of Proximal Interphalangeal Joint Fracture Dislocations

Nicholas M. Caggiano, MD[a], Carl M. Harper, MD[b],
Tamara D. Rozental, MD[c],*

KEYWORDS

- Proximal interphalangeal joint • Fracture-dislocation • Dynamic external fixator
- Volar plate arthroplasty • Hemihamate arthroplasty

KEY POINTS

- Fracture dislocations of the proximal interphalangeal (PIP) joint can have dramatic consequences for hand range of motion, especially when untreated.
- Dorsal fracture dislocations with a volar lip fracture are far more common than volar fracture-dislocations, which occur with a dorsal lip fracture.
- PIP joint fracture dislocations are commonly classified based on the amount of articular involvement on a lateral radiograph (Kiefhaber and Stern classification).
- Treatment of PIP fracture dislocations is based on stability of the joint, the size of the fracture fragment, and associated soft tissue injuries.
- Treatment options for PIP joint fracture dislocations include closed reduction and splint or taping, closed reduction and percutaneous pinning, open reduction with internal fixation, volar plate arthroplasty, hemihamate arthroplasty, and arthrodesis.

INTRODUCTION

Fracture dislocations of the proximal interphalangeal (PIP) joint of the finger are often caused by axial load applied to a slightly flexed joint. The most common injury pattern is a dorsal fracture dislocation with a volar lip fracture of the middle phalanx. Unfortunately, these injuries are too frequently written off by the patient or providers as a so-called jammed finger and are left untreated. The soft-tissue stabilizers of the PIP joint (collateral ligaments, volar plate, central slip of the extensor tendon) are often concomitantly injured, contributing to the swelling, pain, and instability of these fracture patterns. A late-presenting PIP joint fracture dislocation has a poor chance of regaining range of motion equivalent to the unaffected fingers, with unfavorable prognosis for achieving full composite fist formation and normal function of the hand. Thus, the physician must recognize these injury patterns, obtain the proper imaging, and understand the treatment algorithm of PIP joint fracture dislocations. This article is provided as a reference for the current understanding and best practices in treating PIP joint fracture dislocations.

All authors have nothing to disclose.
[a] Department of Orthopaedic Surgery, Beth Israel Deaconess Medical Center, 330 Brookline Avenue–Stoneman 10, Boston, MA 02215, USA; [b] Department of Orthopaedic Surgery, Harvard Medical School, Beth Israel Deaconess Medical Center, 330 Brookline Avenue–Stoneman 10, Boston, MA 02215, USA; [c] Hand and Upper Extremity Surgery, Department of Orthopaedic Surgery, Harvard Medical School, Beth Israel Deaconess Medical Center, 330 Brookline Avenue–Stoneman 10, Boston, MA 02215, USA
* Corresponding author.
E-mail address: trozenta@bidmc.harvard.edu

Hand Clin 34 (2018) 149–165
https://doi.org/10.1016/j.hcl.2017.12.005
0749-0712/18/© 2017 Elsevier Inc. All rights reserved.

ANATOMY

Proper function of the PIP joint is important to normal hand function. This is an inherently stable joint owing to the anatomic constraints that surround it.

The collateral ligament complex of the PIP joint is composed of the proper collateral and the accessory collateral ligaments. The proper collateral ligaments originate from the lateral and slightly dorsal aspect of the proximal phalangeal head just proximal to the articular surface. Its fibers course obliquely distal and volar to insert on a tubercle at the longitudinal axis of the middle phalanx, just distal to the proximal articular surface. The accessory collateral ligament arises slightly proximal and volar to the proper collateral ligament, and takes a more volar course to insert on the lateral aspect of the volar plate. In a simplified sense, the proper collateral ligament tightens with flexion, whereas the accessory collateral tightens with extension.

The anatomy of the volar plate has implications for the joint contractures that commonly occur following PIP joint fracture dislocations. The volar plate is a thick fibrocartilaginous structure that functions to prevent hyperextension of the PIP joint. It is tethered to the proximal phalanx by the checkrein ligaments proximally and laterally. The central and proximal area between these checkrein ligaments is untethered and mobile. With flexion of the PIP joint, this central-proximal part of the volar plate invaginates to allow for a greater flexion amplitude.[1] Thus, prolonged flexion and scarring of the proximal volar plate following fracture dislocation will limit the motion of the volar plate, leading to flexion contracture.[2]

Distally, the volar plate is firmly anchored onto the middle phalanx only at its lateral margins. The central portion between these distal attachments is the relatively thin fibrous portion that does not provide much structural support.

As the extensor tendon traverses the proximal phalanx, it divides into 3 slips: 2 lateral and the medial.[3] The lateral slips progress distally to join the lateral bands, whereas the medial slip (central slip) inserts into the dorsal aspect of the middle phalanx. All 3 slips act in concert to extend the PIP joint. The central slip is often disrupted from the middle phalanx during a volar fracture dislocation because the dorsal lip fragment on which it inserts is sheared off by the proximal phalangeal head. In this injury pattern, the lateral bands are no longer tethered to the extensor tendon via the triangular ligament and are thus permitted to subluxate volarly. As the lateral bands migrate volar, they shorten due to the loss of their tether to the middle phalanx. Their new contracted position volar to the axis of rotation of the PIP joint causes both a flexion at the PIP joint and extension at the distal interphalangeal (DIP) joint, causing the injury pattern known as the acute boutonniere deformity.

The articular surfaces, collateral ligaments, extrinsic tendons, and volar plate all act to confer stability to the joint. The volar plate, collateral ligaments, and central slip form a box around the PIP joint that imparts inherent strength. Each of these restraining structures originates and/or inserts in close proximity to the articular margins of the joint. Therefore, periarticular fractures can dislodge these soft-tissue restraints from the respective phalanx and lead to gross instability.

MECHANISM OF INJURY

PIP joint fracture dislocations can be divided most simply into volar, dorsal, and pilon fracture dislocations. Dorsal fracture dislocations occur far more often than their volar counterparts. As identified by Kiefhaber and Stern,[4] volar and dorsal fractures dislocations result from either shearing or avulsion, or a combination of the 2, whereas pilon fractures are pure axial loading injuries.

Mechanism of Dorsal Fracture Dislocations

Dorsal fracture dislocations (**Fig. 1**) are commonly produced by axial load with the joint held in a mild degree of flexion. The longitudinal force causes the volar lip of the middle phalanx to shear off as it impacts the head of the proximal phalanx. Patients often describe a jammed finger occurring when a ball impacts the tip of an outstretched finger. Unfortunately, these patients often reset the finger themselves and do not seek treatment until the resultant stiffness and swelling becomes unbearable, weeks to months after the initial injury.

Dorsal fracture dislocations can also occur following hyperextension injuries at the PIP joint. Rapid hyperextension leads to separation of the distal volar plate from its insertion on the middle phalanx, often with a bony avulsion.[5] However, disruption of the volar plate is not sufficient to produce dorsal dislocation unless the proper collateral ligament is also disrupted.

Mechanism of Volar Fracture Dislocations

Volar fracture dislocations (**Fig. 2**) occur far less frequently than dorsal dislocations. In these cases, the dorsal lip of the middle phalanx is sheared off by axial force applied to an extended finger, as opposed to the flexed position that leads to volar lip fractures in dorsal dislocations. The mechanism of volar fracture dislocations is thought to include

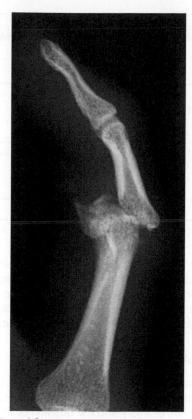

Fig. 1. Dorsal fracture dislocation.

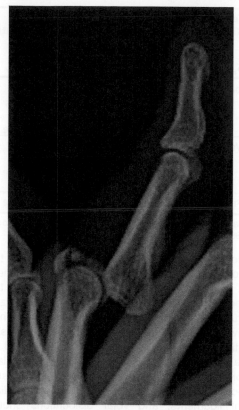

Fig. 2. Volar fracture dislocation. (*From* Meyer ZI, Goldfarb CA, Calfee RP, et al. The central slip fracture: results of operative treatment of volar fracture subluxations/dislocations of the proximal interphalangeal joint. J Hand Surg Am 2017;42(7):572.e3; with permission.)

an element of rotatory force, as well as axial and volar-directed load, onto the middle phalanx.[6] Just as disruption of the volar plate and at least 1 collateral ligament is necessary for a dorsal fracture dislocation, disruption of the central slip and at least 1 collateral ligament is necessary to produce a volar fracture dislocation.[6]

Mechanism of Pilon Fractures

Pilon fractures occur due to longitudinal force placed on the PIP joint sufficient to split the middle phalanx articular surface as it is driven into the head of the proximal phalanx (**Fig. 3**). Both the volar and dorsal lips of the middle phalanx are disrupted. The central articular surface of the middle phalanx may be impacted with metaphyseal compression. The PIP joint is almost always unstable following a pilon fracture.

CLASSIFICATION

Classification systems are most useful when they guide treatment.[7] Because the ultimate goal in treating fracture dislocations of the PIP joint is to provide a mobile, stable, and congruent joint, these injuries are best classified by their stability

and by the size of the articular fracture fragment in the sagittal plane. Stability should thus be assessed immediately following closed reduction of the joint.

The size of the middle phalanx articular involvement can be thought of as a surrogate for stability. Increasing size of the fracture fragment leads to compromised bony and soft tissue constraints and thus decreased stability. A commonly used classification system[4] (**Table 1**) categorizes

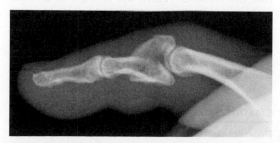

Fig. 3. Pilon fracture.

Table 1
Kiefhaber and Stern stability-based classification of proximal interphalangeal fracture dislocations

Pattern	% Articular Involvement	Stability	Treatment
Dorsal fracture dislocation (volar lip fragment)	<30%	Stable	Splinting
	30%–50%	Tenuous	Splinting if reduced in <30% of flexion Operative fixation otherwise
	>50%	Unstable	Operative fixation
Volar fracture dislocation (dorsal lip fragment)	<50%	Stable	Splinting if no volar subluxation of middle phalanx Operative fixation otherwise
	>50%	Unstable	Operative fixation
Pilon fracture	Any	Unstable	

Adapted from Kiefhaber TR, Stern PJ. Fracture dislocations of the proximal interphalangeal joint. J Hand Surg Am 1998;23(3):373; with permission.

fracture dislocations based on the percent of the middle phalanx articular surface involvement on a lateral radiograph.[4] Understanding the mechanism of injury and potentially traumatized structures is of paramount importance when developing a treatment plan. Thus, fracture dislocations of the PIP joint can also be classified by the direction of the dislocation (dorsal vs volar). Dorsal fracture dislocations should alert the surgeon to assess both the volar plate and the collateral ligaments, and volar dislocations should prompt an assessment of the central slip and collateral ligaments.

Classification of Dorsal Fracture Dislocations

Volar lip fractures occur with dorsal fracture dislocations. According to the Kiefhaber and Stern[4] classification scheme, those that involve 30% or less of the articular surface are generally stable and can be treated with progressive splinting. Fractures involving 50% or more are unstable and will require fixation to provide stability. Those involving 30% to 50% of the joint surface are tenuous and significant consideration should be given to operative fixation.

Classification of Volar Fracture Dislocations

Dorsal lip fractures are associated with volar fracture dislocations. Again, the amount of articular surface involved guides treatment, as well as an assessment of stability. Generally, those that involve less than 50% of the articular surface tend to be stable, whereas a fracture fragment of greater than 50% of the articular surface tends to be unstable.[4]

Classification of Pilon Fractures

Pilon fractures disrupt the entire articular surface and are thus not classified according to the

amount of middle phalanx involved. Classification is based solely on stability: fractures that maintain joint congruency throughout the entire arc of motion are deemed stable, whereas any subluxation or instability renders the fracture pattern unstable.

EVALUATION

The evaluation of a suspected PIP joint fracture dislocation begins with a thorough history. The mechanism of injury and the position of the finger at time of the insult will help to guide diagnosis and treatment. Examination of the finger should be directed at assessing the soft tissue envelope, as well as the neurovascular status of the finger. A significant amount of swelling about the PIP joint is to be expected. Any bleeding necessitates ruling out an open fracture.

Radiographs

After physical examination, imaging is the next most useful adjunct. Generally, posteroanterior and lateral views of the finger will provide enough information to make the diagnosis. The lateral view should be scrutinized not only to assess the approximate percentage of articular involvement but also to assess for avulsions of either the volar plate or the central slip. A V-sign (**Fig. 4**) in which

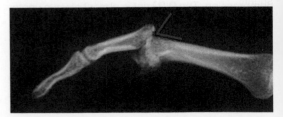

Fig. 4. V-sign as seen on the lateral view of a dorsal fracture dislocation.

gapping of the marginal joint space is noted indicates subluxation of the middle phalanx and thus instability. Similarly, coronal deviation on the posteroanterior view or bony avulsions from either side of the joint implies disruption of the collateral ligament complex.

Advanced Imaging

In the acute setting, computed tomography (CT) scans are rarely necessary. If there is a question about the amount of articular incongruity, a CT scan may provide more information; however, ultimately, the stability of the joint will provide the most guidance with regard to treatment. MRI is not typically used in the setting of an acute injury.

Joint Reduction

After obtaining imaging studies, the joint should be reduced. This can be performed effectively under digital blockade. Although the single subcutaneous injection technique for digital blockade has been shown to provide superior results in comparison with transthecal or dorsal injection techniques,[8] volar injections may not provide adequate analgesia to the dorsum of the PIP joint.[9,10] Therefore, it is recommended that 1 mL of 2% lidocaine be injected into the dorsal webspace on either side of the digit, at a depth of 3 to 4 mm. The use of epinephrine has been shown to be safe in the finger and provides longer duration of analgesic relief.[11]

After successful digital blockade, the joint is reduced based on the direction of dislocation. In the event of a dorsal dislocation, the volar plate may be entrapped in the joint space. Additionally, the use of isolated longitudinal traction will cause the checkrein ligaments of the volar plate to close down, preventing adequate reduction. The middle phalanx should be hyperextended with application of gentle proximally directed force. Longitudinal traction is then applied while holding the middle phalanx in this hyperextended position. Significant soft tissue swelling may make reduction difficult.

When reducing a volar dislocation, the surgeon should keep in mind that the middle phalanx may have button-holed through the flexor tendon sheath. Additionally, the central slip of the extensor tendon may be interposed in the joint space. The reduction technique is analogous to that for dorsal fracture dislocations, with the middle phalanx being flexed instead of extended.

Assessment of Stability

Once the joint is reduced, it should be splinted and reduction confirmed with radiographs. On successful reduction, the joint is then assessed for stability. The patient is asked to actively flex and extend the joint through a full range of motion. The surgeon then observes the joint for evidence of subluxation or dislocation. Fluoroscopy is helpful, as is adequate digital blockade.

While the patient slowly takes the PIP joint through a full range of motion, the surgeon inspects for any signs of instability. Any areas of articular incongruity are noted. The long axis of middle phalanx should always intersect the axis of rotation in the head of the proximal phalanx. The presence of a V-sign indicates some degree of instability.

Dorsal fracture dislocations are generally stable in some degree of flexion along the arc of motion. Stable injuries exhibit concentric reduction without subluxation in full extension. In unstable cases, gradual stability is obtained with increasing PIP joint flexion. Grossly unstable joints will typically demonstrate instability at 30° or more of PIP joint flexion. Volar fracture dislocations and pilon fractures are more binary; they either exhibit stability in full extension or they do not. Those that are stable in extension can be considered stable joints, whereas any instability in extension indicates a globally unstable joint.

The collateral ligaments should also be assessed. Minamikawa and colleagues[12] recommend that lateral stability be assessed in both extension and 30° of flexion to prevent false-negatives; 10° and 20° of angulation, respectively, in full extension and in 30° of flexion indicate proper collateral ligament disruption. Lateral deviation in extension of 15° or 30° in flexion implies additional disruption of the accessory collateral ligament.

TREATMENT
Goals of Treatment

Successful treatment of PIP joint fracture dislocations includes restoring a concentric stable joint while allowing for early range of motion. Delay in diagnosis and/or treatment will predictably lead to stiffness of the PIP joint, greatly compromising the normal function of the hand. Any treatment algorithm must strike a balance between providing adequate stability of the joint while allowing for early mobilization.

In addition to fixation of articular fracture fragments, soft tissue injuries must be recognized and treated. Collateral ligament damage results in coronal plane instability. The volar plate is commonly disrupted in dorsal fracture dislocations; failure to recognize and manage these injuries can lead to a swan-neck deformity. Central slip avulsions, seen with volar fracture dislocations, will progress to boutonniere deformity.

Treatment Algorithm

Treatment of fracture dislocations is based on stability of the joint, the size of the fracture fragment, and associated soft tissue injuries. Stable injuries can be treated in a closed manner, whereas unstable joints can be treated in a variety of fashions, including closed treatment, dynamic traction, external fixation, open reduction and internal fixation, advanced joint reconstruction, or arthrodesis. Any treatment should achieve joint stability and articular congruity, allowing early mobilization when possible. **Figs. 5–7** outline treatment algorithms for dorsal, volar, and pilon fracture dislocations.

Treatment of Stable Dorsal Fracture Dislocations

Buddy taping
Stable dorsal fracture dislocations generally disrupt less than 30° of the middle phalanx articular surface and are stable in extension. Because stability is present throughout the full range of motion of the PIP joint, buddy taping or strapping (**Fig. 8**) to an unaffected neighboring finger is the preferred treatment. This allows for early active range of motion while limiting the risk of hyperextension. The fingers are taped together for 3 to 4 weeks, at which time passive flexion and strengthening can begin.

Treatment of Tenuous Dorsal Fracture Dislocations

Extension block splinting
Tenuous fracture dislocations generally involve 30% to 50% of the middle phalanx articular surface and are stable between 0° and 30° of flexion. The goal of treatment is to take advantage of the stable range of motion between 30° and 90°. Extension block splinting (**Fig. 9**) allows for immediate active range of motion while preventing extension that could separate the volar lip fragment from the remainder of the middle phalanx. Repeat radiographs are required for the first 2 to 3 weeks to ensure no subsequent loss of reduction. The splint should be initially fabricated in the least amount of flexion that exhibits joint stability (maximum of 30°). The splint should be serially adjusted to decrease flexion by about 10° weekly, with a goal of full extension at 3 to 4 weeks.

Treatment of Unstable Dorsal Fracture Dislocations

Unstable dorsal fracture dislocations generally involve greater than 50% of the middle phalanx articular surface. Treatment focuses on providing concentric reduction and stability to the fracture fragment, allowing early range of motion while the fracture unites. The various surgical procedures described, as well as the lack of strong level-of-evidence studies, make surgical decision-making difficult.

Closed reduction and transarticular pinning
Perhaps the simplest method of surgical fixation is closed reduction and transarticular percutaneous pinning. The PIP joint is held in 30° to 60° of flexion while reduction of the fracture fragment is confirmed under fluoroscopy. A Kirschner (K)-wire is driven either retrograde or anterograde across the PIP joint, from the dorsum of the proximal phalanx to the dorsum of the middle phalanx. The wire is left in place for 4 weeks, at which time progressive extension block splinting is performed to a goal of full extension at 6 weeks. At that time, the splint is removed and therapy is begun for range of motion and strengthening.

de Haseth and colleagues retrospectively reviewed the results of 9 patients with unstable dorsal PIP joint fracture dislocations treated with transarticular K-wires. Their patients had an average articular involvement of 36%. By the end of their 6-month follow-up, the patients achieved a mean PIP joint flexion of 104° and an extension lag of 4°.[13]

Barksfield and colleagues[14] performed a similar review of 12 patients treated with transarticular pinning of unstable dorsal PIP joint fracture dislocations. Their series included an average 40% articular fracture fragment and 3-month follow-up. The patients had considerable loss of PIP joint range of motion, with a 56° arc of motion and a 15° flexion contracture. The endpoint of flexion was 73°. However, they note that their study included a relatively short follow-up period.

Closed reduction and percutaneous pinning
A variation of closed reduction and percutaneous pinning published by Vitale and colleagues[15] involves direct fixation of the fracture fragment to the middle phalanx (**Fig. 10**). The fracture is reduced with a towel clip under fluoroscopic guidance. After adequate reduction is achieved, a K-wire is driven from volar to dorsal (through the flexor tendon) to secure the fragment to the middle phalanx. The K-wire can be used to elevate the central impaction, and is then driven across the phalanx and out the dorsum of the finger. The wire is withdrawn from the dorsal side until the volar aspect is flush with the volar cortex of the fracture fragment. A second K-wire is inserted on the opposite side of the phalanx, resulting in 2 dorsal-to-volar pins, 1 in the radial half of the phalanx and 1 in the ulnar half. The K-wires are then

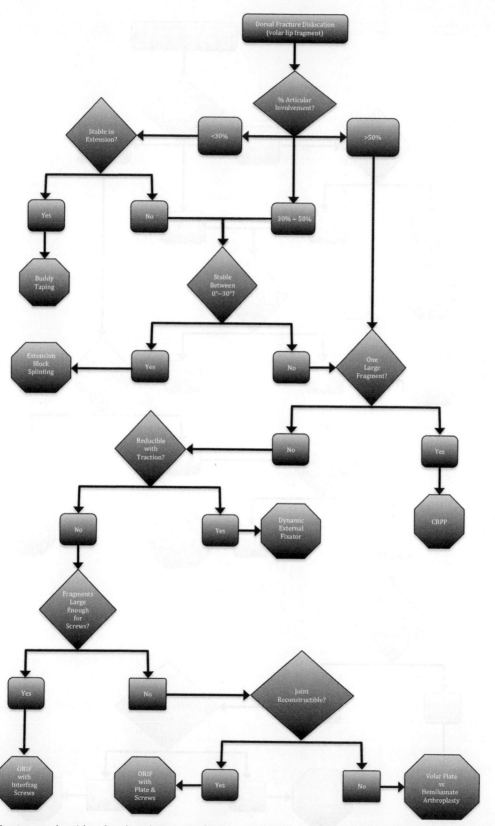

Fig. 5. Treatment algorithm for dorsal PIP joint fracture dislocations. CRPP, closed reduction and percutaneous pinning; ORIF, open reduction and internal fixation.

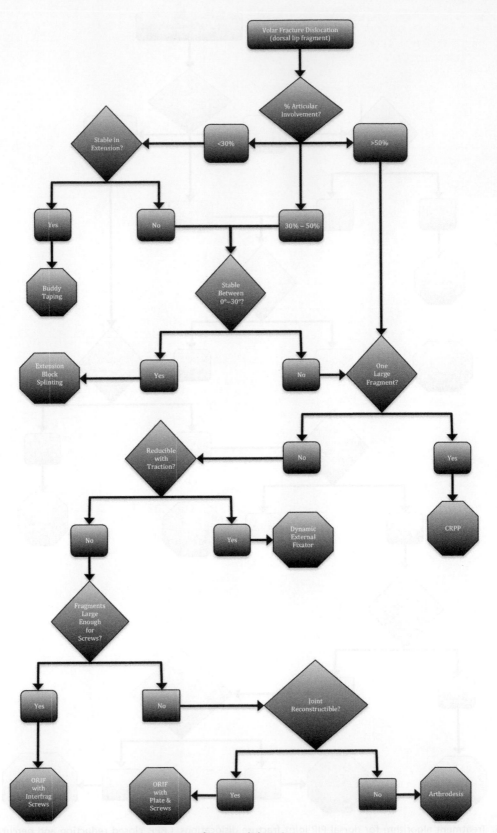

Fig. 6. Treatment algorithm for volar PIP joint fracture dislocations.

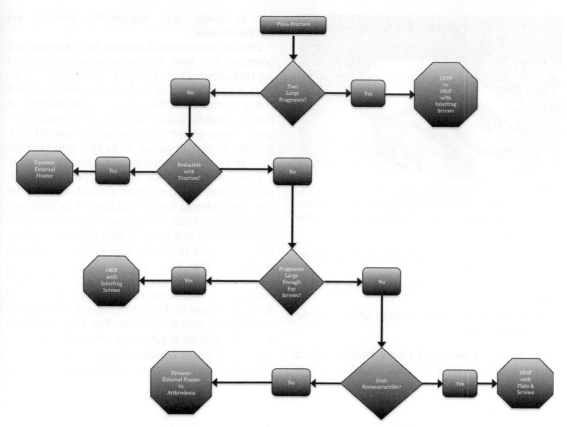

Fig. 7. Treatment algorithm for pilon-type PIP joint fracture dislocations.

bent and cut and a dorsal blocking K-wire is inserted dorsally to prevent extension of the PIP joint. The pins are kept in place for 4 weeks, at which time therapy is started. The Vitale and colleagues[15] series on 6 subjects treated in this manner demonstrated an 89° arc of motion (4°–93°), a Disability of the Arm, Shoulder, and

Hand (DASH) score of 8 and a visual analog (VAS) score of 1.4 out of 10.

Dynamic external fixation

Several K-wire–based dynamic external fixation devices have been developed that take advantage of ligamentotaxis to provide joint reduction. Concentric articular congruity must be achievable via a combination of longitudinal traction and translation to obtain a successful outcome.[16] In 1987, Agee[17] devised a 3-pin force couple splint that uses rubber bands to correct the sagittal plane deformity while allowing for full range of motion of the PIP joint. His series of 16 subjects followed for an average of 21 months had an average of 42% articular involvement. Although his cohort included chronic subluxations in addition to acute unstable fracture dislocations, the acute injuries averaged a 95° PIP joint arc of motion. Although he noted that only 6 subjects regained full extension, it is not clear whether those were chronic or acute cases.

Ruland and colleagues devised an external fixator using 3 0.045-in longitudinal K-wires and dental-grade rubber bands[18] (**Fig. 11**). The wires are placed

Fig. 8. Buddy strapping. (*From* Jensen C, Rayan G. Buddy strapping of mismatched fingers: the offset buddy strap. J Hand Surg Am 1996;21(2):317; with permission.)

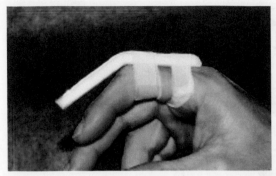

Fig. 9. Extension block splinting. (*From* Williams CS. Proximal interphalangeal joint fracture dislocations: stable and unstable. Hand Clin 2012;28(3):413; with permission.)

1. Through the center of rotation of the proximal phalangeal head
2. Through the middle phalanx just distal to the fracture
3. Through the center of rotation of the middle phalangeal head.

The wires are bent and rubber bands applied such that the proximal pin acts to pull the finger out to length and reduce the fracture via ligamentotaxis.

Ellis and colleagues published the outcomes of 8 unstable PIP joint fracture-dislocations treated with the external fixator described by Slade.[16] Subjects were allowed to perform immediate limited range of motion of the PIP joint after surgery. In their admittedly small treatment group, the investigators were able to achieve an average 88° PIP joint arc of motion (range: 1° to 89°), grip strength 92% of the unaffected side, and a pain VAS of 0.6.

Badia and colleagues[19] recently published a series in which they performed a modification of the dynamic external fixator popularized by Gaul and Rosenberg in 1998.[20] This design does not involve rubber bands but uses longitudinal traction between the pins to induce ligamentotaxis and joint reduction. This frame is created by applying a 0.045-in K-wire transversely through the axis of rotation of the proximal phalanx. A second 0.045-in K-wire is driven transversely through the head of the middle phalanx. The proximal wires are bent 3 times to provide a cradle for the distal wires. This cradle provides the longitudinal traction necessary to maintain a congruent and reduced

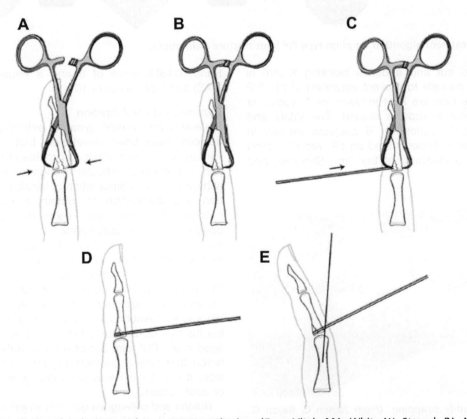

Fig. 10. (*A–E*) Closed reduction and percutaneous pinning. (*From* Vitale MA, White NJ, Strauch RJ. A percutaneous technique to treat unstable dorsal fracture-dislocations of the proximal interphalangeal joint. J Hand Surg Am 2011;36(9):1455–6; with permission.)

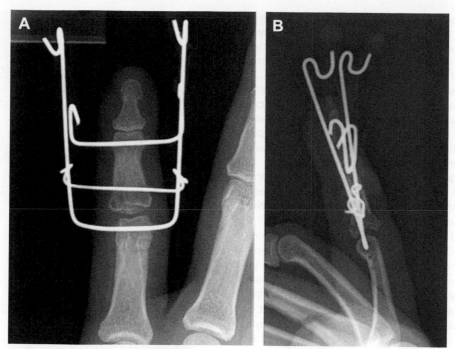

Fig. 11. (*A*, *B*) Dynamic external fixator.

joint through full PIP joint range of motion. The series by Badia and colleagues[19] followed 6 subjects over 24 months with 48% middle phalanx articular involvement. The subjects demonstrated an average 89° PIP joint arc of motion with a 5° extensor lag. No instability was noted at final follow-up.

Open reduction and internal fixation with interfragmentary screws
Dorsal fracture dislocations with large fracture fragments and minimal comminution are amenable to open reduction and internal fixation. This can be performed with either lag screws or plate and screw constructs. Headless compression screws provide stable fixation with minimal tendon irritation and stability to start early range of motion (**Fig. 12**).

Open reduction and interfragmentary screw fixation can be performed from either a volar or dorsal approach, or with a combined approach. If using a dorsal approach alone, care must be taken to avoid disruption of the central slip of the extensor tendon. Subperiosteal dissection is performed to gain lateral exposure to the level of the deep flexor tendon, taking care to preserve the neurovascular bundle.

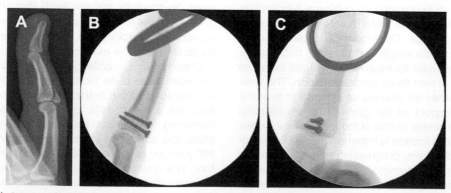

Fig. 12. (*A*) Open reduction internal fixation with (*B*, *C*) interfragmentary screws. (*Courtesy of* P. Blazar, MD, Boston, MA.)

Once the volar aspect of the middle phalanx is exposed, a freer-elevator or hypodermic needle can be used to disimpact and reduce the fracture fragment. Cancellous autograft or allograft can be used to fill any void in the metaphyseal region. After reduction is achieved, a headless compression screw is inserted from dorsal to volar, taking care to limit the amount of screw penetrating the volar cortex to avoid flexor tendon irritation. A splint is applied with the fingers in extension; however, the patient can come out of the splint for daily range of motion exercises. Passive range of motion exercises can be started at 2 weeks and strengthening can begin at 4 to 6 weeks postoperatively.

Lee and Tech[21] fixed 12 dorsal fracture dislocations in 10 hands with either 1.3-mm or 1.5-mm interfragmentary screws alone. All joints were unstable; 4 subjects had 21% to 40% articular surface involvement, whereas 8 had greater than 40% involvement. Results were obtained at an average of 8 months of follow-up. All fractures achieved union with an average 85° PIP joint arc of motion. However, 7 subjects developed an extensor lag averaging 20°.

Open reduction and internal fixation with plate and screws

Open reduction and volar plating is an option for fixation of the volar lip fragment seen with dorsal fracture dislocations. A Bruner-style incision is made on the volar aspect of the middle phalanx, exposing the A3 and C2 pulleys. The A4 pulley can be vented for additional exposure. The flexor tendons are retracted laterally, which should provide access to the volar lip fragment. The volar plate is often still attached to the fragment and can be carefully retracted proximally to expose the fracture site.

The fragment is reduced and a 3-hole plate is applied with cortical screw fixation. The plate can be a cut-down T-plate or a mini-hook plate (**Fig. 13**) can be created by cutting a 3-hole plate in the middle of the distal hole and bending the remaining prongs. Care must be taken to select the correct plate length that provides buttress fixation of the volar lip fragment, while not being so long as to create flexor tendon irritation. The volar plate provides an element of protection over the proximal aspect of the plate. The rehabilitation protocol is similar to that of independent lag screw fixation. Early motion is important to prevent flexor tendon adhesions, progressing to passive motion at 2 weeks and strengthening at 4 to 6 weeks.

Ikeda and colleagues[22] reported on a series of 18 subjects with unstable dorsal fracture dislocations involving greater than 40% of the articular

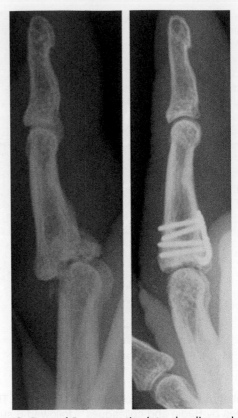

Fig. 13. Pre and Post-operative lateral radiographs of volar hook plate. (*From* Cheah AE, Tan DM, Chong AK, et al. Volar plating for unstable proximal interphalangeal joint dorsal fracture-dislocations. J Hand Surg Am 2012;37(1):30; with permission.)

surface. They used a T-plate cut to 3 holes and applied the plate in buttress fashion. At 16 months of follow-up, they identified no major complications or nonunions. PIP joint arc of motion averaged 85° with a 5° flexion contracture. They emphasized that early passive and active extension is important to prevent tendon adhesions. Additionally, they identified that screw length must be carefully chosen such that the screws gain purchase in the dorsal cortex to prevent the screws from backing out, while not being proud so as to irritate the extensor tendon.

Cheah and colleagues[23] retrospectively reviewed volar plate fixation of 13 subjects over an average of 25 months. The volar lip fractures involved a mean 44% of the articular surface. Following volar plate fixation with a mini-hook plate, the study group exhibited an average 75° PIP joint arc of motion with 10° of flexion contracture. The investigators identified the need to place the plate distal enough that the hooks do not interfere with joint function but not so distal as to irritate the flexor tendon.

Volar plate arthroplasty

Comminuted volar lip fractures are not amenable to interfragmentary screws or plate fixation. Restoration of the buttressing effect of the volar lip is necessary to preserve concentric reduction. Volar plate arthroplasty was first described by Eaton and Malerich[24] in 1980 to solve this problem (**Fig. 14**). The premise behind this procedure is to use the volar plate to resurface the PIP joint. The indications for this procedure are acute and chronic PIP joint dorsal fracture dislocations in which congruous reduction is not possible due to loss of the volar buttress.

The PIP joint is approached through a standard Bruner incision. The neurovascular bundles are mobilized and protected, and the A3 pulley is reflected laterally, exposing the flexor tendons that are, in turn, reflected laterally. The volar plate is reflected proximally and any comminuted fracture fragments are debrided away. A trough is made in the volar aspect of the middle phalanx to accept the volar plate as it is advanced.

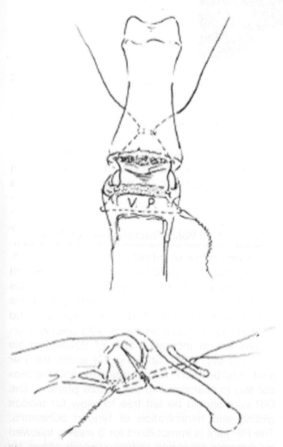

Fig. 14. Volar plate arthroplasty. (*From* Eaton RG, Malerich MM. Volar plate arthroplasty of the proximal interphalangeal joint: a review of 10 years' experience. J Hand Surg Am 1980;5(3):262; with permission.)

Stout nonabsorbable sutures are placed through the distal volar plate both radially and ulnarly. Keith needles and a wire driver are used to pass the sutures through the middle phalanx, emerging dorsally. The sutures can be passed through the skin in the case of a tie-over button, or an incision can be made to tie the sutures over the periosteum.[25] Under fluoroscopic guidance, the volar plate is advanced to the middle phalanx until the joint is concentrically reduced, at which time the sutures are secured dorsally. Concentric reduction is again confirmed under fluoroscopy before final suture tying. Care must be taken to not overtighten and create a flexion contracture. An extension block splint or pin is placed to maintain the volar plate position and is removed after 2 to 3 weeks.

The initial account of volar plate arthroplasty by Eaton and Malerich[24] described 7 subjects treated for acute unstable dorsal PIP joint fracture dislocations. These subjects achieved a 95° PIP joint arc of motion and a 6° flexion contracture at a follow-up of 38 months. Twenty years later, Dionysian and Eaton reported[26] on 11 acute dorsal fracture dislocations treated with volar plate arthroplasty. These subjects demonstrated an 85° arc of motion with 100° of flexion and 15° extensor lag. It is unclear why this second group had less motion with greater flexion contracture.

Lee and colleagues[27] reported a modification of this procedure, using a suture anchor in lieu of transosseous sutures. Fourteen subjects were treated for acute unstable dorsal fracture dislocations. At 25 months postoperatively, the subjects had a 100° of flexion and 11° of extensor lag. It is interesting that this study showed similar range of motion, considering that their protocol seemingly involved immobilization of the digits (including the DIP joint) for 2 weeks postoperatively.

Hemihamate autograft

Unstable, comminuted volar lip fractures can be treated with hemihamate resurfacing arthroplasty. The PIP joint is approached volarly as described in the volar plate arthroplasty technique. Once the fracture site is exposed, the volar and distal margins of the recipient site are prepared with a saw or rongeur (**Fig. 15**). The size of the defect is measured, taking note of the location of the interarticular ridge.

The wrist is then pronated to harvest the autograft. A transverse incision is made over the dorsum of hand, overlying the base of the 4th and 5th metacarpals. The extensor digiti minimi and extensor digitorum communis are retracted to expose the carpometacarpal capsule, which is then reflected off of the metacarpals distally. The

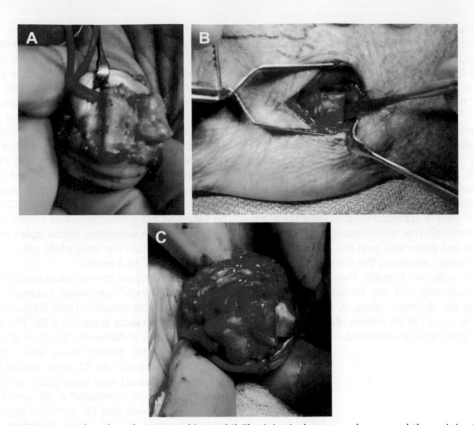

Fig. 15. Hemihamate arthroplasty harvest and inset. (*A*) The joint is shotgunned open and the recipient site prepared. (*B*) The hemihamate is harvested. (*C*) The hemihamate is inset to recreate the articular surface. (*Courtesy of* P. Blazar, MD, Boston, MA.)

donor bone is taken from the distal articular surface of the hamate, where it articulates with both the 4th and 5th metacarpals. A ridge exists between the 2 carpometacarpal articulations, which will be used to recreate the proximal articular surface of the middle phalanx. The donor tissue is harvested with a saw or osteotome, taking slightly more donor tissue than measured. The capsule is reapproximated and the wound is irrigated and closed.

The graft is then placed into the recipient bed and fixed with 1.1-mm or 1.3-mm interfragmentary screws (**Fig. 16**). The joint is reduced and range of motion assessed. The originators of this technique highlight that the hamate has thicker articular cartilage than the middle phalanx, so imaging may give the appearance of an articular stepoff[28]; articular congruity is assessed with direct visualization. Once satisfied with the concentric reduction in full range of motion, the wound is closed and the joint is rehabilitated as for open reduction and interfragmentary screw fixation. The hamate donor site does not require any rehabilitation over and above the brief immobilization for the PIP joint.

Williams and colleagues[29] evaluated the outcome of hemihamate autograft resurfacing on 11 subjects for unstable volar lip fractures averaging 60% of the articular surface. At an average of 16 months, average PIP joint arc of motion was 85° with 9° flexion contracture. Two subjects developed a recurrent dorsal subluxation of the PIP joint without functional complaints. All autografts went on to union.

Treatment of Volar Fracture Dislocations

Extension block splinting
Stable volar fracture dislocations can be treated with extension block splinting. Kang and colleagues[30] advocated that only dorsal lip fractures with less than 2 mm of fragment separation be treated closed because those with greater than 2 mm are at increased risk of developing an extensor lag. When applying the splint, the PIP joint must be held in full extension to allow the central slip to scar down to the middle phalanx. The DIP joint should be left free to allow for tendon gliding and minimization of tendon adhesions. The PIP joint is immobilized for 3 weeks, followed by dynamic extension splinting, which allows for active flexion for another 2 weeks. Afterward, passive flexion and strengthening exercises are started.

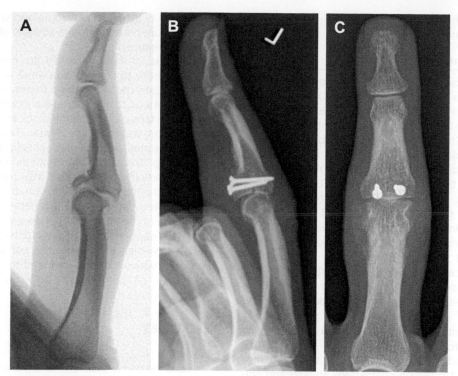

Fig. 16. (*A–C*) Hemihamate arthroplasty fixation. (*Courtesy of* P. Blazar, MD, Boston, MA.)

Closed reduction and transarticular pinning

Unstable joints and stable joints with greater than 2 mm of fragment separation are at risk of extensor lag due to the inability of the central slip to reliably heal to the middle phalanx. If the fracture fragment can be reduced and the dorsal aspect of the middle phalanx is restored so as to allow the central slip to heal to it, closed reduction and transarticular pinning is an option. Rosenstadt and colleagues[6] published a series on 9 subjects with acute volar fracture dislocations treated with transarticular pinning. Although the final range of motion of the PIP joints was 87% of the unaffected side, there was a considerable amount of extensor lag seen at the DIP joint, presumably due to tendon adhesions secondary to prolonged immobilization of the DIP joint.

Dynamic external fixation

Volar fracture dislocations that exhibit articular congruity with longitudinal traction and translation can be treated with a dynamic external fixator, as described for dorsal fracture dislocations. Abou Elatta and colleagues[31] treated 13 volar PIP joint fracture dislocations with dynamic external fixation for 5 to 6 weeks. Their subjects achieved average PIP joint motion of 90° (range 80° to 100°) and total active motion averaging 256°. The investigators noted that the DIP joint had a

tendency to hyperextend, possibly indicating an early boutonniere deformity; they recommended keeping the DIP joint flexed throughout the traction period.

Open reduction and internal fixation with interfragmentary screws

An alternative, if the fracture fragment is large enough, is to fix the fracture to the middle phalanx with a mini-fragment screw. Tekkis and colleagues[32] reported on 2 cases in which a single 1-mm lag screw was used to fix each fracture. Range of motion exercises were started after 1 week postoperatively. At 16-month follow-up, subjects had greater than 100° of flexion but a 10° extension lag. This technique has the advantage of early motion; however, the fracture fragment must be large enough to hold a lag screw, and there is a risk of extensor tendon irritation.

Open reduction and internal fixation with plate and screws

Open reduction and internal fixation with a hook plate can be used to treat these injuries when the fracture fragment is too small to accept a lag screw. Komura and colleagues[33] published a case report of a rugby player treated in this manner who had 100° of flexion at the PIP joint and no extensor lag at 4-month follow-up. Care must be taken to avoid screw penetration into the flexor tendon sheath, as well as plate irritation of the lateral bands distally.

Treatment of Pilon Fractures

Pilon fractures can be treated with many of the modalities previously described. Open reduction and internal fixation is useful if the fracture fragments are large enough to accept interfragmentary screws. Stern and colleagues[34] published a series on 9 subjects treated with open reduction and K-wire fixation for pilon fractures of the PIP joint. Seven of their subjects achieved 70° PIP joint arc of motion with 10° flexion contracture. Four subjects had pain with axial loading, 1 had pain with heavy lifting, and 2 had continuous pain. The investigators noted that the results of open reduction and internal fixation were inferior their experience with dynamic external fixation.

Pilon fractures with severe comminution can be treated with dynamic external fixation. Hynes and Giddins[35] presented a series of 8 pilon fractures treated with dynamic external fixation, albeit with a short follow-up averaging 7.5 months. Their cohort had a final average 88° PIP joint arc of motion with 12° flexion contracture. Ruland and colleagues[18] reported on a series of 8 subjects with PIP joint pilon fractures treated in this manner. That study included unstable dorsal fracture dislocations, as well as pilon fractures, making it difficult to assess the results for pilon fractures alone; however, the subjects had a PIP joint arc of motion of 88° with extension from 10° of hyperextension to 25° of flexion contracture.

SUMMARY

PIP joint fracture dislocations threaten the normal use of the hand if not recognized and managed in a timely manner. The soft tissues that stabilize the uninjured joint are commonly disrupted, leading to significant pain, swelling, and instability. Fracture dislocations that present late are at very high risk of chronic stiffness and loss of motion that leads to loss of function of the hand.

The treating physician should be suspicious of a PIP joint injury whenever a patient presents with a swollen finger or complaint of a jammed finger. Plain films should be obtained to aid in diagnosis, with the knowledge that these injuries may self-reduce, and radiographs should be scrutinized for evidence of fracture dislocation.

An understanding of the anatomy, as well as the mechanism of injury, will help to guide treatment. Once the fracture pattern is recognized, it can be classified into either a volar or dorsal fracture dislocation, or a pilon fracture. Plain films as well as physical examination will help to determine the stability of the joint. The combined knowledge of the fracture pattern and the stability of the joint will guide treatment.

The goals of treatment are to preserve or restore stability to the joint to permit early range of motion. Early motion will help to prevent the adhesions that lead to contractures and loss of function. Buddy taping or extension block splinting are both tolerated well for stable injuries. Tenuous and unstable injuries may require closed reduction with pinning. Truly unstable fractures with a high degree of articular involvement may benefit from open reduction and internal fixation, or even joint reconstruction with a hemihamate autograft. Regardless of the intervention, however, the goal should be early motion. It is incumbent on the treating physician to educate the patient on the guarded prognosis of this joint and the absolute importance of compliance with the therapy protocol.

REFERENCES

1. Lee SW, Ng ZY, Fogg QA. Three-dimensional analysis of the palmar plate and collateral ligaments at the proximal interphalangeal joint. J Hand Surg Eur Vol 2014;39(4):391–7.
2. Green DP, Wolfe SW, Harold Lefkoe Memorial Book Fund. Green's operative hand surgery. 6th edition. Philadelphia: Elsevier/Churchill Livingstone; 2011.
3. Schmidt H-M, Lanz U. Surgical anatomy of the hand. New York: Thieme; 2004.
4. Kiefhaber TR, Stern PJ. Fracture dislocations of the proximal interphalangeal joint. J Hand Surg Am 1998;23(3):368–80.
5. Bowers WH, Wolf JW Jr, Nehil JL, et al. The proximal interphalangeal joint volar plate. I. An anatomical and biomechanical study. J Hand Surg Am 1980; 5(1):79–88.
6. Rosenstadt BE, Glickel SZ, Lane LB, et al. Palmar fracture dislocation of the proximal interphalangeal joint. J Hand Surg Am 1998;23(5):811–20.
7. Bernstein J, Monaghan BA, Silber JS, et al. Taxonomy and treatment–a classification of fracture classifications. J Bone Joint Surg Br 1997;79(5):706–7 [discussion: 708–9].
8. Hung VS, Bodavula VK, Dubin NH. Digital anaesthesia: comparison of the efficacy and pain associated with three digital nerve block techniques. J Hand Surg Br 2005;30(6):581–4.
9. Williams JG, Lalonde DH. Randomized comparison of the single-injection volar subcutaneous block and the two injection dorsal block for digital anesthesia. Plast Reconstr Surg 2006;118(5):1195–200.
10. Yin ZG, Zhang JB, Kan SL, et al. A comparison of traditional digital blocks and single subcutaneous palmar injection blocks at the base of the finger

and a meta-analysis of the digital block trials. J Hand Surg Br 2006;31(5):547–55.

11. Lalonde D, Bell M, Benoit P, et al. A multicenter prospective study of 3,110 consecutive cases of elective epinephrine use in the fingers and hand: the Dalhousie Project clinical phase. J Hand Surg Am 2005;30(5):1061–7.

12. Minamikawa Y, Horii E, Amadio PC, et al. Stability and constraint of the proximal interphalangeal joint. J Hand Surg Am 1993;18(2):198–204.

13. de Haseth KB, Neuhaus V, Mudgal CS. Dorsal fracture-dislocations of the proximal interphalangeal joint: evaluation of closed reduction and percutaneous Kirschner wire pinning. Hand (N Y) 2015; 10(1):88–93.

14. Barksfield RC, Bowden B, Chojnowski AJ. Hemihamate arthroplasty versus transarticular Kirschner wire fixation for unstable dorsal fracture-dislocation of the proximal interphalangeal joint in the hand. Hand Surg 2015;20(1):115–9.

15. Vitale MA, White NJ, Strauch RJ. A percutaneous technique to treat unstable dorsal fracture-dislocations of the proximal interphalangeal joint. J Hand Surg Am 2011;36(9):1453–9.

16. Ellis SJ, Cheng R, Prokopis P, et al. Treatment of proximal interphalangeal dorsal fracture-dislocation injuries with dynamic external fixation: a pins and rubber band system. J Hand Surg Am 2007;32(8): 1242–50.

17. Agee JM. Unstable fracture dislocations of the proximal interphalangeal joint. Treatment with the force couple splint. Clin Orthop Relat Res 1987;(214): 101–12.

18. Ruland RT, Hogan CJ, Cannon DL, et al. Use of dynamic distraction external fixation for unstable fracture-dislocations of the proximal interphalangeal joint. J Hand Surg Am 2008;33(1):19–25.

19. Badia A, Riano F, Ravikoff J, et al. Dynamic intradigital external fixation for proximal interphalangeal joint fracture dislocations. J Hand Surg Am 2005;30(1): 154–60.

20. Gaul SJ, Rosenberg SN. Fracture-dislocation of the middle phalanx at the proximal interphalangeal joint: repair with a simple intradigital traction-fixation device. Am J Orthop (Belle Mead NJ) 1998;27(10): 682–8.

21. Lee JY, Tech LC. Dorsal fracture dislocations of the proximal interphalangeal joint treated by open reduction and interfragmentary screw fixation: indications, approaches and results. J Hand Surg Br 2006;31(2):138–46.

22. Ikeda M, Kobayashi Y, Saito I, et al. Open reduction and internal fixation for dorsal fracture

23. dislocations of the proximal interphalangeal joint using a miniplate. Tech Hand Up Extrem Surg 2011;15(4):219–24.

23. Cheah AE, Tan DM, Chong AK, et al. Volar plating for unstable proximal interphalangeal joint dorsal fracture-dislocations. J Hand Surg Am 2012; 37(1):28–33.

24. Eaton RG, Malerich MM. Volar plate arthroplasty of the proximal interphalangeal joint: a review of ten years' experience. J Hand Surg Am 1980;5(3): 260–8.

25. Blazar PE, Robbe R, Lawton JN. Treatment of dorsal fracture/dislocations of the proximal interphalangeal joint by volar plate arthroplasty. Tech Hand Up Extrem Surg 2001;5(3):148–52.

26. Dionysian E, Eaton RG. The long-term outcome of volar plate arthroplasty of the proximal interphalangeal joint. J Hand Surg Am 2000;25(3):429–37.

27. Lee LS, Lee HM, Hou YT, et al. Surgical outcome of volar plate arthroplasty of the proximal interphalangeal joint using the Mitek micro GII suture anchor. J Trauma 2008;65(1):116–22.

28. Williams RM, Hastings H 2nd, Kiefhaber TR. Pip fracture/dislocation treatment technique: use of a hemi-hamate resurfacing arthroplasty. Tech Hand Up Extrem Surg 2002;6(4):185–92.

29. Williams RM, Kiefhaber TR, Sommerkamp TG, et al. Treatment of unstable dorsal proximal interphalangeal fracture/dislocations using a hemihamate autograft. J Hand Surg Am 2003;28(5): 856–65.

30. Kang R, Stern PJ. Fracture dislocations of the proximal interphalangeal joint. J Hand Surg 2002; 2(2):47–59.

31. Abou Elatta MM, Assal F, Basheer HM, et al. The use of a simple dynamic external fixator for the treatment of volar fracture subluxation of proximal interphalangeal joints of the fingers. Tech Hand Up Extrem Surg 2016;20(4):161–5.

32. Tekkis PP, Kessaris N, Gavalas M, et al. The role of mini-fragment screw fixation in volar dislocations of the proximal interphalangeal joint. Arch Orthop Trauma Surg 2001;121(1–2):121–2.

33. Komura S, Yokoi T, Nonomura H. Mini hook plate fixation for palmar fracture-dislocation of the proximal interphalangeal joint. Arch Orthop Trauma Surg 2011;131(4):563–6.

34. Stern PJ, Roman RJ, Kiefhaber TR, et al. Pilon fractures of the proximal interphalangeal joint. J Hand Surg Am 1991;16(5):844–50.

35. Hynes MC, Giddins GE. Dynamic external fixation for pilon fractures of the interphalangeal joints. J Hand Surg Br 2001;26(2):122–4.

Treating the Proximal Interphalangeal Joint in Swan Neck and Boutonniere Deformities

Paige M. Fox, MD, PhD*, James Chang, MD

KEYWORDS

- Boutonniere • Swan neck • RA • Central slip • Lateral bands

KEY POINTS

- Proper preoperative assessment of active and passive distal interphalangeal (DIP), proximal interphalangeal (PIP), and metacarpophalangeal (MP) joint motion is critical to treatment of PIP joint injuries.
- Radiographs are important to identify underlying arthritis.
- Multiple soft tissue procedures exist for the treatment of swan neck and boutonniere deformities.
- Soft tissue procedures will not be successful in restoring active joint motion if passive joint motion is not present.
- Before surgery, patients should be counseled on the likelihood of incomplete correction and recurrence of PIP joint deformities.

The proximal interphalangeal (PIP) joint is a hinge joint stabilized by collateral ligaments on its radial and ulnar aspect, the volar plate on its ventral surface, and the central slip and lateral bands of the extensor mechanism dorsally.[1] The multiple stabilizing structures of the joint allow for flexion and extension only, without radial or ulnar deviation or circumduction about the joint. In most patients, there is minimal hyperextension at the PIP joint but flexion to approximately 100°. Disruption of the delicate balance of flexion and extension forces on the PIP joint can result in deformity over time. Although flexion and extension at the PIP and distal interphalangeal (DIP) joints are closely linked, here the authors focus on management of the PIP joint in swan neck and boutonniere deformities.

SWAN NECK DEFORMITIES
Introduction: Nature of the Problem

A swan neck deformity refers to a DIP joint in flexion with a PIP joint in hyperextension (**Fig. 1**). There are 3 primary causes of swan neck deformities: trauma, rheumatoid arthritis (RA), and cerebral palsy (CP). The deformity can originate at the metacarpophalangeal (MP) joint, the PIP joint, or the DIP joint. Swan neck deformities can be aesthetically unpleasing, but, more importantly, they can lead to difficulty initiating functional grasp as the patient attempts to overcome hyperextension at the PIP joint.

In 1979, Zancolli[2] classified traumatic swan neck deformities into 3 categories: extrinsic,

Disclosure Statement: None.
Department of Surgery, Division of Plastic Surgery, Stanford University, 770 Welch Road, Suite 400, Palo Alto, CA 94304, USA
* Corresponding author.
E-mail address: Pfox@Stanford.Edu

Hand Clin 34 (2018) 167–176
https://doi.org/10.1016/j.hcl.2017.12.006
0749-0712/18/Published by Elsevier Inc

hand.theclinics.com

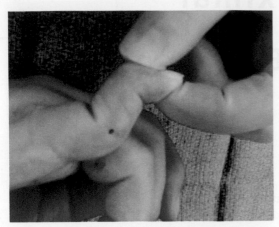

Fig. 1. Small finger swan neck deformity. A hyperextension deformity at the PIP joint and flexion deformity at the DIP joint are seen.

intrinsic, and articular. Extrinsic causes include disruption of the terminal tendon (mallet deformity) and wrist or MP flexion contractures. Intrinsic causes are chronic MP joint volar subluxation, ischemic contracture, and tendon adhesions. Articular causes include disruption of the flexor digitorum superficialis (FDS) or a volar plate/capsule injury.

Extrinsic causes result in a swan neck deformity due to extension forces on the middle phalanx. For example, a mallet finger injury results in disruption of the terminal tendon and flexion of the DIP joint. The flexion allows the lateral bands to migrate proximally and, in doing so, extend the middle phalanx, resulting in PIP joint hyperextension. In contrast, an MP or wrist flexion contracture causes increased tension on the extensor digitorum communis (EDC), which inserts as the central slip on the dorsal aspect of the middle phalanx. As tension on the EDC increases, the middle phalanx is pulled into an extended position and PIP joint hyperextension occurs.

Intrinsic causes refer to those resulting from tightness of the intrinsic muscles, such as occur after an ischemic insult to the hand because of a compartment syndrome or crush injury. Chronic volar subluxation of the MP joint can also lead to intrinsic tightness. The Bunnell test can be valuable to assess for intrinsic tightness. The examiner places the MP joint in mild hyperextension and assesses maximal PIP joint flexion. The examiner then moves the MP joint to a flexed position, putting the intrinsics in a more relaxed position. If PIP joint flexion improves (increases), intrinsic tightness

is contributing. If the PIP joint flexion does not improve, dorsal capsule or extensor tendon contracture may be the cause.

Articular causes refer to those that originate on the volar surface of the PIP joint. A volar dislocation of the PIP joint can lead to volar plate laxity, allowing for PIP joint hyperextension. The FDS acts as a volar stabilizer of the PIP joint. If this tendon insertion is disrupted owing to trauma or in a tendon transfer procedure, a swan neck deformity can occur.

In RA, swan neck deformities can occur because of chronic volar subluxation of the MP joints, resulting in extension of the middle phalanx, as discussed above. In addition, a swan neck can occur because of periarticular inflammation at the PIP joint, leading to volar plate and capsule laxity. The terminal tendon can become stretched and lax over the DIP joint, resulting in a mallet deformity, which can initiate a swan neck deformity if left untreated. As for CP, swan neck deformities can be caused by tension on the EDC due to wrist flexion contractures or to spasticity of the intrinsic muscles of the hand.[3]

Treatment options depend not only on the cause of the deformity but also on the duration of symptoms, disability, and condition of the joint. Nalebuff classified swan neck deformities into 4 types (**Table 1**).[4] Classification can help guide surgical management. Nonsurgical options include figure-of-8 ring splints or custom splints that block PIP joint hyperextension (**Fig. 2**). These options are good for patients with full active range of motion (ROM) of the PIP joint but resting hyperextension. Before considering surgical intervention, the surgeon should obtain radiographs of the finger to assess the DIP and PIP joints. Severe arthritis at the PIP joint will limit results from a soft tissue procedure, and an arthroplasty or arthrodesis may be indicated, whereas a DIP fracture may warrant fixation to rebalance the extensor mechanism.

INDICATIONS/CONTRAINDICATIONS

The indications and contraindications to surgical soft tissue procedures to limit hyperextension of the PIP joint are shown in **Table 2**.

SURGICAL TECHNIQUE/PROCEDURE

Multiple techniques have been described for soft tissue rebalancing of the PIP in the setting of swan neck deformity. One option, the FDS tenodesis or FDS sling, is addressed in later

Table 1
Classification and management of swan neck deformities

Type	Characteristics	Joint Management		
		MP	PIP	DIP
I	Full ROM, no functional limitations	None	Splint or soft tissue procedure to limit hyperextension (considering cause)	Nonsurgical management vs arthrodesis
II	Intrinsic tightness	Intrinsic release, reconstruction if required	Soft tissue procedure to limit hyperextension	Nonsurgical management vs arthrodesis
III	Limited PIP motion in all positions of MP, joint preserved	Intrinsic release, reconstruction if required	Stepwise approach to restore joint motion + soft tissue procedure	Nonsurgical management vs arthrodesis
IV	Severe arthritic changes	Intrinsic release, reconstruction if required	Arthroplasty + soft tissue procedure OR arthrodesis	Nonsurgical management vs arthrodesis

Data from Strauch RJ. Extensor Tendon Injury. In: Wolfe SW, Hotchkiss RN, Pederson WC, et al., eds. Green's Operative Hand Surgery, 6th edition. Philadelphia: Elsevier; 2011.

discussion. The goal of the procedure is to establish a restraint against hyperextension and rebalance the forced on the joint. MP and DIP joint procedures are beyond the scope of this article.

Preoperative Planning

- Preoperative radiographs of the affected digit or digits
- Medication review, which is especially important for RA patients, whose immunosuppressive medications should be optimized for surgery by working with the patient's rheumatologist
- AROM and PROM of DIP, PIP, and MP joints measured
- Bunnell test performed to assess intrinsic tightness

- Plan for staged or simultaneous procedures on the DIP and MP joints
- Assess for the presence of an FDS in the digit of interest (especially important in the small finger). Assess for a functioning FDP tendon that will remain.

Preparation and Patient Positioning

The patient is placed supine on the operating table with the operative extremity on the hand table. Ideally, the shoulder is placed at 90° and centered on the hand table. However, some patients, especially RA patients, may have limited ROM of the shoulder and elbow, making positioning more difficult. A nonsterile biceps level tourniquet is padded and placed. The patient's hand and arm are prepared in a standard fashion up to the elbow.

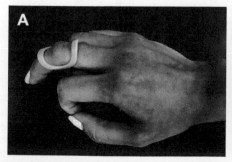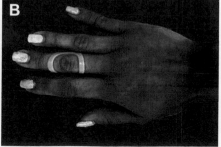

Fig. 2. Figure-of-8 splint. Splint (*A*) Lateral view allows for PIP joint flexion while (*B*) Dorsal view limiting joint hyperextension (*A*) Lateral view. (*B*) Dorsal view.

Table 2
Indications and contraindications to soft tissue procedures to treat swan neck deformities

Indications	Contraindications
Difficulty initiating grasp	Severe arthritis of the PIP joint
Pain due to snapping of the lateral bands	Poorly optimized medical management of RA
Progressive hyperextension deformity	No PROM of PIP joint[a]
Limited AROM of PIP joint with full PROM	Unstable proximal joints (RA)

Abbreviations: AROM, active range of motion; PROM, passive range of motion. RA, rheumatoid arthritis.
[a] PROM of the joint must be restored before soft tissue procedures.

Surgical Approach

The PIP joint can be approached volarly through a variety of incisions, including a standard Bruner, a half-Bruner, or a midlateral approach.[5] The surgeon will need access to the FDS tendon at the location of division and planned inset. As multiple insertions can be used for tenodesis, the surgeon may need to make an additional incision for fixation. If using the A1 pulley for FDS attachment, an incision in the palm can be used and an incision on the digit can be avoided. The authors' preferred technique of tenodesis to the A2 pulley is addressed in later discussion.

Surgical Procedure

1. Design a Bruner style incision over the proximal phalanx, extending from the metacarpal head to the PIP joint (**Fig. 3**)

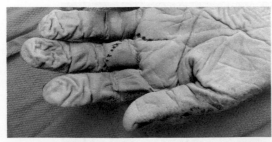

Fig. 3. Volar Bruner incision. An incision that allows clear visualization of the A2 pulley and access to the FDS distal to the A2 pulley is designed.

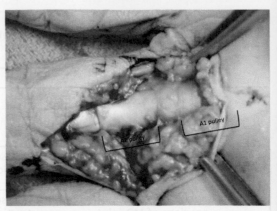

Fig. 4. A2 pulley. The A2 pulley can be seen at the central portion of the dissection with the distal aspect of the A1 pulley visible at the far right of the image.

2. Exsanguinate the hand and inflate the tourniquet
3. Secure the digits in a lead hand
4. Incise the skin and dissect down to expose the flexor tendon sheath, protecting the neurovascular bundles
5. Identify the A2 pulley (**Fig. 4**)
6. Identify both slips of the FDS and choose one for tenodesis
7. The A3 pulley can be incised laterally and lifted to allow better access to the FDS
8. Pull the slip of FDS distally and cut as proximal as possible just distal to the A2 pulley. This creates a distally based slip of FDS of the length needed for securing around the A2 pulley
9. Identify the center of the A2 pulley from proximal to distal (**Fig. 5**)

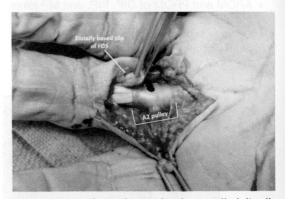

Fig. 5. FDS tenodesis. The FDS has been pulled distally and cut proximally. A purple line marks the midpoint of the A2 pulley. The FDS can be passed through a slip in the pulley and secured to itself, fixated to the lateral aspect of the pulley, or a bone anchor can be used.

10. Make a small slit in the pulley to allow for tendon passage through the pulley
11. The cut end of the slip of the FDS is then passed from distal to proximal and deep to superficial through the slit in A2
12. Secure the tendon on to itself using several nonabsorbable sutures holding the PIP joint in 20° to 30° of flexion
13. Alternatively, the FDS slips can be sutured to the lateral edges of the tendon sheath, with care not to block the passage of the remaining FDP tendon
14. Assess passive flexion and extension of the joint (**Fig. 6**)
15. Pin the PIP joint temporarily in 20° of flexion for 2 weeks
16. Deflate the tourniquet and obtain hemostasis
17. Close the skin
18. Place the patient in a well-padded dorsal blocking splint

COMPLICATIONS AND MANAGEMENT

There are 2 primary complications after the above procedure:

- Recurrent hyperextension deformity: This can be due to undertensioning the initial tenodesis or stretching over time. The repair can be revised. An alternative tenodesis location can be considered into bone if A2 pulley stretch was responsible.
- Creation of a flexion contracture greater than desired at the PIP joint: This can result from poor compliance with rehabilitation postoperatively or overtensioning of the initial repair. Repairs tend to stretch over time, so this can be monitored or surgically adjusted depending on the time since surgery.

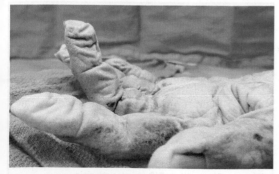

Fig. 6. Resting digit position after securing the FDS slip. The FDS has been secured around the distal half of the A2 pulley creating flexion of the PIP joint at rest.

Postoperative Care

- *At 10 to 14 days postoperatively:* Remove sutures, remove pin, and inspect incision. Place into a custom dorsal blocking splint that maintains desired PIP flexion. Patients are taught active flexion and extension while in the confines of the splint. The splint can be hand or finger based depending on the number of digits involved.
- *6 weeks postoperatively:* Patient is weaned from the splint.
- *Special considerations:* For CP patients, some investigators recommend temporarily pinning the PIP joint in flexion for 4 weeks after swan neck deformity correction.[3]

Outcomes

Outcomes after swan neck deformity are difficult to generalize because of limited studies, a variety of causes, and the diversity of treatment options. Based on the data presented in **Table 3**, results are stable for 2 years postoperatively. However, they may be less stable in CP patients because of ongoing deforming forces after surgical correction.[9] In addition, surgery does not improve the overall ROM of the joint, but it improves the resting position of the joint for initiation of grasp making the joint more functional.[7,10]

BOUTONNIERE DEFORMITIES
Introduction: Nature of the Problem

A boutonniere deformity is defined as a flexion deformity at the PIP joint with a hyperextension deformity at the DIP joint. The deformity results from disruption or attenuation of the central slip and triangular ligament of the extensor mechanism. The central slip is the termination and insertion of the EDC on the middle phalanx. The triangular ligament is formed between the distal aspect of the central slip proximally, the terminal tendon distally, and the lateral bands laterally. The central slip acts to extend the PIP joint, whereas the triangular ligament prevents volar subluxation of the lateral bands. When both are disrupted or significantly attenuated, the PIP joint moves into flexion and the lateral bands sublux volarly and proximally, causing DIP joint hyperextension. Initially, this deformity will be passively correctable but, over time, the deformity becomes fixed.

A true boutonniere deformity must be distinguished from a pseudo–boutonniere deformity. The Elson test for central slip integrity can be used to distinguish between the 2. A digital block

Table 3
Outcomes after correction of swan neck deformity

First Author, y	Cause	Technique	Outcome
Brulard et al,[6] 2012	RA	FDS tenodesis (A2 pulley)	23 digits at 61 mo Avg postoperative arc −4° to 65° 1 patient (4 digits) with unsatisfactory results
Carlson et al,[3] 2007	CP	Central slip tenotomy	Avg 32° improvement in PIP position at 23 mo postoperatively
Kiefhaber and Strickland,[7] 1993	RA	Dorsal capsulotomy + lateral band mobilization	Preoperative arc of motion 32 (−16° to 16°) Postoperative arc of motion 53° (21°–74°) 11 of 92 digits required revision 15 digits at 54 mo avg arc 15°–54°
Charruau et al,[8] 2016	All	Lateral band mobilization (secured in volar plate/FDS pulley)	41 fingers at 8 y: Avg active flexion of 86° Avg loss of extension of 15° Avg patient satisfaction 7.5/10
de Bruin et al,[9] 2010	CP	Lateral band mobilization (secured to flexor tendon sheath)	69 fingers, avg age 21 No recurrent HE in 84% at 1 y No recurrent HE in 60% at 5 y
Sirotakova et al,[10] 2008	RA	Same as Charruau but lateral band fixed to PP with bone anchor	101 digits No recurrence of deformity 20 mo Avg preoperative PIP arc −13° to 40° Avg postoperative PIP arc 13°–62°

Abbreviations: avg, average; CP, cerebral palsy; HE, hyperextension; RA, rheumatoid arthritis.

may be necessary if the joint is tender. The examiner will place the finger in 90° of flexion at the PIP joint and ask the patient to extend the PIP joint against resistance. If the DIP joint remains in a neutral position and is lax, the central slip is intact. If the DIP joint moves into a hyperextended position with attempted extension of the PIP joint, the central slip is not intact and the patient is pulling though the lateral bands in an attempt to extend the PIP joint. In a true boutonniere deformity, the central slip is not intact. In a pseudo–boutonniere deformity, the inability to extend the PIP joint is due to scarring between the volar plate and flexor tendons. The treatment of this entity is mobilization, serial casting or splinting, and hand therapy.[4]

It is important to determine the duration of deformity and prior trauma to the joint. In addition to a thorough history and physical examination, plain radiographs of the digit are useful to assess for bony central slip avulsions in acute injuries as well as joint space narrowing and arthritis in the chronic setting. The DIP joint should also be examined.

Acute central slip injuries are treated with splinting or pinning the PIP joint in full extension for 6 weeks. DIP joint exercises are performed throughout immobilization to move the lateral

bands into their proper dorsal position. Night splinting is continued for an additional 4 to 6 weeks.

Chronic boutonniere deformities are usually secondary to missed traumatic injuries, failed acute traumatic treatment, RA, or volar contractures (eg, Dupuytren contractures, burn scars). Burton classified chronic boutonniere deformities into multiple stages, as summarized in **Table 4**.[11] The stages can be used to help guide treatment.

Table 4
Burton classification of chronic boutonniere deformities

Stage	Description
I	Supple, passively correctable deformity
II	Fixed contracture + contracted lateral bands
III	Fixed contracture + joint fibrosis + collateral and volar plate contractures
IV	Stage III + PIP joint arthritis

Data from Burton RI. Extensor Tendons - late reconstruction. In: Green DP, ed. Operative Hand Surgery. 2nd ed. New York: Churchill Livingstone; 1988.

Stage I deformities can be treated with hand therapy and are managed similar to acute central slip injuries. The patient is started in a PIP joint extension splint for approximately 6 weeks with DIP joint exercises. PIP joint flexion exercises are then initiated with additional night splinting of the PIP joint in extension. Stage II treatment is also nonsurgical with serial casting or splinting to achieve PIP joint extension while exercising the DIP joint. Once achieved, the stage I pathway is adopted.

Stage III deformities often require surgical intervention, which may need to be staged. The PIP joint contracture may need to be addressed first to restore PROM of the joint. The surgeon can then proceed with soft tissue rebalancing. For stage IV disease, arthrodesis or arthroplasty is indicated.

Indications/Contraindications

The indications and contraindications to surgical soft tissue procedures to improve PIP joint extension through tendon rebalancing are shown in **Table 5**.

Surgical Technique/Procedure

If the patient's primary limitation is due to DIP joint hyperextension limiting grasp of small objects, a terminal tendon release (distal Fowler or Dolphin tenotomy) alone may be sufficient. The terminal tendon is divided over the middle phalanx proximal to the insertion of the oblique retinacular ligament. A mallet deformity may occur but is usually well tolerated.[12,13]

Multiple soft tissue procedures have been described for PIP joint contractures caused by both traumatic insults and RA.[12,14,15] In 1983, Curtis and colleagues[16] described a staged technique for the repair of traumatic boutonniere deformities. Stage I is tenolysis of the extensor tendon over the dorsal capsule of the PIP joint and transverse retinacular ligament (TRL), which tethers the lateral bands volarly. Stage II is sectioning of the TRL. Stage III is step-cut lengthening of the lateral bands, and stage IV is scar excision from the central tendon and readvancement. Stages I and II are performed in a stepwise fashion assessing the patient's progress after each procedure to see of the next is required. The surgeon then chooses between stages III and IV. If the patient has an extensor lag of greater than 20°, the surgeon will proceed to stage IV. If the lag is <20°, the surgeon will proceed with stage III.

Here, the authors discuss central slip reattachment and lateral band mobilization in detail. The goal of the procedure is to restore the appropriate length of the central slip and free the lateral bands from their volarly subluxed position. A terminal tenotomy is performed to correct DIP joint hyperextension.

Preoperative Planning

- Preoperative radiographs of the affected digit or digits
- Medication review, which is especially important for RA patients, whose immunosuppressive medications should be optimized for surgery by working with the patient's rheumatologist
- Measure active and passive ROM of DIP, PIP, and MP joints
- Plan for staged or simultaneous procedures on the DIP joint

Preparation and Patient Positioning

The patient is placed supine on the operating table with the operative extremity on the hand table. Ideally, the shoulder is placed at 90° and centered on the hand table. A nonsterile biceps level tourniquet is padded and placed. The patient's hand and arm are prepared in a standard fashion up to the elbow.

Surgical Approach

A dorsal approach to the PIP and DIP joints is used. A curvilinear incision is designed over the dorsal aspect of the PIP joint extending

Table 5
Indications and contraindications to tendon rebalancing to treat chronic boutonniere deformities

Indications	Contraindications
Failed conservative management	Severe arthritis of the PIP joint
Progressive fixed flexion deformity	Poorly optimized medical management of RA
Able to achieve good PROM at the PIP joint	No PROM of PIP joint[a]
Limited grasp of large objects	Full flexion and normal grip strength

[a] PROM of the joint must be restored or arthroplasty/arthrodesis of the joint performed before soft tissue procedures.

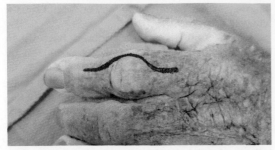

Fig. 7. Dorsal incision over PIP. A curvilinear incision over the PIP joint is shown. The midline is intentionally avoided to prevent the central slip and lateral band repairs from occurring deep to the incision.

proximally to the middle of the proximal phalanx and distally to the distal aspect of the middle phalanx.

Surgical Procedure

1. Design a curvilinear incision over the dorsal aspect of the PIP joint (**Fig. 7**)
2. Exsanguinate the hand and inflate the tourniquet
3. Rest the digits on a rolled towel
4. Incise the skin and dissect down to the extensor mechanism
5. Identify the central slip, lateral bands, TRL, and terminal tendon (**Fig. 8**)
6. Incise the TRL radially and ulnarly to allow dorsal subluxation of the lateral bands
7. Identify the stretched or scarred segment of the central slip and excise (**Fig. 9**)
8. Primarily repair the central slip. If limited distal tendon is available, use a bone anchor in the middle phalanx to secure the tendon
9. Check the DIP joint. If it remains hyperextended or cannot be passively flexed beyond 15°, perform a terminal tenotomy proximal to the DIP joint

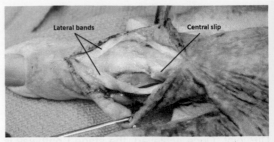

Fig. 9. The central slip and lateral bands are separated. The redundant central slip can be excised. The central slip can then be repaired or reinserted into the middle phalanx with a bone anchor.

10. Assess PIP joint position. If position is acceptable, no fixation of the lateral bands is required. However, if reinforcement is needed, the lateral bands are sutured together dorsally over the central slip (**Fig. 10**)
11. Use a 0.045 K-wire to pin the PIP joint in extension
12. Deflate the tourniquet and obtain hemostasis
13. Close the skin
14. Place the patient in a well-padded volar splint with the PIP and DIP in neutral and the MP joints in slight flexion

Complications and Management

There are 3 primary complications after soft tissue rebalancing:

- Recurrent flexion deformity: This can be due to underlying joint damage or stretch of the rebalancing. Arthrodesis is indicated if underlying joint damage is suspected. The lateral bands can be used to reinforce the repair if not previously used. The central slip can be readvanced if inadequate correction was obtained.
- Limited flexion of the PIP joint: This can result from poor compliance with rehabilitation postoperatively or overtensioning of the initial repair. Repairs tend to stretch over time, so

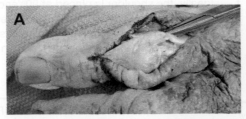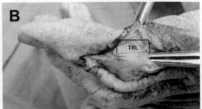

Fig. 8. TRL. (A) From a dorsal view, the clamp is passed deep to the TRL, which is located volar to the lateral bands at the PIP joint. (B) From a lateral view, the TRL can be seen overlying the clamp.

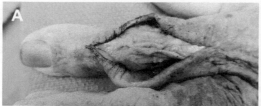
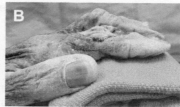

Fig. 10. Centralizing the lateral bands. (*A*) If more extension of the PIP is needed, the lateral bands can be sutured together in the midline. (*B*) Resting extension of the PIP joint is obtained.

this can be monitored or surgically adjusted depending on the time since surgery. If the lateral bands were sutured centrally, this can be released.

- Mallet deformity of the DIP joint: If a greater than 15° extensor lag is noted after terminal tenotomy, postoperative splinting is indicated. If not improved, DIP joint arthrodesis should be considered.

Postoperative Care

- *0 to 2 weeks postoperatively*: Bulky volar resting splint preventing PIP joint flexion and keep the DIP joint at neutral.
- *At 10 to 14 days postoperatively:* Remove sutures and inspect incision. Place into a custom splint that maintains PIP joint extension. Inspect the DIP joint for an extensor lag greater than 15°. If seen, consider a DIP joint extension splint. Otherwise, the DIP joint can

remain free and the patient can begin active flexion and extension.

- *4 weeks postoperatively:* Pin is removed and PIP joint exercises are begun. Dynamic extension splint is maintained when not exercising during the day and a static splint is used at night.[13]
- *8 weeks postoperatively:* Patient is weaned from the splint.

Outcomes

The ability to determine predictable outcomes is limited. The authors have listed a few case series in **Table 6**. However, the large variety of techniques used in these cases and the very small number of patients in each series make generalizations difficult. The Dolphin tenotomy is reliable.[19] Results at the PIP joint are less reliable, and incomplete correction is common. Recurrence was common in Kiefhaber and Strickland's[7]

Table 6			
Outcomes after correction of boutonniere deformity			
First Author, y	**Cause**	**Technique**	**Outcome**
Kiefhaber and Strickland,[7] 1993	RA	Central tendon reconstruction (2 different techniques with similar results)	19 digits, avg FU 22 mo Avg ext lag 67° pre to 39° post 4 digits with recurrent lag ≥ 70° Avg 12° loss of flexion
Caroli et al,[17] 1990	Trauma	Central slip excision and repair	18 pts, avg age 29, avg FU 26 mo 72% with excellent results (≤10° ext lag and ≥80° flexion)
Curtis et al,[16] 1983	Trauma	Curtis procedure	23 pts followed up to 1 y 17 pts avg ext lag 41° pre to 10° post (stages I–III) 6 pts avg ext lag 55° pre to 17° post (stages I–IV)
El-Sallakh et al,[18] 2012	Trauma	Lateral band mobilized, secured centrally and Dolphin tenotomy	12 digits, avg age 32, avg FU 33 mo PIP: Avg ext lag 60° pre to 7° post DIP: Avg 10°HE pre to 75° active flexion post

Abbreviations: avg, average; ext, extension; FU, follow-up; HE, hyperextension; pre, preoperative; post, postoperative; Pts, patients.

experience but less common in the series by El-Sallakh and colleagues[18] and Caroli and colleagues.[17]

SUMMARY

Treating swan neck and boutonniere deformities of the PIP joint is a difficult challenge. Understanding the cause of the deformity, the associated biomechanical changes of the adjacent joints, the functional limitations of the patient, and the articular status of the joint will improve decision making and outcomes. It is important to properly counsel the patient on expected continued limited ROM at the PIP joint and the possibility of repeat procedures in the future.

REFERENCES

1. Kuczynski K. The proximal interphalangeal joint. Anatomy and causes of stiffness in the fingers. J Bone Joint Surg Br 1968;50(3):656–63.
2. Zancolli E. Structural and dynamic bases of hand surgery. 2 edition. Philadelphia: Lippincott; 1979. p. 64–79, 92–103.
3. Carlson MG, Gallagher K, Spirtos M. Surgical treatment of swan-neck deformity in hemiplegic cerebral palsy. J Hand Surg Am 2007;32(9):1418–22.
4. Strauch RJ. Extensor tendon injury. In: Wolfe SW, Hotchkiss RN, Pederson WC, et al, editors. Green's operative hand surgery, 1, 6th edition. Philadelphia: Elsevier; 2011. p. 159–88.
5. Wei DH, Terrono AL. Superficialis sling (flexor digitorum superficialis tenodesis) for swan neck reconstruction. J Hand Surg 2015;40(10):2068–74.
6. Brulard C, Sauvage A, Mares O, et al. Treatment of rheumatoid swan neck deformity by tenodesis of proximal interphalangeal joint with a half flexor digitorum superficialis tendon. About 23 fingers at 61 months follow-up. Chir Main 2012;31(3):118–27 [in French].
7. Kiefhaber TR, Strickland JW. Soft tissue reconstruction for rheumatoid swan-neck and boutonniere deformities: long-term results. J Hand Surg 1993; 18(6):984–9.
8. Charruau B, Laulan J, Saint-Cast Y. Lateral band translocation for swan-neck deformity: outcomes of 41 digits after a mean follow-up of eight years. Orthop Traumatol Surg Res 2016;102(4 Suppl): S221–4.
9. de Bruin M, van Vliet DC, Smeulders MJ, et al. Long-term results of lateral band translocation for the correction of swan neck deformity in cerebral palsy. J Pediatr Orthop 2010;30(1):67–70.
10. Sirotakova M, Figus A, Jarrett P, et al. Correction of swan neck deformity in rheumatoid arthritis using a new lateral extensor band technique. J Hand Surg Eur Vol 2008;33(6):712–6.
11. Burton RI. Extensor tendons-late reconstruction. In: Green DP, editor. Operative hand surgery. New York: Churchill Livingstone; 1988. p. 2073–116.
12. Boyer MI, Gelberman RH. Operative correction of swan-neck and boutonniere deformities in the rheumatoid hand. J Am Acad Orthop Surg 1999;7(2): 92–100.
13. Williams K, Terrono AL. Treatment of boutonniere finger deformity in rheumatoid arthritis. J Hand Surg 2011;36(8):1388–93.
14. Littler JW, Eaton RG. Redistribution of forces in the correction of Boutonniere deformity. J Bone Joint Surg Am 1967;49(7):1267–74.
15. Dolphin JA. Extensor tenotomy for chronic boutonni'ere deformity of the finger; report of two cases. J Bone Joint Surg Am 1965;47:161–4.
16. Curtis RM, Reid RL, Provost JM. A staged technique for the repair of the traumatic boutonniere deformity. J Hand Surg 1983;8(2):167–71.
17. Caroli A, Zanasi S, Squarzina PB, et al. Operative treatment of the post-traumatic boutonniere deformity. A modification of the direct anatomical repair technique. J Hand Surg 1990;15(4):410–5.
18. El-Sallakh S, Aly T, Amin O, et al. Surgical management of chronic boutonniere deformity. Hand Surg 2012;17(3):359–64.
19. Stern PJ. Extensor tenotomy: a technique for correction of posttraumatic distal interphalangeal joint hyperextension deformity. J Hand Surg 1989;14(3): 546–9.

Proximal Interphalangeal Joint Fusion
Indications and Techniques

James Jung, MD[a], Brandon Haghverdian, MD[b],
Ranjan Gupta, MD[a,*]

KEYWORDS

- Proximal interphalangeal joint arthrodesis • Surgical techniques • Indications • Treatment
- Contraindications

KEY POINTS

- Proximal interphalangeal joint (PIPJ) arthritis leads to significant hand impairment; both nonoperative and operative treatment modalities are available.
- PIPJ arthrodesis is the mainstay of treatment with few contraindications.
- Several surgical techniques are available to perform the arthrodesis: tension band, compression screw, dorsal plate, and 90/90 wiring.
- PIPJ arthrodesis has excellent postoperative outcomes with an extremely high success rate.

INTRODUCTION

The proximal interphalangeal joint (PIPJ) of the finger is a bicondylar joint critical to motion and function. Injury and arthritis to the PIPJ lead to considerable hand impairment because flexibility and stability of the joint are important in maintaining finger motion and hand function. Osteoarthritis of the hand is extremely common and has been shown to be prevalent in 67% of women and 55% of men aged 55 years or older. PIPJ arthritis is the second leading cause of hand pain after thumb carpometacarpal joint arthritis.[1] Degenerative changes of the PIPJ secondary to trauma, osteoarthritis, or inflammatory arthritis can lead to pain, instability, and deformity.[2] Initial treatment involves anti-inflammatories and activity modification; however, if these measures fail, operative interventions need to be considered and offered to the patient.

Surgical interventions of the PIPJ are taken with immense caution, because the joint is prone to severe and irreversible postoperative stiffness, leading to procedures beyond volar plate arthroplasty to hemi-hamate reconstruction. Moreover, there have been substantial changes in arthrodesis of the PIPJ over the past few decades. Understanding the specific disease process that initiated the joint destruction aids in determining the value of an arthrodesis. Moreover, significant consideration must be taken into account to appreciate the functional limitation with an isolated posttraumatic digit versus arthritis involving all of the fingers. Patients need to be counseled that a single joint arthrodesis may not present a significant alteration in hand function. In contrast, multiple digits with fused PIPJs may provide significant limitations. Positioning of the PIPJ is critical to success in these patients. Many investigators suggest the index finger PIPJ be fused at

---

Disclosure Statement: No disclosures.
[a] Orthopaedic Surgery, University of California, 101 The City Drive South, Pavilion 3, 2nd Floor, Orange, CA 92868, USA; [b] Orthopaedic Surgery, University of Pennsylvania, Philadelphia, PA, USA
* Corresponding author. 101 The City Drive South, Pavilion 3, 2nd Floor, Orange, CA 92868.
E-mail address: ranjang@uci.edu

Hand Clin 34 (2018) 177–184
https://doi.org/10.1016/j.hcl.2017.12.007

40°, with an increasing cascade radially to ulnarly by an additional 5°.[3,4] Although arthroplasty options are available, the one-stage solution for achieving pain relief and stability for arthritic PIPJ remains arthrodesis.[5] There are multiple techniques to perform the arthrodesis. The tension band technique is a fast, reliable, and inexpensive way to fuse the PIPJ.[6–10] Headless compression screw fixation and intramedullary screw fixation for PIPJ arthrodesis have demonstrated consistent success with relatively low complication rates.[5,11] Dorsal plating techniques as well as 90/90 wiring have been used for revision arthrodesis.[5,12]

INDICATIONS AND CONTRAINDICATIONS

Surgical interventions remain the mainstay for treatment of PIPJ arthritis. The classic indications for arthrodesis of the PIPJ are pain that is refractory to conservative measures, deformity, and stiffness. Alternative options that may be considered before arthrodesis are arthroplasty, osteochondral reconstruction, and soft-tissue reconstruction.[4]

Indications

- Painful primary osteoarthritis (**Table 1**)
- Posttraumatic osteoarthritis refractory to nonoperative and conservative treatment
- Chronic PIPJ dislocations, chronic instability
- Fractures and fracture dislocations
- Chronic septic arthritis
- Significant loss of bone stock
- Fixed joint contractures

Table 1
Indications and contraindications for proximal interphalangeal joint arthrodesis

Indications		Contraindications
Painful primary osteoarthritis	Posttraumatic osteoarthritis refractory to conservative treatment	Recent infection
Chronic PIPJ dislocations and instability	Fractures and fracture dislocations	Soft tissue compromise/ loss
Chronic septic arthritis	Significant loss of bone stock	
Fixed joint contracture	Poor soft tissue	
Tendon injuries	PIPJ arthroplasty revision	

- Poor skin coverage (as compared with arthroplasty)
- Irreparable tendon injuries
- Salvage for failed PIPJ arthroplasty[13]

Contraindications

- Recent infection
- Soft tissue compromise/loss

SURGICAL TECHNIQUE/PROCEDURE
Preoperative Planning

- Dedicated posterior anterior and lateral radiographs of the finger (**Fig. 1**)[4,11,14]
- Identify appropriate implant for arthrodesis
- Identify presence of bone deficiency
- Assess individual patient function to determine proper fusion angles
- Encourage patients to wear custom fabricated orthoplast splints at different angles to determine most functional angle

Preparation

- Upper arm tourniquet

Surgical Approach

- Dorsal curvilinear incision[11,14] (**Figs. 2 and 3**)
- Dorsal serpentine incision can be used if atrophic or compromised skin to create flaps for closure
- Incise extensor mechanism longitudinally
- The central slip should NOT be detached from P2 but elevated subperiosteally
- The lateral bands are left undisturbed to allow function of the dorsal interphalangeal joints
- Expose articular surfaces subperiosteally
- Release collateral ligaments both radially and ulnarly to allow free range of motion of PIPJ; in addition, the volar plate can be partially excised as needed
- Flex the PIPJ to expose the entire distal condyle of the proximal phalanx
- Perform osteotomy of head of proximal phalanx and base of middle phalanx to remove articular surfaces using an oscillating saw or rongeur so that the ends of the bone mate
- Bone is resected on proximal phalanx at desired angle of fusion
- Positioning of PIPJ arthrodesis is critical at this juncture, usually 30° to 40° for the index finger, 35° to 45° for the middle finger, 40° to 50° for the ring finger, and 45° to 55° for the small finger

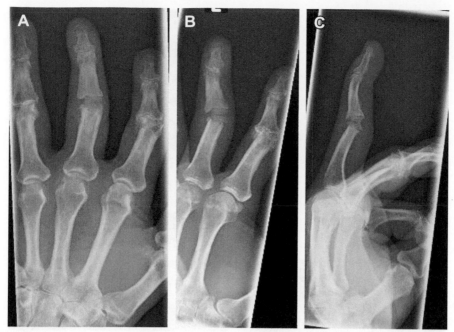

Fig. 1. A 68-year-old man who previously underwent left middle finger PIPJ arthroplasty. He was observed in clinic for approximately 1 year as he began having increased stiffness and deformity. (*A–C*) Radiographic images obtained preoperatively are shown here.

Surgical Procedure

Once the bony surfaces are prepared, the arthrodesis is performed. There are multiple techniques to performing the arthrodesis, as mentioned in later discussion.

Tension band technique

- A 0.045-in (1.4 mm) K-wire is used to drill transversely in the dorsal aspect of the middle phalanx[9,10,14] (**Figs. 4** and **5**)

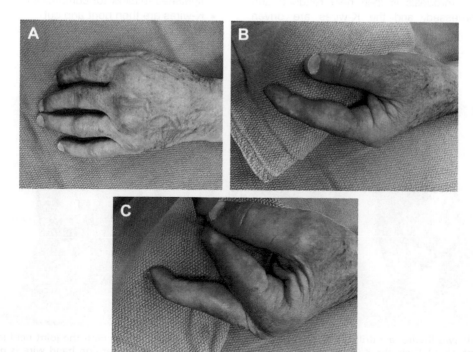

Fig. 2. (*A–C*) Intraoperative images of the left hand.

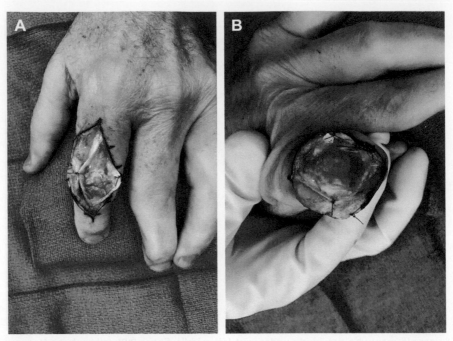

Fig. 3. (A, B) Left index finger PIPJ exposure.

- A 24-gauge wire is then passed through the drill hole
- Two parallel K-wires are drilled retrograde through the proximal phalanx perpendicular and central to the osteotomy site (see **Fig. 4**)
- The arthrodesis is then held reduced and compressed, and the K-wires are driven anterograde into the middle phalanx. Rotation

and alignment of the digit are confirmed at this stage
- The 24-gauge wire is then looped around the proximal end of the pins in a figure-of-8 fashion with a double-loop technique. The loop is then tightened to allow for compression
- K-wires are then bent and cut
- Joint capsule is closed over the hardware

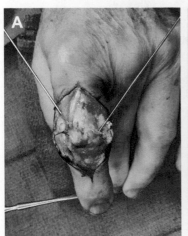
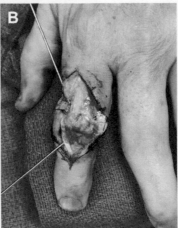
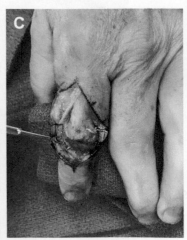

Fig. 4. (A) Two K-wires are drilled from proximal to distal in a cross-bar fashion with the joint held in proper alignment. (B, C) Then, the K-wire is driven across the arthrodesis site and a tension band wire is placed to hold the fusion in place as described.

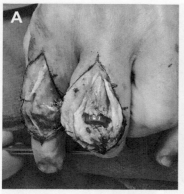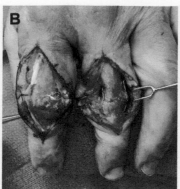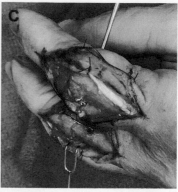

Fig. 5. (*A*) Prior silicon arthroplasty is removed from the middle finger. (*B, C*) K-wire tension banding technique is used to perform the arthrodesis.

Compression screw technique

- Screw is inserted anterograde at the dorsal aspect of proximal phalanx[11,15]
- The dorsal entry site *must* be at least 5 to 7 mm proximal to the joint surface to avoid fracture of the dorsal cortical bridge
- The proximal phalanx is drilled using a larger drill bit. The middle phalanx is then drilled with a smaller drill bit (lag technique)
- The dorsal hole in the proximal phalanx must be enlarged to prevent fracture
- Usually, 2.4-mm screws between 16 and 22 mm in length are chosen
- The arthrodesis is then held reduced and compressed while the screw is advanced
- If the fracture occurs or there is no compression, another technique *must* be used

Dorsal plate technique

- An 8-hole 2.0-mm titanium plate is placed dorsally over the PIPJ after exposure[5,16]
- The plate is bent slightly more than the desired angle of arthrodesis to induce compression across the bony surfaces
- Drill holes are placed eccentrically to provide firm axial compression when the screws are driven into the plate
- Adequate closure of extensor tendons and skin over the plate is necessary to prevent future infection

90/90 wiring technique

- A 0.035-in K-wire is used to drill in both the proximal and the middle phalanx in the coronal and sagittal planes[5,12]
- Two 22-gauge or 26-gauge circular wires are then inserted through the drill holes

- The wires are then tightened around the PIPJ in both the coronal and the sagittal planes
- Both wires are then tightened and twisted on the ulnar and dorsal aspect of the phalanx

COMPLICATIONS AND MANAGEMENT

- Nonunion: ~3%[4,10,12] (**Table 2**)
- Malunion: ~1%
- Hardware prominence: ~9% require hardware removal
- Fracture
- Infection and skin necrosis: ~3.5%

Management of Complications

PIPJ arthrodesis has been shown to carry a nonunion rate of 0% to 15%.[9,10,15–18] For revision purposes, the most utilized techniques used in the literature were 90/90 wiring or dorsal plating.[5,12] For successful revision, bone grafting is often necessary to avoid overshortening of the digit. Bone graft can be obtained from the distal radius, olecranon, or iliac crest. Additional complications that may arise are superficial or deep infections that can be treated with antibiotics, local wound care, or hardware removal.

Table 2	
Complications of proximal interphalangeal joint arthrodesis	
Nonunion	3%
Malunion	1%
Hardware prominence	9%
Infection	3.5%

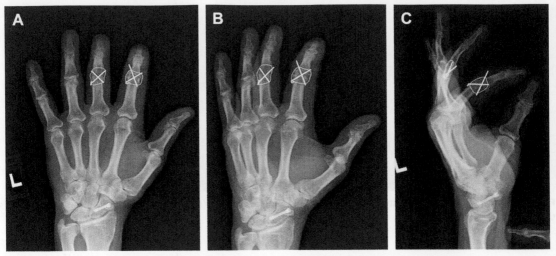

Fig. 6. (*A–C*) Final postoperative radiographs show index and middle finger PIPJ arthrodesis.

POSTOPERATIVE CARE

- Transition to rigid finger-based splint 1 week postoperatively or after suture removal (**Figs. 6–9**)
- Allow for gentle active range of motion of adjacent joints early

- Return to activities of daily living at approximately 4 weeks postoperatively
- Radiographic imaging used at 6 and 12 weeks postoperatively to assess fusion
- Once fusion is visualized radiographically, allow for return to normal function

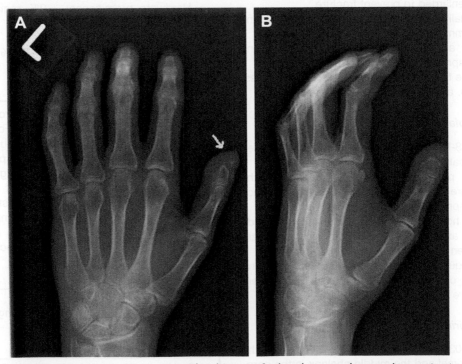

Fig. 7. Radiographs of a 47-year-old woman with a history of scleroderma and worsening contractures of her PIPJs. She had extremely limited range of motion preoperatively in her index PIPJ from 100° to 105°. (*A, B*) Preoperative radiographs of the left hand show anteroposterior and oblique views of the left index finger PIPJ arthritis.

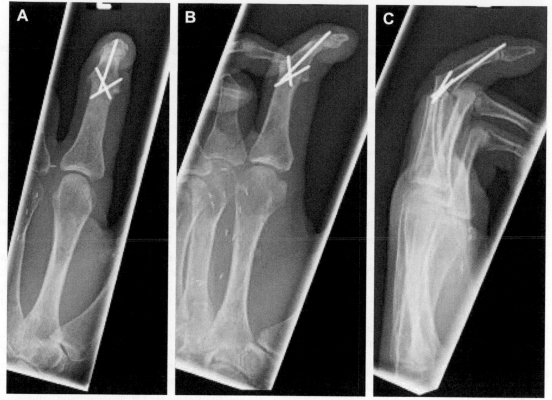

Fig. 8. (A–C) Radiographs of a 47-year-old woman who had undergone PIPJ arthrodesis.

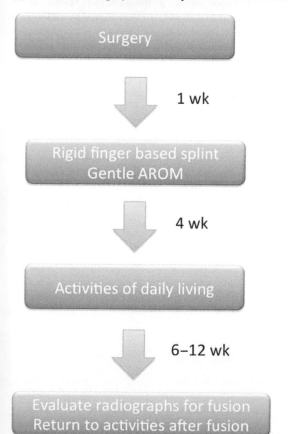

Fig. 9. Postoperative plan. AROM, active range of motion.

OUTCOMES

- High union rates: ~95% to 98%
- Alterations in precision pinch in index finger PIPJ

SUMMARY

PIPJ arthritis leads to significant hand impairment in the general population. In patients who fail nonoperative management of the disease, surgical options exist, including arthrodesis. PIPJ arthrodesis has very few contraindications, with an excellent overall success rate, making it an excellent option for surgical management. However, there are a multitude of surgical fixation devices to perform PIPJ arthrodesis and fusion. As outlined in this review, these various methods can provide the proper stability to allow for fusion.

REFERENCES

1. Dahaghin S, Bierma-Zeinstra SMA, Ginai AZ, et al. Prevalence and pattern of radiographic hand osteoarthritis and association with pain and disability (the Rotterdam study). Ann Rheum Dis 2005;64(5): 682–7.
2. Pellegrini VD, Burton RI. Osteoarthritis of the proximal interphalangeal joint of the hand: arthroplasty or fusion? J Hand Surg Am 1990;15(2):194–209.

3. Beldner S. Arthrodesis of the metacarpophalangeal and interphalangeal joints of the hand: current concepts. J Am Acad Orthop Surg 2016;24(5):290–7.

4. Wolfe SW, Hotchkiss RN, Pederson WC, et al. Revision of: Green DP. Green's operative hand surgery.

5. Capo JT, Melamed E, Shamian B, et al. Biomechanical evaluation of 5 fixation devices for proximal interphalangeal joint arthrodesis. J Hand Surg Am 2014; 39(10):1971–7.

6. IJsselstein CB, van Egmond DB, Hovius SE, et al. Results of small-joint arthrodesis: comparison of Kirschner wire fixation with tension band wire technique. J Hand Surg Am 1992;17(5):952–6.

7. Khuri SM. Tension band arthrodesis in the hand. J Hand Surg Am 1986;11(1):41–5.

8. Kovach JC, Werner FW, Palmer AK, et al. Biomechanical analysis of internal fixation techniques for proximal interphalangeal joint arthrodesis. J Hand Surg Am 1986;11(4):562–6.

9. Stahl S, Rozen N. Tension-band arthrodesis of the small joints of the hand. Orthopedics 2001;24(10): 981–3.

10. Stern PJ, Gates NT, Jones TB. Tension band arthrodesis of small joints in the hand. J Hand Surg Am 1993;18(2):194–7.

11. Leibovic SJ. Arthrodesis of the interphalangeal joints with headless compression screws. J Hand Surg Am 2007;32(7):1113–9.

12. Satteson ES, Langford MA, Li Z. The management of complications of small joint arthrodesis and arthroplasty. Hand Clin 2015;31(2):243–66.

13. Jones DB, Ackerman DB, Sammer DM, et al. Arthrodesis as a salvage for failed proximal interphalangeal joint arthroplasty. J Hand Surg Am 2011;36(2):259–64.

14. Uhl RL. Proximal interphalangeal joint arthrodesis using the tension band technique. J Hand Surg Am 2007;32(6):914–7.

15. Ayres JR, Goldstrohm GL, Miller GJ, et al. Proximal interphalangeal joint arthrodesis with the Herbert screw. J Hand Surg Am 1988;13(4):600–3.

16. Büchler U, Aiken MA. Arthrodesis of the proximal interphalangeal joint by solid bone grafting and plate fixation in extensive injuries to the dorsal aspect of the finger. J Hand Surg Am 1988;13(4): 589–94.

17. Leibovic SJ, Strickland JW. Arthrodesis of the proximal interphalangeal joint of the finger: comparison of the use of the Herbert screw with other fixation methods. J Hand Surg Am 1994;19(2):181–8.

18. Uhl RL, Schneider LH. Tension band arthrodesis of finger joints: a retrospective review of 76 consecutive cases. J Hand Surg Am 1992;17(3): 518–22.

Advances in Proximal Interphalangeal Joint Arthroplasty
Biomechanics and Biomaterials

Andy F. Zhu, MD[a], Paymon Rahgozar, MD[b],
Kevin C. Chung, MD, MS[c],*

KEYWORDS

- Proximal interphalangeal joint • Biomechanics • Arthritis • Silicone arthroplasty
- Surface replacement arthroplasty • Pyrocarbon arthroplasty

KEY POINTS

- Proximal interphalangeal (PIP) joint arthritis is a debilitating condition. The complexity of the joint makes management particularly challenging.
- Treatment of PIP arthritis requires an understanding of the biomechanics of the joint.
- PIP joint arthroplasty is one treatment option that has evolved over time.
- Advances in biomaterials have improved and expanded arthroplasty design. This article reviews biomechanics and arthroplasty design of the PIP joint.

INTRODUCTION

Proximal interphalangeal (PIP) joint arthritis is a painful, debilitating condition causing significant joint deformity and loss of motion. Common causes of arthritis include osteoarthritis, post-traumatic arthritis, and rheumatoid arthritis. Each has its own unique treatment challenges. Surgical management of painful PIP arthritis ranges from arthroplasty to fusion to amputation.[1] Replacement arthroplasty aims to relieve pain, restore motion, and maintain stability of the affected joint. Designing an effective replacement arthroplasty requires a thorough understanding of current biomaterials and an appreciation of the complex PIP joint biomechanics.

BIOMECHANICS

The PIP joint is a ginglymus, hinged joint composed of the proximal phalanx, middle phalanx, and supporting soft tissue structures. Its principal motion is in the sagittal plane but small amounts of motion also occur in the coronal and axial plane. The distal articular surface of the proximal phalanx is composed of two concentric condyles separated by an intercondylar ridge. The condyles are not identical in size and vary in relationship from finger to finger. In the coronal plane, the index and long finger have a more prominent ulnar condyle compared with the ring and small finger, which have a more prominent radial condyle (**Fig. 1**).[2] The head of the proximal phalanx

Disclosure Statement: A Midcareer Investigator Award in Patient-Oriented Research (2 K24-AR053120-06) awarded to Dr K.C. Chung supported this work. The content is solely the responsibility of the authors and does not necessarily represent the official views of the National Institutes of Health.

[a] Department of Orthopaedic Surgery, University of Michigan, 2912 Taubman Center, 1500 East Medical Center Drive, Ann Arbor, MI 48109, USA; [b] Section of Plastic Surgery, Department of Surgery, University of Michigan, 2130 Taubman Center, 1500 East Medical Center Drive, Ann Arbor, MI 48109-0340, USA; [c] Section of Plastic Surgery, University of Michigan, 2130 Taubman Center, SPC 5340, 1500 East Medical Center Drive, Ann Arbor, MI 48109-5340, USA
* Corresponding author.
E-mail address: kecchung@med.umich.edu

Hand Clin 34 (2018) 185–194
https://doi.org/10.1016/j.hcl.2017.12.008
0749-0712/18/© 2018 Elsevier Inc. All rights reserved.

hand.theclinics.com

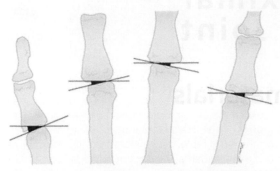

Fig. 1. In the coronal plane, the proximal phalanx of the index and long finger has a more prominent ulnar condyle. The ring and small finger have a more prominent radial condyle. (*Courtesy of* N. Fujihara, MD, Nagoya, Japan.)

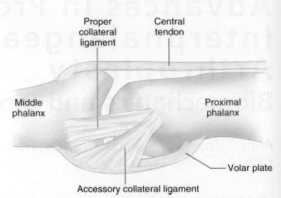

Fig. 2. Origin and attachment of the proper collateral ligament and accessory collateral ligament. (*Adapted from* Chung KC, Brown M. Capsulotomy for proximal interphalangeal contracture. In: Chung KC, editor. Operative techniques: hand and wrist surgery. 3rd edition. Philadelphia: Elsevier; 2018. p. 70; with permission.)

is trapezoidal in shape when viewed in cross-section. The volar aspect is approximately twice the length of the dorsal aspect. These anatomic relationships allow rotation of the joint in addition to flexion and extension.[3]

The base of the middle phalanx consists of a ridge separating the condylar recesses that articulate with the condyles of the proximal phalanx. The PIP joint is not perfectly congruent because the base of the middle phalanx has a larger radius of curvature than the head of the proximal phalanx. This incongruity permits additional motion outside the sagittal plane. On the volar aspect of the joint, the thick volar plate and its associated checkrein ligaments prevent hyperextension. Stability is also provided by the dorsal capsule of the joint that is largely comprised of fibers of the central tendon.[4] The combination of bony anatomy and soft tissue constraints allows for approximately 100° of motion at the PIP joint in the sagittal plane.[3]

Stability of the PIP joint in the coronal plane is derived from congruity of the bony anatomy along with the strong collateral ligaments. The collateral ligaments are divided into two distinct portions: the proper collateral ligament and accessory collateral ligament. The proper collateral ligament is the thicker of the two collateral ligaments and provides the most lateral stability. Both collateral ligaments originate in pits on either side of the proximal phalanx head and insert into the middle phalanx (**Fig. 2**). The accessory collateral ligament attaches volar to the proper collateral ligament blending with the volar plate and suspending the volar plate to the joint.[3]

The finger is composed of a kinetic chain of joints including the PIP, metacarpophalangeal (MCP), and distal interphalangeal (DIP) joints. These joints work in concert through a complex network of tendons and ligaments to produce coordinated and purposeful movement. In the 1960s, Landsmeer[5–7] provided an in-depth description of PIP joint motion. Rotation of a joint is a product of relative shortening and lengthening of flexor and extensor tendon units. The degree of rotation produced is a function of tendon excursion and distance from the center of rotation of the joint. The excursion of the extensor tendon is a linear function of the radius of curvature of the head of the proximal phalanx and maintains a constant distance from the center of rotation. In contrast, the flexor system runs through a tendon sheath and its distance to the center of rotation increases with progressive flexion of the joint.[7] Understanding and recreating these anatomic relationships in replacement arthroplasty is required to preserve normal joint biomechanics and restore anatomic joint range of motion.

The flexor and extensor system span multiple joints and thus motion at the PIP joint is dictated by the position of the adjacent joints. DIP and PIP joint flexion is determined by laxity of the lateral bands and central slip, respectively. The extensor complex moves as a single unit and is comprised of the central slip and terminal tendon, which is formed by the convergence of the lateral bands. The lateral bands are closer than the central slip to the center of rotation of the PIP joint; therefore, more laxity is produced at the DIP joint per unit excursion than PIP joint. The relative increase in flexion of the DIP with PIP flexion allows for a coordinated flexion movement to grasp objects. This relationship is disrupted in deformities, such as swan-neck and boutonnieres. and replacement arthroplasty alone without soft tissue correction is insufficient treatment.

Construction of an anatomically accurate implant that does not recreate normal joint kinematics provides no benefit. To design an implant successfully, one must consider not only the structural design but also the effect on biomechanics of the native soft tissue structures and adjacent joints.

ARTHROPLASTY DESIGN

Arthroplasty design continues to evolve because past implants have had variable success. Several basic requirements have been proposed for developing a successful arthroplasty implant. An implant should restore functional range of motion, restore normal mechanical advantage, provide stability, facilitate easy implantation, and have good wear characteristics.[8,9] Replacement arthroplasty has developed into two general categories: constrained and unconstrained implants.

Normal PIP joint motion ranges from 0 to 100°.[3] Flexibility of the joint is achieved through the bicondylar articulation of the proximal phalanx head with the concave bicondylar articulation of the base of the middle phalanx. The two condylar heads of the proximal phalanx are not identical in size and the base of the middle phalanx has a larger curvature of radius than that of the proximal phalanx condyles.[2] Surface replacement arthroplasty (SRA), also known as unconstrained arthroplasty, aims to recreate both components of the PIP joint to restore full native joint range of motion. Constrained and single implant arthroplasty are alternative designs that are used in PIP joint arthroplasty. Constrained arthroplasty has traditionally involved a hinge element, which allows for motion in the plane of the hinge but limits motion in all other planes. The most commonly used constrained single implant arthroplasty is the silicone arthroplasty.[10] Implant flexibility provides motion in multiple planes but the constrained hinge design does not reproduce the native PIP articulation.

Proper biomechanics of a joint must be restored to achieve full, functional range of motion. The implant should reestablish the joint center of rotation while maintaining the anatomic distances between muscle and tendon units of the finger. This recreates the normal force couple relationships of the joint. Factors influencing center of rotation include type of prosthesis, offset of prosthesis articulation relative to stem, and placement of the prosthesis within the bone.[11] In a hinged arthroplasty design, flexion of the joint causes dorsal translation of the center of rotation increasing the mechanical advantage to the flexor unit. However, dorsal translation of the center of rotation shortens the distance to the extensor unit creating a mechanical disadvantage and predisposing the joint to develop flexion contractures (**Fig. 3**A).[12] SRA aims to recreate the center of rotation of the native joint, which allows for a

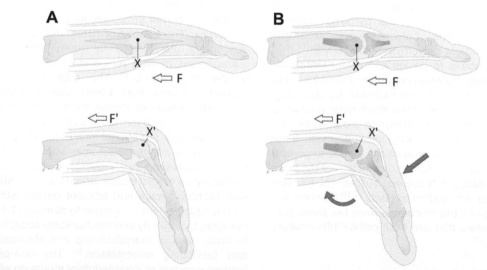

Fig. 3. Moment about the PIP joint axis. (A) In hinged arthroplasty, flexion moment about the PIP joint requires force (F) with moment arm (X). The moment arm from a flexed position (X′) decreases because of dorsal displacement of the center of rotation requiring an increase in extension force (F′) to return the PIP joint to neutral. (B) In SRA arthroplasty the center of rotation is maintained so flexion force (F) is equal extension force (F′) and the moment arm remains unchanged (X = X′). SRA arthroplasty also allows for rolling and translation in addition to rotation (*solid arrows*). (*Courtesy of* N. Fujihara, MD, Nagoya, Japan.)

combination of rolling and sliding at the terminal ends of motion providing the extensor units the required mechanical advantage for reversal of motion (Fig. 3B).[11]

Implant stability is achieved through preservation of soft tissue structures, implant-bone-interface integration, and inherent implant design. Preservation of previously described surrounding soft tissue structures decreases the forces on the implant. Thinner and flexible implants require less exposure, which facilitates preservation of soft tissue, whereas large multicomponent implants require wider exposures.[11] Currently, implant bone stability is achieved most effectively through an intramedullary stem design. The stem provides a large surface area for contact, dispersing forces that may otherwise lead to implant loosening. An ideal stem should match the contour of the intramedullary canal and quickly incorporate into the bone. Different types of stem incorporation include osseous ingrowth, osseous on-growth, and fibrocapsular formation.[13–15] Cement is a common adjunct used to strengthen the implant tissue interface but may result in thermal injury and difficulties in revision surgery; therefore, the use of cement for the PIP joint is not in favor.[11] Constrained implants rely less on surrounding soft tissue and more on inherent stability of the implant. Unconstrained implants have some inherent stability provided by joint congruency but rely heavily on soft tissues for stability.

Developments in material engineering have provided numerous biocompatible materials suitable for implantation including metallic alloys and nonmetallic alloys, such as pyrolytic carbons, ceramics, silicone polymers, and ultrahigh-molecular-weight polyethylene (UHMWPE).[11,16,17] The challenge is to design an implant that maximizes certain material properties while minimizing the effects of others. For example, pyrolytic carbon has demonstrated excellent wear properties but it has not been shown to incorporate into bone.[13,18] Titanium readily integrates with bone and has a modulus of elasticity similar to cortical bone by facilitating stress distribution at the bone implant interface; however, it does not function well as an articulation surface.[13,19] Silicone implants replace the articular surface but cause particulate debris that can elicit painful inflammatory reactions.[20]

SILICONE ARTHROPLASTY

Swanson[21] first introduced the concept of a silicone rubber spacer for joint replacement in 1962. To this day the Swanson finger joint silicone arthroplasty implant is the most used small joint arthroplasty.[10] Swanson graduated from the University of Illinois medical school in 1947 and subsequently underwent orthopedic training at Illinois, Northwestern, and Indiana University. He was interested in treating children with polio, cerebral palsy, congenital limb differences, and arthritic deformities of the hand. While using silicone to develop an internal pad for below-knee amputations, he discovered that silicone would be an ideal implant material for joint arthroplasty.[22] Similar silicone-based implants have been designed without comparable success.[23]

Silicon is a chemical element and in its pure state forms a hard, brittle crystalline solid. It is more commonly found as silicon dioxide or silicate, an anionic silicon-containing compound that makes up most of the rocks, sand, and minerals found on Earth. Silicones are polymers composed of repeating siloxane units, chains of alternating silicon and oxygen atoms. Silicone elastomers are created by three-dimensional cross-linking of linear silicone polymer chains.[16] These elastomers have found widespread use within the medical field ranging from catheters to drains to implants. Desirable material properties of the elastomer include biocompatibility, heat stability, and durability.[16,24–27] Additional benefits specific to silicone implant arthroplasty include flexibility, force dampening properties, and ability to withstand various sterilization techniques (heat, gamma ray, ethylene oxide).[16]

Silicone elastomers are generally classified by the curing mechanism and condition. Vulcanization is the chemical process of adding curatives to modify polymer cross-linking, altering material properties. The two major categories of silicone elastomers are formed by room temperature vulcanization or high temperature vulcanization, greater than 100°C.[16] The original Swanson implant was made from a heat-vulcanized, medical-grade silicone elastomer stock. The implants were one piece and formed in a mold at 250°F under 325 pounds per square inch of pressure.[28]

Swanson's silicone elastomer implant fulfilled most of his criteria for an ideal joint replacement: maintenance of joint space, preservation of stable joint motion, simple and efficient design, simple and durable fixation, resistance to stress and deterioration, biologically and mechanically acceptable to host, ease of manufacturing and sterilization, and facilitating rehabilitation.[28] The one-piece implant consists of intramedullary stems on either side bridged by a hinge. The inherent flexibility of the silicone elastomer allows flexion and extension at the hinge of the implant and provides a dampening effect on the bone. The implant is stiff enough to maintain joint alignment after bony resection and soft tissue balancing. Silicone implants have been machine tested for more than 130 million cycles without evidence of breakdown.[28]

A biocompatible implant coexists in the body without inflicting harm to the host system. Implant design that generates a host response but does no damage to the host is considered biocompatible. Stability of the silicone elastomer implant occurs through the well-described host response process of joint encapsulation. Within 3 days of implantation a fibrous capsule envelops the new implant maturing to a well-developed capsule consisting of predominately type III collagen.[15] The firm capsule is surrounded by new bone formation further stabilizing the joint. The stems are not transfixed to the bone and allow small amounts of piston motion at the stem, decreasing the forces and prolonging life of the implant.

Silicone arthroplasty has reproducibly demonstrated pain improvement in the arthritic PIP joint. Swanson and coworkers[29] reported on his experience with his implant on 424 arthroplasties with 98% of patients reporting improvement or complete pain relief. Subsequent series have demonstrated similar results in providing pain relief.[30–35] In these series, pain was improved consistently regardless of the cause of the arthritis. Chan and colleagues[36] performed a systematic review of 718 silicone arthroplasties with 76% patients reporting complete resolution of pain.

Unfortunately, improvements in range of motion have been met with variable amounts of success. In 1973 Swanson[21] reported an average postoperative arc of motion of 63°, which decreased to 51° in a later follow-up study.[29] Conolly and Rath[37] performed 39 arthroplasties for post-traumatic pain and stiffness with 52% of patients achieving greater than 40° of motion and 18% achieving between 15% and 40°. Thirty four of the 39 patients showed improvement. Bales and colleagues[34] reviewed 38 arthroplasties performed for osteoarthritis and demonstrated a decrease in arc of motion from 55° preoperatively to 50° postoperatively. Ashworth and colleagues[31] performed 99 arthroplasties for post-traumatic arthritis and found a decrease in arc of motion from 38° to 29°. It is important to consider functional range of motion when evaluating success of an arthroplasty. Normal functional range of motion for the PIP joint is between 23° and 87°.[38] Transposing the arc of motion into a functional zone improves joint function even if total arc of motion remains unchanged.

Silicone arthroplasty for correction of deformity has proven to be ineffective. The destructive nature of rheumatoid arthritis in particular can cause severe deformities including boutonniere, swan-neck, subluxation, radial deviation, and ulnar deviation. The process involves damage to the surrounding tissues, destabilizing the joint. Post-traumatic arthritic joints may be associated with fixed flexion and extension contractures that can also be challenging to correct. Takigawa and colleagues[33] performed silicone arthroplasty on 33 of 70 rheumatoid joints. There were 30 severe flexion contractures (greater than 30°), 14 boutonniere deformities, six swan-neck deformities, four dislocations, three subluxations, and four unstable joints. No joint with flexion contractures achieved full extension. Twenty joints had partial improvement and six joints were unimproved. Of the 14 joints with boutonniere deformities, three joints had improved range of motion (greater than 40°), four joints had functional range of motion improvement, six joints had no improvement of contracture, and one joint dislocated. All six swan-neck deformities recurred and three additional swan-neck deformities developed. Nineteen joints had recurrence of ulnar deviation with only one improvement, but also one developed de novo. Overall, there was no significant change in arc of motion.

Adamson and colleagues[39] treated 40 rheumatoid PIP joints with 22 boutonniere and 16 swan-neck deformities. The boutonniere deformity group had no change in arc of motion. Fourteen of the 22 joints had recurrence of deformity and two developed a swan-neck deformity. Of the swan-neck deformity group, there was a loss of 18° arc of motion with 14 of the 16 joints developing recurrence of the deformity. Conolly and Rath[37] demonstrated that preoperative contracture was inversely related to the arc of motion that could be restored. Flexion contractures greater than 60° improved 17° compared with 41° of improvement in contractures less than 20°. Adamson and colleagues[39] suggested that silicone arthroplasty not be performed in cases of swan-neck deformity. However, there is a role for silicone arthroplasty in treatment of boutonniere deformity if the arc of motion lies outside the functional range of motion. Patients should be cautioned that recurrence of deformity is common.

Implant fracture is a complication unique to silicone arthroplasty. Fractures are typically caused by a tear in the implant from excessive wear from a sharp bone edge. Swanson and coworkers[29] original study reported a 5.2% fracture rate, 22 fractures out of 424 implants. Twelve of the fractured implants were symptomatic and required revision. In the literature, implant fractures are reported to range from 0% to 55%.[30,31,33,34,39]

A fractured implant is not necessarily correlated with pain and disability. Bales and colleagues[34] reviewed 21 fractures (55%), noting that only three joints required revision for symptomatic pain. They concluded that the formation of fibrous tissue around the implant provides stability and may prevent joint pain. Radiographic changes including radiolucency, prosthetic settling, and abnormal bone formation were common in their study and did not correlate with outcome.

Long-term survivorship (8–10 years) of silicone implants in the PIP joint has been reported between 80% and 90%.[33,34,39] In a systematic review performed by Chan and colleagues[36] 4% of all implants required revision surgery and 2% required a salvage procedure. Lateral joint instability is a concern particularly in the index finger given the large forces experienced with pinch grip and alternative treatments should be considered.[40] Overall silicone arthroplasty has remained a good treatment option for PIP joint arthritis and has the most reported long-term follow-up of all available implant arthroplasties.

SURFACE REPLACEMENT ARTHROPLASTY

The concept of SRA was first introduced to treat hip pathology in the early 1900s. Smith-Petersen was a pioneer of hip arthroplasty and developed the first Vitallium, cobalt chromium (CoCr) alloy cup arthroplasty between 1937 and 1939.[41] Inspired by this design, Burman[42] designed a Vitallium cap hemiarthroplasty in 1940 for an arthritic MCP joint. The development of metal implant arthroplasty led Brannon and Klein[43] to design a metal hinged arthroplasty for the MCP and PIP joint in 1959. Complications with prosthetic loosening became prevalent and modifications of the stem design to combat loosening were largely unsuccessful.[44,45]

The modern day SRA was introduced by Linscheid and Dobyns in 1979.[12] Their aim was to reproduce a physiologic articulation while preserving bone stock and collateral ligaments for stability. It was believed that approximation of the original center of rotation would restore balanced forces and proper moments to the joint. Preservation of the collateral ligaments would also decrease endosteal contact forces, minimizing osteolysis and subsidence.[46] The original implant consisted of a proximal CoCr alloy component and a distal hand-machined UHMWPE component.[12] The release of pyrolytic carbon-based implants in 2002 provided an alternative bearing surface to the traditional CoCr and UHMWPE combination for SRA.[14] Currently, these two materials represent the most common and studied SRA implants used today.

COBALT CHROMIUM AND ULTRAHIGH-MOLECULAR-WEIGHT POLYETHYLENE

To date, large joint hip and knee arthroplasty are one of the most successful and well-established procedures performed by orthopedic surgeons. Unfortunately, this success has not directly translated to small joint arthroplasty. Difficulties encountered include small joint size, complicated kinetic chain movements, unique function of each individual finger, and soft tissue balancing. Nonetheless, the advances in large joint arthroplasty have guided the development of small joint arthroplasty.

The CoCr and UHMWPE articulation is a frequently used combination in hip arthroplasty. Linscheid and Dobyns[12] developed the first small joint SRA using this articulation.[12] The wear-resistant and corrosion-resistant properties of CoCr were first discovered in the early 1900s.[47] The alloys are extracted from cobalt oxide and chromium oxide ores, prepared, and fused together using a vacuum process.[48] Polyethylene is formed from ethylene ($C2H4$) gas. The process involves polymerizing ethylene (reactive gas), hydrogen, and titanium tetra chloride (catalyst) in a solvent suitable for mass and heat transfer producing a UHMWPE powder.[49] The powder is consolidated under high temperatures and pressure. The final product is typically produced by compression molding and ram extrusion because of its high melt viscosity.[49]

The original design contained a CoCr alloy proximal component with a tapered stem, rectangular cross-section, and dorsal longitudinal groove. The articular surface of the proximal component consisted of a bicondylar head and was angled slight palmarly relative to the stem to simulate the native proximal phalanx. The distal component consisted of a single piece of UHMWPE with a 2-mm-thick bifacet, biconcave articular surface with a square stem.[46] Linscheid and coworkers[46] reviewed 66 SRAs performed over a 14-year period for degenerative arthritis (37), traumatic arthritis (16), and inflammatory arthritis (13). According to the author, all implants were cemented for several reasons: variation in endosteal configuration, porous ingrowth material cannot be easily applied to UHMWPE, and ease of proper alignment with cement application. Postoperatively 56 of 66 joints were pain free, whereas 10 joints had mild to moderate ache with activity. Postoperative range of motion improved to 47° compared with 35° preoperatively. Twenty-one joints had either ulnar or radial deviation of greater than 10° preoperatively with only four joints having deformity postoperatively. Complications included instability (five), swan-neck deformity (five), stiffness (22), infection (one), and swelling (one) with 12 secondary operations. The author concluded that the procedure is indicated for degenerative arthritis without static deformity including in the index finger.

In 2000 the implant stem was modified to a titanium distal component to allow press-fit, cementless fixation of the UHMWPE articulating surface.[50] Johnstone and colleagues[50] compared the results of the original cemented arthroplasty (27) with the new cementless version (21) through a dorsal central slip elevating approach. Postoperatively there was a significant improvement in pain across both groups compared with preoperatively but no difference between the two groups. No significant difference in arc of motion was found postoperatively or between the two groups. However, there was a significant increase in subsidence of the uncemented implants (13) compared with the cemented implants (one). Overall, there was no association between implant fixation and joint failure with five failures in the cemented group and two failures in the uncemented group. The author concluded that cement fixation provides more durable stability. Jennings and Livingston[51] had similar results with loosening of 16 of the 41 (39%) uncemented implants compared with only 2 of 45 (4%) in the cemented group. Ten of the 11 revisions performed in their series were for loosening of uncemented prosthesis. Both groups demonstrated good pain relief with no significant improvement in range of motion. A 10-year follow-up of the same cohort revealed an 8° decrease in range of motion, no further radiographic evidence of loosening, and no additional revisions.[52] The authors recommended that all implants should be inserted with cement. Additionally, patients with rheumatoid arthritis were found to have less satisfactory outcomes and no differences in outcomes were observed in arthroplasty of the index finger compared with the other fingers.

CoCr and UMWPE implants have demonstrated good pain relief with minimal improvement in range of motion.[46,50,52–54] There are conflicting data with regards to implant cementation.[50,51,53] A recent modification of implant design involved the addition of hydroxyapatite coating to the stems of the implant. Short-term 2-year follow-up of this implant is promising with no radiographic evidence of loosening or subsidence but long-term follow-up is needed.[54] Complications, however, remain high ranging from 21% to 40%.[46,50,51,53–55] The most common complications include loosening, deformity, and stiffness. CoCr and UMWPE remains a suitable treatment of degenerative joints with intact soft tissue and sufficient bone stock. Caution is advised when treating inflammatory conditions that are often associated with soft tissue disruption.

PYROLYTIC CARBON

Pyrolytic carbon (Pyrocarbon) MCP joint arthroplasty was first introduced in 1983.[56] However, pyrolytic carbon implant arthroplasty for the PIP joint is new and was initially introduced in Europe in 2000. It was approved for use in the United States in 2002 by the Food and Drug administration through a humanitarian device exemption.[14] The use of pyrolytic carbon in implants is not a novel concept. In 1969, pyrolytic carbon was first incorporated into mechanical heart valves.[57] The excellent material properties, biocompatibility, and wear characteristics demonstrated in heart valves spurred interest in its use in surface bearing arthroplasty.[17]

Carbon is a nonmetallic, tetravalent chemical element. The physical forms, allotropes, of carbon vary widely depending on the bonding pattern. The most well-known allotropes of carbon include diamond, graphite, and amorphous carbon. The varying physical properties of carbon compounds is attributed to the flexibility of its valence electrons that allow for a spectrum of structural organization from haphazard carbon array stacking to complex, precise carbon array stacking sequences.[58]

Pyrolytic carbon belongs to a group of carbon compounds known as turbostratic carbons that lack structural organization. These are composed of parallel layers of carbon with no spatial relationship between layers. The haphazard layers form small (<100 Å) organized units known as crystallites.[58] Modification of crystallite size, crystallite density, and preferred orientation (relationship between layers) presents pyrolytic carbon to have a low modulus of elasticity while still possessing high strength.[59] Pyrolysis is the decomposition of organic material by heat. Pyrolysis of hydrocarbons in a fluidized bed at high temperatures (>1000°C) releases carbon gas.[58,60] The carbon gas forms a thin coat over the implant. Implants are generally made of high-strength graphite, a carbon-based material.

The low modulus of elasticity and high breaking strength are ideal for joint arthroplasty for several reasons. This combination provides a relative high strain to failure compared with other bearing surfaces, such as ceramic, and requires greater energy to fracture. Unlike metals and polymers, pyrolytic carbon does not undergo degradation caused by cyclic loading. Pyrolytic carbon surfaces are able to withstand large amounts of elastic strain without deformation. Under concentrated loads, the elastic strain redistributes localized high abrasive forces preventing galling, a type of adhesion wear. In vivo testing of pyrolytic carbon implants has demonstrated negligible wear with more than 5 million cycles of testing.[18] Ex vivo implant retrieval data demonstrated similar amounts of minimal wear.[61] Long-term clinical data from MCP pyrolytic carbon implants have also confirmed the superior wear resistance and durability of the implant.[19]

The primary indication for PIP arthroplasty is pain. Overall the literature suggests that pyrolytic carbon implants have been successful in improving pain.[62–69] Unfortunately, improvement of range of motion has been unreliable. Some studies have demonstrated increases in range of motion with variable significance,[14,62,66,67] whereas others have demonstrated no change or even decreases in range of motion.[63,65,69,70] The variability in the effect on range of motion is attributable to the heterogeneity of the study populations with regards to approach, arthritis pathology, and previous deformity.

Overall high complication rates, up to 68%,[69] have been observed with pyrolytic carbon implants.[14,62,64,66–68,70] Daecke and colleagues[71] performed a prospective randomized comparison of silicone, CoCr and UHMWPE, and pyrolytic carbon implants and discovered increased complications in the pyrolytic carbon group. Radiographic lucency, loosening, and subsidence are all common complications found with pyrolytic carbon implant use. The difficulty in assessing radiographic change lies in its subjective nature and clinical relevance. Pyrolytic carbon does not readily osteointegrate and the coating itself is radiolucent, which leaves a 0.5-mm rim around the implant on radiographs.[71,72] Bravo and colleagues[14] reported 40% (20 implants) of implants demonstrated radiographic migration, of which four required a revision surgery. They concluded that after initial postoperative settling, implants become stable with sclerotic bone on-growth to the implant. However, Sweets and Stern[70] observed progressive loosening over time in 15 of 31 (48%) with five requiring revisions.

Other common complications found with pyrolytic carbon arthroplasty include contracture, implant squeaking, implant dislocation, and stiffness. The high number of complications has also resulted in higher revision rates with pyrolytic carbon implants. Midterm studies have demonstrated fair implant survival. Dickson and colleagues[69] performed a Kaplan-Meier assessment on implant survival revealing an 85% survival rate at 5 and 10 years. All but two of the revisions fell within the first 2 years of surgery leading to a Kaplan-Meier curve that was not consistent with progressive loosening. The authors suggested that the early failures may represent technical issues, such as soft tissue balancing. Pyrolytic carbon arthroplasty remains an option for PIP arthritis. Patients should be cautioned regarding the high complication rates associated with use of the implant. Improved techniques and long-term follow-up are needed to determine the role and outcome of pyrolytic carbon arthroplasty in PIP joint arthroplasty.

The advancements in PIP joint arthroplasty have provided patients and physicians more options in treating this joint. The improvements in implant materials have spurred the development of SRA, which aims to recreate normal joint mechanics. Early results have demonstrated improvements in pain but long-term follow-up and a decrease in complication rate are required. Silicone arthroplasty has had a long track record and reliably improves pain but has its own complications and shortcomings. Great strides have been made in treatment of PIP joint arthritis but it continues to remain a difficult problem to treat with no clear consensus in arthroplasty option.

ACKNOWLEDGMENTS

The authors thank Dr Nasa Fujihara, MD for her generous figure contribution.

REFERENCES

1. Carroll RE, Taber TH. Digital arthroplasty of the proximal interphalangeal joint. J Bone Joint Surg Am 1954;36(5):912–20.
2. Ash HE, Unsworth A. Proximal interphalangeal joint dimensions for the design of a surface replacement prosthesis. Proc Inst Mech Eng H 1996; 210(2):95–108.
3. Leibovic SJ, Bowers WH. Anatomy of the proximal interphalangeal joint. Hand Clin 1994;10(2):169–78.
4. Hotchkiss RN. Treatment of the stiff finger and hand. In: Wolfe SW, editor. Green's operative hand surgery. 7th edition. Philadelphia: Elsevier; 2017. p. 338–44.
5. Landsmeer JM. Studies in the anatomy of articulation. I. The equilibrium of the "intercalated" bone. Acta Morphol Neerl Scand 1961;3:287–303.
6. Landsmeer JM. Studies in the anatomy of articulation. II. Patterns of movement of bi-muscular, bi-articular systems. Acta Morphol Neerl Scand 1961; 3:304–21.
7. Landsmeer JM. The coordination of finger-joint motions. J Bone Joint Surg Am 1963;45:1654–62.
8. Flatt AE, Fischer GW. Biomechanical factors in the replacement of rheumatoid finger joints. Ann Rheum Dis 1969;28(5 Suppl):36–41.

9. Swanson AB. A flexible implant for replacement of arthritic or destroyed joints in the hand. N Y Univ Inter-Clin Inf Bull 1966;6:16–9.

10. Murray PM. New-generation implant arthroplasties of the finger joints. J Am Acad Orthop Surg 2003; 11(5):295–301.

11. Linscheid RL. Implant arthroplasty of the hand: retrospective and prospective considerations. J Hand Surg 2000;25(5):796–816.

12. Linscheid RL, Dobyns JH. Total joint arthroplasty. The hand. Mayo Clin Proc 1979;54(8):516–26.

13. Daecke W, Veyel K, Wieloch P, et al. Osseointegration and mechanical stability of pyrocarbon and titanium hand implants in a load-bearing in vivo model for small joint arthroplasty. J Hand Surg 2006;31(1): 90–7.

14. Bravo CJ, Rizzo M, Hormel KB, et al. Pyrolytic carbon proximal interphalangeal joint arthroplasty: results with minimum two-year follow-up evaluation. J Hand Surg 2007;32(1):1–11.

15. Vistnes LM, Ksander GA, Kosek J. Study of encapsulation of silicone rubber implants in animals. A foreign-body reaction. Plast Reconstr Surg 1978; 62(4):580–8.

16. Jerschow P. Silicone elastomers. Shawbury, UK: Smithers Rapra; 2001.

17. Leuer LH, Gross JM, Johnson KM. Material properties, biocompatibility, and wear resistance of the Medtronic pyrolytic carbon. J Heart Valve Dis 1996;5(Suppl 1):S105–9 [discussion: 110].

18. Naylor A, Bone MC, Unsworth A, et al. In vitro wear testing of the PyroCarbon proximal interphalangeal joint replacement: five million cycles of flexion and extension. Proc Inst Mech Eng H 2015;229(5): 362–8.

19. Cook SD, Beckenbaugh RD, Redondo J, et al. Long-term follow-up of pyrolytic carbon metacarpophalangeal implants. J Bone Joint Surg Am 1999;81(5): 635–48.

20. Naidu SH, Beredjiklian P, Adler L, et al. In vivo inflammatory response to silicone elastomer particulate debris. J Hand Surg 1996;21(3):496–500.

21. Swanson AB. Implant resection arthroplasty of the proximal interphalangeal joint. Orthop Clin North Am 1973;4(4):1007–29.

22. Swanson AB. Improving end-bearing characteristics of lower-extremity amputation stumps. N Y Univ Inter-Clin Inf Bull 1966;5:1–7.

23. Niebauer JJ, Shaw JL, Doren WW. Silicone-Dacron hinge prosthesis. Design, evaluation, and application. Ann Rheum Dis 1969;28(5 Suppl):56–8.

24. Swanson AB. Flexible implant arthroplasty for arthritic finger joints: rationale, technique, and results of treatment. J Bone Joint Surg Am 1972; 54(3):435–55.

25. Nalbandian RM, Swanson AB, Maupin BK. Long-term silicone implant arthroplasty. Implications of animal and human autopsy findings. JAMA 1983; 250(9):1195–8.

26. Swanson AB, Nalbandian RM, Zmugg TJ, et al. Silicone implants in dogs. A ten-year histopathologic study. Clin Orthop Relat Res 1984;(184): 293–301.

27. DeHeer DH, Owens SR, Swanson AB. The host response to silicone elastomer implants for small joint arthroplasty. J Hand Surg 1995;20(3 Pt 2): S101–9.

28. Swanson AB. Finger joint replacement by silicone rubber implants and the concept of implant fixation by encapsulation. Ann Rheum Dis 1969; 28(5Suppl):47–55.

29. Swanson AB, Maupin BK, Gajjar NV, et al. Flexible implant arthroplasty in the proximal interphalangeal joint of the hand. J Hand Surg 1985;10(6 Pt 1): 796–805.

30. Lin HH, Wyrick JD, Stern PJ. Proximal interphalangeal joint silicone replacement arthroplasty: clinical results using an anterior approach. J Hand Surg 1995;20(1):123–32.

31. Ashworth CR, Hansraj KK, Todd AO, et al. Swanson proximal interphalangeal joint arthroplasty in patients with rheumatoid arthritis. Clin Orthop 1997; 342:34–7.

32. Herren DB, Simmen BR. Palmar approach in flexible implant arthroplasty of the proximal interphalangeal joint. Clin Orthop Relat Res 2000;(371):131–5.

33. Takigawa S, Meletiou S, Sauerbier M, et al. Long-term assessment of Swanson implant arthroplasty in the proximal interphalangeal joint of the hand. J Hand Surg 2004;29(5):785–95.

34. Bales JG, Wall LB, Stern PJ. Long-term results of Swanson silicone arthroplasty for proximal interphalangeal joint osteoarthritis. J Hand Surg 2014;39(3): 455–61.

35. Hage JJ, Yoe EP, Zevering JP, et al. Proximal interphalangeal joint silicone arthroplasty for posttraumatic arthritis. J Hand Surg 1999;24(1):73–7.

36. Chan K, Ayeni O, McKnight L, et al. Pyrocarbon versus silicone proximal interphalangeal joint arthroplasty: a systematic review. Plast Reconstr Surg 2013;131(1):114–24.

37. Conolly WB, Rath S. Silastic implant arthroplasty for post-traumatic stiffness of the finger joints. J Hand Surg Br 1991;16(3):286–92.

38. Bain GI, Polites N, Higgs BG, et al. The functional range of motion of the finger joints. J Hand Surg Eur Vol 2015;40(4):406–11.

39. Adamson GJ, Gellman H, Brumfield RH, et al. Flexible implant resection arthroplasty of the proximal interphalangeal joint in patients with systemic inflammatory arthritis. J Hand Surg 1994;19(3):378–84.

40. Minamikawa Y, Imaeda T, Amadio PC, et al. Lateral stability of proximal interphalangeal joint replacement. J Hand Surg 1994;19(6):1050–4.

41. Hernigou P. Smith-Petersen and early development of hip arthroplasty. Int Orthop 2014;38(1):193–8.

42. Burman M. Vitallium cap arthroplasty of metacarpophalangeal and interphalangeal joints of the fingers. Bull Hosp Jt Dis 1940;1:79–89.

43. Brannon EW, Klein G. Experiences with a finger-joint prosthesis. J Bone Joint Surg Am 1959;41(1):87–102.

44. Flatt AE. Restoration of rheumatoid finger-joint function. J Bone Joint Surg Am 1961;43(5):753–74.

45. Girzadas DV, Clayton ML. Limitations of the use of metallic prosthesis in the rheumatoid hand. Clin Orthop 1969;67:127–32.

46. Linscheid RL, Murray PM, Vidal MA, et al. Development of a surface replacement arthroplasty for proximal interphalangeal joints. J Hand Surg 1997;22(2):286–98.

47. Haynes E. Metal alloy. IN: US Patent Office; 1913.

48. Hyslop DJS, Abdelkader AM, Cox A, et al. Electrochemical synthesis of a biomedically important Co–Cr alloy. Acta Mater 2010;58(8):3124–30.

49. Kurtz SM. Chapter 2-from ethylene gas to UHMWPE component: the process of producing orthopedic implants. In: The UHMWPE handbook. San Diego (CA): Academic Press; 2004. p. 13–36.

50. Johnstone BR, Fitzgerald M, Smith KR, et al. Cemented versus uncemented surface replacement arthroplasty of the proximal interphalangeal joint with a mean 5-year follow-up. J Hand Surg 2008;33(5):726–32.

51. Jennings CD, Livingstone DP. Surface replacement arthroplasty of the proximal interphalangeal joint using the PIP-SRA implant: results, complications, and revisions. J Hand Surg 2008;33(9):1565.e1-11.

52. Jennings CD, Livingstone DP. Surface replacement arthroplasty of the proximal interphalangeal joint using the SR PIP implant: long-term results. J Hand Surg 2015;40(3):469–73.e6.

53. Murray PM, Linscheid RL, Cooney WP, et al. Long-term outcomes of proximal interphalangeal joint surface replacement arthroplasty. J Bone Joint Surg Am 2012;94(12):1120–8.

54. Flannery O, Harley O, Badge R, et al. MatOrtho proximal interphalangeal joint arthroplasty: minimum 2-year follow-up. J Hand Surg Eur Vol 2016;41(9):910–6.

55. Luther C, Germann G, Sauerbier M. Proximal interphalangeal joint replacement with surface replacement arthroplasty (SR-PIP): functional results and complications. Hand (N Y) 2010;5(3):233–40.

56. Beckenbaugh RD. Preliminary experience with a noncemented nonconstrained total joint arthroplasty for the metacarpophalangeal joints. Orthopedics 1983;6(8):962–5.

57. Haubold AD. On the durability of pyrolytic carbon in vivo. Med Prog Technol 1994;20(3–4):201–8.

58. Bokros JC. Carbon biomedical devices. Carbon 1977;15(6):353–71.

59. Kaae JL. Relations between the structure and the mechanical properties of fluidized-bed pyrolytic carbons. Carbon 1971;9(3):291–9.

60. Haubold AD, Shim HS, Bokros JC. Developments in carbon prosthetics. Biomater Med Devices Artif Organs 1979;7(2):263–9.

61. Bone MC, Giddins G, Joyce TJ. An analysis of explanted pyrolytic carbon prostheses. J Hand Surg Eur Vol 2014;39(6):666–7.

62. Herren DB, Schindele S, Goldhahn J, et al. Problematic bone fixation with pyrocarbon implants in proximal interphalangeal joint replacement: short-term results. J Hand Surg Br 2006;31(6):643–51.

63. Nunley RM, Boyer MI, Goldfarb CA. Pyrolytic carbon arthroplasty for posttraumatic arthritis of the proximal interphalangeal joint. J Hand Surg 2006;31(9):1468–74.

64. Meier R, Schulz M, Krimmer H, et al. Proximal interphalangeal joint replacement with pyrolytic carbon prostheses. Oper Orthop Traumatol 2007;19(1):1–15.

65. Wijk U, Wollmark M, Kopylov P, et al. Outcomes of proximal interphalangeal joint pyrocarbon implants. J Hand Surg 2010;35(1):38–43.

66. Ono S, Shauver MJ, Chang KWC, et al. Outcomes of pyrolytic carbon arthroplasty for the proximal interphalangeal joint at 44 months' mean follow-up. Plast Reconstr Surg 2012;129(5):1139–50.

67. McGuire DT, White CD, Carter SL, et al. Pyrocarbon proximal interphalangeal joint arthroplasty: outcomes of a cohort study. J Hand Surg Eur Vol 2012;37(6):490–6.

68. Storey PA, Goddard M, Clegg C, et al. Pyrocarbon proximal interphalangeal joint arthroplasty: a medium to long term follow-up of a single surgeon series. J Hand Surg Eur Vol 2015;40(9):952–6.

69. Dickson DR, Nuttall D, Watts AC, et al. Pyrocarbon proximal interphalangeal joint arthroplasty: minimum five-year follow-up. J Hand Surg 2015;40(11):2142–8.e4.

70. Sweets TM, Stern PJ. Pyrolytic carbon resurfacing arthroplasty for osteoarthritis of the proximal interphalangeal joint of the finger. J Bone Joint Surg Am 2011;93(15):1417–25.

71. Daecke W, Kaszap B, Martini AK, et al. A prospective, randomized comparison of 3 types of proximal interphalangeal joint arthroplasty. J Hand Surg 2012;37(9):1770–9.e1-3.

72. Ascension orthopedics, vol. 1. Austin (TX): Ascension Orthopedics; 2005.

Implant Arthroplasty
Selection of Exposure and Implant

Michiro Yamamoto, MD, PhD[a,b,*], Kevin C. Chung, MD, MS[c]

KEYWORDS

- Proximal interphalangeal joint • Arthroplasty • Implant • Approach • Exposure

KEY POINTS

- Outcomes after implant arthroplasty for osteoarthritis of the proximal interphalangeal joint are different according to the selection of surgical exposure and implant design.
- Silicone implants with the volar approach show the best arc of motion and fewer complications after surgery among all combinations of exposure and implant design.
- Reconstruction of appropriate soft tissue balance and alignment of the finger are essential to success with surface replacement arthroplasty.
- Future directions for implants should focus on osteointegration and durability.

INTRODUCTION

The prevalence of symptomatic proximal interphalangeal (PIP) joint osteoarthritis (OA) ranged from 0.7% to 2.0% in the Framingham Offspring and Community cohort study,[1] which is the equivalent of 2.3 million people in the United States in 2000. Current treatment options for PIP OA include silicone, metal, pyrocarbon, and ceramic arthroplasties using a volar, lateral, or dorsal approach. Many hand surgeons have been putting substantial effort into the development of these small joint prostheses. However, there is not yet a standard for PIP implant arthroplasties and various types of implants and approaches have been reported (**Fig. 1**). For this article, we reviewed studies on PIP implant arthroplasties that used different exposures and implants. We compared the reported arc of motion (AOM), extension lag, and complication rates among different type of implants and exposures because,

unlike PIP arthrodesis, the goal of PIP implant arthroplasty is to maintain or improve joint motion.

METAL HINGED IMPLANT ARTHROPLASTY

In 1959, Brannon and Klein[2] reported on the use of a metal, hinge-joint, finger prosthesis in 14 patients with posttraumatic conditions; the longest follow-up period was 3 years. The prostheses were originally made of stainless steel, but were later changed to titanium. This design consists of 2 parts along with an intramedullary stem that are locked by a screw. All cases were operated on using a lateral approach. Although pain relief was achieved in all 14 patients, complications involving bone resorption around the stems, sinking in of the prosthesis with rotation, and loosening of the screw were found more often in the earlier version made with stainless steel. These complications result in shortening of the finger and loss of motion.[2]

Disclosure Statement: A Midcareer Investigator Award in Patient-Oriented Research (2 K24-AR053120-06) awarded to Dr K.C. Chung supported this work. The content is solely the responsibility of the authors and does not necessarily represent the official views of the National Institutes of Health.

[a] Section of Plastic Surgery, Department of Surgery, University of Michigan, 2130 Taubman Center, 1500 E. Medical Center Drive, Ann Arbor, MI 48109, USA; [b] Department of Hand Surgery, Nagoya University Graduate School of Medicine, 65 Tsurumai-cho, Showa-ku, Nagoya, Aichi 466-8550, Japan; [c] Section of Plastic Surgery, Department of Surgery, University of Michigan, 2130 Taubman Center, SPC 5340, 1500 E. Medical Center Drive, Ann Arbor, MI 48109, USA
* Corresponding author. Department of Hand Surgery, Nagoya University Graduate School of Medicine, 65 Tsurumai-cho, Showa-ku, Nagoya, Aichi 466-8550, Japan.
E-mail address: michi-ya@med.nagoya-u.ac.jp

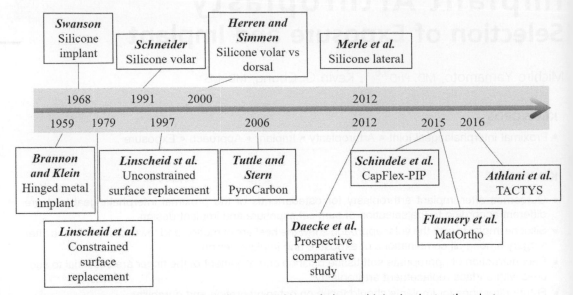

Fig. 1. Chronology of outstanding reports for proximal interphalangeal joint implant arthroplasty.

To prevent the rotational instability seen in the prosthesis of Brannon and Klein,[2] Flatt[3] developed another hinged, metal prosthesis with 2-pronged stems and implanted them into 20 patients with rheumatoid arthritis. The study had a mean follow-up time of 6.2 years, during which 11 implants (15%) were removed because of infection, implant failure, or soft tissue problems. Extraction of the prosthesis was difficult because of bone absorption around the prosthesis, scarring, and heterotopic bone formation surrounding the hinge.[4]

Recently, results from a 17-year longitudinal study were published, reporting the effects of hinged, piston-based DIGITOS (Osteo AG, Selzach, Switzerland) PIP prostheses inserted using a lateral approach. The DIGITOS prosthesis exhibited radiolucent lines at the bone-cement junction and periprosthetic osteophytes stemming from instability in the first 7 years. However, radiolucent lines around the implants had not increased in the longer follow-up, and all 12 patients showed good pain relief and expressed high satisfaction.[5] Some motion between the metal hinge and a polyethylene cuff might be effective in preventing implants from loosening, because the pistonlike motion between the hinge and cuff absorbs stress to the bone. However, DIGITOS prosthesis was taken off the market because of the early osteolysis and the formation of large osteophytes.

Although several types of metal, hinged implants have been developed, they all share common problems of bone absorption, implant loosening, and osteophyte formation. Metal, hinged implants are used much less often than silicone implants and surface replacement arthroplasties.

SILICONE ARTHROPLASTY

After Swanson and colleagues[6] introduced the silicone implant to treat PIP joint arthritis in 1968, they reported rewarding results for dorsal approach arthroplasty with good pain relief in 98% of patients. Except in cases of swan-neck deformities, average AOM improved after surgery. Swanson and colleagues[6] also reported 88 (11%) surgical revisions with a minimum 1-year follow-up. Of these revision surgeries, 41 cases were because of stiffness or deformity.[6] Most surgeons favored a dorsal approach for silicone implants because of easier joint exposure,[7–9] but the revision surgery rate after silicone arthroplasties using a dorsal approach is higher compared with that of using a volar approach. In our search, more than a few patients required secondary tenolysis or revision surgeries for stiffness after undergoing a dorsal approach arthroplasty, but none were reported after a volar approach arthroplasty.[6,8,10]

Beneficial outcomes have been reported since Schneider[11] first published his method for silicone arthroplasty with a volar approach for PIP joint OA in 1991. An 8-year follow-up study of volar approach PIP joint silicone arthroplasty demonstrated their lasting effects with only 1 revision surgery (3%) performed.[12] Secondary tenolyses or arthrolyses were quite rare using this approach as well. The volar approach has the advantage of preserving the extensor mechanism. It enables early and aggressive postoperative exercise to avoid extensor tendon adhesion and joint contracture. It also results in a better restoration of extension in the AOM without extension lag (**Fig. 2**). The

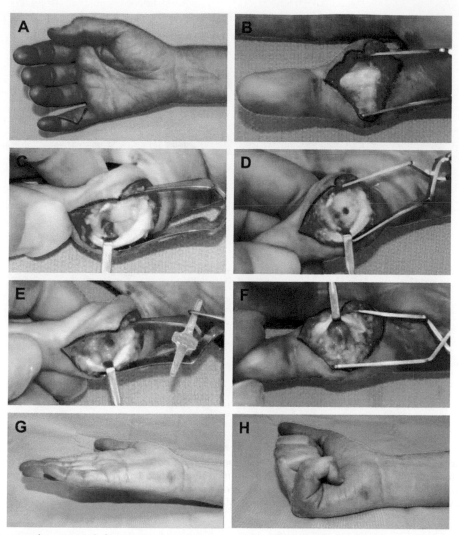

Fig. 2. Silicone volar approach for proximal interphalangeal joint degenerative osteoarthritis. (*A*) Incision design. (*B*) Skin flap was elevated and neurovascular bundle was identified. (*C*) The A3 pulley was opened and the volar plate was released after retracting the flexor digit superficialis tendon volarly. (*D*) The head of the proximal phalanx was removed using a saw and the medullary cavity was broached. (*E, F*) The #00 implant was placed and sat within the medullary cavity. (*G, H*) Good motion of the little finger was gained at 4 months postoperative.

dorsal approach has advantages of wide exposure and easy access to the joint, but risks extensor tendon adhesion that causes joint contracture or reduced AOM of the finger (**Fig. 3**). Extensor tenolysis is occasionally effective for these conditions, but it is more important to try to prevent these complications. Although a comparative study of dorsal and volar approaches showed no significant difference in the 2 groups with regard to postoperative AOM, the investigators stated that the volar approach for silicone arthroplasty of PIP joints is preferable in cases for which no dorsal bony or extensor tendon correction was necessary, because the volar approach enables early active and more aggressive rehabilitation.[13]

A lateral approach for PIP arthroplasties also has been reported. Merle and colleagues[14] published a series of 51 cases using a lateral approach. The mean AOM of the PIP joint improved from 38° to 63° after surgery. Subjective outcomes like visual analog scale (VAS) and Quick Disability of the Arm, Shoulder, and Hand (DASH) also improved from means of 5.1 and 69.2 to 1.9 and 12.3, respectively. Although axial deviation is not an issue in most cases using a volar or dorsal approach, there was an average axial deviation of 17° (range 10°–30°) after arthroplasty with a lateral approach.[14] This approach needs to release the capsule and collateral ligaments of the PIP joint at their proximal insertion to open the joint, and a contralateral

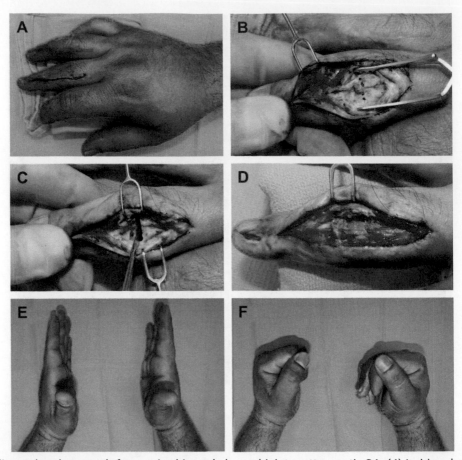

Fig. 3. Silicone dorsal approach for proximal interphalangeal joint posttraumatic OA. (*A*) Incision design. (*B*) A central extensor tendon splitting approach was performed and cutting line of the head of proximal phalanx was drawn. (*C*) The head of proximal phalanx was cut using a saw. (*D*) A silicone implant was seated and collateral ligaments were preserved. (*E*, *F*) The range of motion of the middle finger at 2 months postoperative.

incision and ligament reinforcement are required to improve lateral stability. Outcomes with a lateral approach are still uncertain, because there are few articles reporting on this approach.[14–16]

Minamikawa and colleagues[17] reported on the significant lateral laxity in cadaver PIP joints of silicone implants compared with surface replacement arthroplasty. Swanson[18] immediately responded, writing that silicone implants become stable under the correct procedures when they are encapsulated in vivo, including reattachment of collateral ligaments. Previous articles report silicone arthroplasties in index and middle fingers along with ulnar little and ring fingers despite concerns over lateral pinch stability.

The type of silicone implant may affect the outcomes after PIP joint arthroplasty. Swanson flexible finger joint implants (Wright Medical Technology Inc, Arlington, TN) have been used most frequently.[6,19] Recently, the use of the NeuFlex silicone implant (Depuy, Warwaw, IN) and the Avanta

silicone implant (Avanta Orthopaedice, San Diego, CA) were introduced with favorable outcomes. The NeuFlex silicone implant has a 15° prebend at the PIP hinge to improve postoperative flexion and durability against implant fracture.[20,21] Using the NeuFlex implant and a dorsal approach, Namdari and Weiss[20] reported a mean postoperative AOM of 61° and only 1 (6%) implant fracture at the mean 49-month follow-up. Merle and colleagues,[14] also using NeuFlex implants, showed a mean gain in AOM of 25°, and revision surgery was performed in only 1 (2%) patient because of implant fracture. Bouacida and colleagues,[22] using a volar approach, reported a mean postoperative AOM of 58°, a gain in AOM of 29°, and 3 (11%) implant fractures at the mean follow-up of 39 months. The longevity of the NeuFlex implants is comparable with Swanson implants. A review of Swanson PIP implants showed 39 fractures among 2463 PIP implants (2%).[23]

The Avanta silicone implant has a volarly shifted center of flexion compared with the Swanson silicone implant to improve the postoperative flexion angle.[24] Proubasta and colleagues[24] reported a mean postoperative AOM of 72°, gained AOM of 35°, and 2 (6%) implant fractures at the mean follow-up time of 18 months using Avanta implants with a volar approach. These are not significant differences between types of silicone implants in terms of postoperative flexion and implant fracture rates; however, modifications for improving implants are important for future advancement.

SURFACE REPLACEMENT ARTHROPLASTY

SR-PIP (Small Bone Innovations, Inc, Morrisville, PA) and PyroCarbon (Ascension Orthopedics, Inc, Austin, TX) arthroplasties are currently the most commonly used and reported implants for surface replacement arthroplasty.

The first anatomic surface replacement arthroplasty developed by Linscheid and colleagues[25] was a cobalt-chrome (CoCr) proximal component and high-molecular-weight polyethylene distal component in 1979. At the time, a prosthetic design from the Mayo Clinic was based on the 6 concepts:

1. Maintain adequate bone length
2. Adjust the position of the distal component to influence the center of rotation
3. Secure an internal constraint mechanism to forces outside the sagittal plane
4. Conform to the rounded dorsal contour for lateral volar translation of the lateral bands during flexion
5. Provide a normal range of motion of the joint
6. Provide relative ease of insertion

In 67 fingers of 45 patients, the PIP joint was replaced with a Mayo-type prosthesis through a variety of dorsal incisions. The initial diagnoses were rheumatoid arthritis (72%), degenerative arthritis (18%), or other (10%). Results with an average 15 months of follow-up were disappointing; satisfactory results, as rated by the examining physician, were obtained in only 20 fingers (30% success rate). Progressive erosion of the device into cortical bone appeared to be a factor of the unsatisfactory results.[25] The size of the proximal component necessitates removal of the head of the proximal phalanx. This results in disruption of the collateral ligaments and has a deteriorating effect on the resistance of the cortical bone to migration and erosion by the prosthetic components. This is because the initial Mayo-type surface replacement arthroplasty used a mated, internally constrained prosthesis.[25]

Eighteen years later, Linscheid and colleagues[26] reported on the development of an unconstrained surface replacement (SR) arthroplasty for the PIP joint. This was based on their assumption that an unconstrained SR prosthesis would give a more physiologic articulation and, if it was inserted with minimal bony excision and proper preservation of the collateral ligaments, would provide a more stable joint. The proximal component was made of CoCr, and the distal component was made of ultrahigh-molecular-weight polyethylene (UHMWPE) with a truncated square stem and a bifaceted biconcave articular alignment.[26] In a 14-year period, a total of 66 PIP joints from 47 patients were replaced with this unconstrained SR prosthesis using lateral (n = 13), volar (n = 10), and dorsal (n = 43) approaches with cement. Of these patients, 24 had degenerative OA, 15 had traumatic arthrosis, and 8 had rheumatoid arthritis. The results, based on pain relief, motion, and deformity, were good in 32 fingers, fair in 19, and poor in 15 at a mean follow-up of 4.5 years. Outcomes using a dorsal approach were better than those of lateral or volar approaches. More satisfactory results were gained in patients with degenerative OA compared with traumatic arthrosis and rheumatoid arthritis.[26] In a longer follow-up study, complication rates after surgery also differed according to the approach used. SR-PIP prostheses implanted using a volar approach failed more often than those implanted using a dorsal approach during a mean of 8.8 years of follow-up.[27] Current SR-PIP prostheses have a titanium alloy stem that has an external surface to promote bone growth rather than using cement.

The PyroCarbon implant is iso-elastic to cortical bone with assumed higher durability and wear resistance.[28] PyroCarbon has been used for components of heart valves and is currently the most popular implant biomaterial, used in more than 4 million heart valves annually.[29] The PyroCabon PIP implant is an unconstrained resurfacing device without cement. Joint stability is gained by the tongue and groove–like surface, and preservation of the collateral ligaments at the surgery. PyroCarbon PIP implants were introduced with a high expectation to be used for successful PIP arthroplasties.[30] PyroCarbon PIP arthroplasty has the potential to attain pain relief, good AOM, and correction of deformity; however, the results were unpredictable and not better compared with other arthroplasties.[30] Furthermore, frequent complications with implant dislocation and subsidence were observed.[19,31,32] Loosening of the PyroCarbon implant was frequently reported at longer follow-up; on histologic examination, it was found that PyroCarbon has poor implant-bone contact in vivo.[31,33] Although the volar approach for this implant was suggested recently,[34] there is little evidence of favorable outcomes using this approach.

Unlike for silicone implants, a dorsal approach to the PIP joint was commonly used for these surface replacement arthroplasties (**Fig. 4**).[35,36]

Osteointegration of the implant is one of the key factors to achieve satisfactory results after surface replacement arthroplasty to prevent subsidence or migration. The MOJE ceramic implant (MOJE ceramic implants, Petersburg, Germany) is coated with hydroxyapatite to promote bony ingrowth against loosening of the prosthesis, and favorable results were reported.[37,38] Although the follow-up period was short (12 months), loosening was seen in only 2 cases (10%).[37] More recently, a novel surface PIP joint prosthesis named CapFlex-PIP (KLS Martin Group, Tuttlingen, Germany) was developed. The CapFlex-PIP is an unconstrained, modular gliding surface PIP joint prosthesis. The proximal component is a bicondylar cap of CoCr

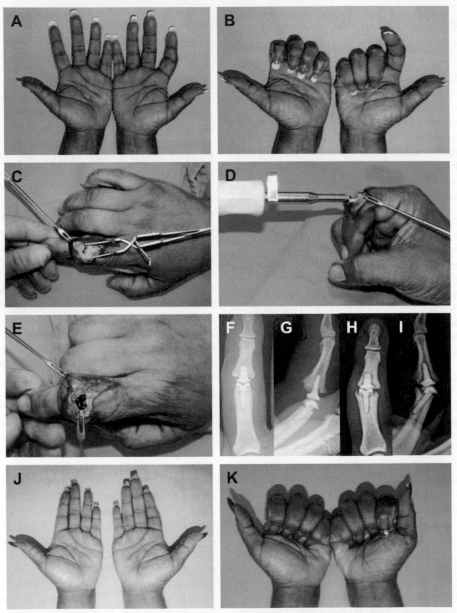

Fig. 4. PyroCarbon arthroplasty with dorsal approach for PIP degenerative OA. (*A*, *B*) Preoperative motion of finger. (*C*) A central extensor tendon splitting approach. (*D*) The medullary cavity was broached after removing the head of the proximal phalanx. (*E*) After the base of the middle phalanx was broached, PyroCarbon implant was placed. (*F–I*) The posterior-anterior and lateral views of 2 weeks and 2 years postoperative radiographs. Subsidence of both proximal and distal implants was noted. (*J*, *K*) Motion of finger at 2 years postoperatively. (*Courtesy of* Integra Japan, Toyko, Japan.)

alloy, and the distal component has an articular surface of UHMWPE, similar to the prostheses currently available for total knee arthroplasty. The CapFlex-PIP also has a titanium pore base for cement-free osteointegration, as does another recent version of the SR-PIP implant. One of the characteristics of this implant design is a shorter stem in both components than in the SR-PIP implant. Schindele and colleagues[39] published a prospective case series with a 1-year follow-up. They used the dorsal Chamay approach in all 10 PIP joints studied. Lateral instability was minimal in 9 joints, and all 10 implants remained intact with no migration or osteolysis. Although 2 patients required tenolysis due to stiffness and dorsal ossification, both patients were successfully treated with secondary tenolysis.[39] Because a dorsal approach has a risk of extensor tendon problems, the investigators used a volar approach with improved results after their preliminary report.[39]

Flannery and colleagues[40] reported on the MatOrtho PIPR (Mole Business Park, Leatherhead, UK) arthroplasties with a minimum 2-year follow-up. The MatOrtho PIPR is a CoCr, metal-on-polyethylene, mobile-bearing, cementless surface replacement arthroplasty prosthesis with a hydroxyapatite coating to hasten osteointegration. A total of 109 implants were inserted in 56 patients using a dorsal approach. Although good pain relief and improved grip strength were achieved, the mean AOM after surgery did not improve. In terms of radiographic outcomes, there was evidence of new bone formation around the components and no circumferential loosening. Surgical revision was performed in 13 cases because of stiffness in 5, instability in 4, swan-neck deformity in 3, and dislocation in 1. The investigators were somewhat disappointed because there was no overall improvement in AOM, and adjusted their surgical approach from dorsal to lateral.[40]

More recently, PIP joint arthroplasty using the TACTYS (Stryker-Memometal, Bruz, France) prosthesis was reported.[41] The TACTYS is a fully modular, gliding, unconstrained total PIP joint prosthesis; its proximal and distal stems are anatomic titanium alloy with a hydroxyapatite coating on the epiphyseal-metaphyseal portion. The proximal and distal bearing surfaces are made from polyethylene and CoCr, respectively. TACTYS consists of these 4 components with size variations. Athlani and colleagues[41] implanted these prostheses via a dorsal approach into the PIP joint of 22 patients with a mean age of 64 years for primary OA (18 cases), posttraumatic OA (3 cases), and rheumatoid arthritis (1 case). Good pain relief and increases in AOM were observed during the mean follow-up of 34 months. The mean pain score decreased

from 6.5 to 1.9 on the VAS, and the mean AOM increased from 39° to 58° after surgery. Surgical revisions were reported in 4 patients (18%) because of dorsal tenolysis (3 cases) and resection of the anterior osteophyte (1 case). These results are comparable to other existing surface replacement arthroplasties.[41]

The volar approach for surface replacement arthroplasty does not always provide satisfactory results. Shirakawa and Shirota[42] reported on postoperative contracture of the PIP joint using the Ishizuki Total Finger System (Nakashima Medical, Okayama, Japan) in 12 cases, or the Self-Locking Finger Joint System (Nakashima Medical) in 3 cases. Eight of 15 fingers operated on required salvage surgery due to contracture during the average 73 months of follow-up. In addition, the mean AOM was 46° preoperatively and 40° at the final follow-up. They concluded that intraoperative fracture or fragility of the central slip insertion were risk factors for contracture.[42] Unlike silicone implants, surface replacement arthroplasty needs to remove the base of the middle phalanx. Particularly in the volar approach, the central slip insertion in the deep site might be at risk of fracture during resection of the articular surface of the middle phalanx.

Appropriate selection of implant design, surgical approach, and patient conditions are all essential factors for successful PIP joint arthroplasty. Unlike hinged implants, these unconstrained surface replacement arthroplasties have a risk of joint dislocation or instability. Careful soft tissue rebalancing and reconstruction of good finger alignment are necessary for promising results. There are few comparative studies of various types of implants and surgical approaches. Daecke and colleagues[19] reported a prospective, randomized comparative study of silicone, SR-PIP, and Pyro-Carbon arthroplasty for degenerative PIP joint OA using a dorsal approach. Although there was no significant improvement for AOM of the PIP joint in all 3 types, implant explantations were required in 11% of silicone, 27% of SR-PIP, and 39% of PyroCarbon arthroplasty at the mean follow-up 35 months. Silicone arthroplasties had the fewest complications among the 3 groups.[19] A systematic review can summarize all the available evidence on the selection of implants and surgical approach and their outcomes for PIP joint arthroplasty.

A SYSTEMATIC LITERATURE REVIEW FOR ARC OF MOTION, EXTENSION LAG, AND COMPLICATION

We searched the PubMed and EMBASE databases for articles reporting on outcomes of implant arthroplasty for PIP joint OA from 1970 to

Table 1
Summary of arc of motion (AOM) from published articles

Implant Type and Approach	Number of Fingers	Mean Follow-up Period, mo	Mean Postoperative AOM, degree	Gained AOM, degree
Silicon volar	235	41	58	17
Silicone lateral	120	37	54	16
Silicone dorsal	541	58	51	12
Surface replacement volar	27	77	47	1
Surface replacement dorsal	881	48	51	8

2016. A total of 882 articles were screened, of which 42 were included in our review. Articles were screened for information on the primary outcomes (AOM of the PIP joint and complications) and follow-up period. In our analysis, we combined brands of prostheses based on the type of arthroplasty and surgical exposure method.

Seventeen studies reported on the use of silicone implants. Of these, 6 used a volar, 3 used a lateral, and 8 used a dorsal approach. Three studies reported on surface replacement arthroplasty using a volar approach, whereas 26 used a dorsal approach. Two articles used both volar and dorsal approaches with separately extractable data. One article used silicone, PyroCarbon, and SR-PIP prostheses with separately extractable data. Finally, we reviewed 46 studies from 42 articles.

ARC OF MOTION

Silicone implants with a volar approach showed the best gain in AOM among all implant designs and exposures. The mean gain in AOM from large to small was silicone volar (17°), silicone lateral (16°), silicone dorsal (12°), surface replacement dorsal (8°), and surface replacement volar (1°) (**Table 1**).

EXTENSION LAG

Silicone implants with a volar approach showed the least extension lag postoperatively among all implant designs and exposures. The extension lag, from small to large, was silicone volar (5°),

silicone dorsal (8°), silicone lateral (12°), surface replacement dorsal (14°), and surface replacement volar (17°) (**Table 2**).

COMPLICATION

Silicone arthroplasties with a volar approach had the lowest surgical revision rate (all revisions including minor and salvage procedures) of 6% at the mean of 41 months of follow-up. The surgical revision rate of surface replacement with a dorsal approach was 18% at the mean 51 months of follow-up. The surgical revision rate, from low to high, was silicone volar (6%), silicone lateral (10%), silicone dorsal (11%), surface replacement dorsal (18%), and surface replacement volar (37%) (**Table 3**).

Among silicone arthroplasties using a volar approach, only 13 revision surgeries were reported, including revision to silicone (54%), arthrodesis (15%), amputation (8%), and other procedures (23%).

In total, 157 revision surgeries were reported after surface replacement arthroplasties with a dorsal approach. These revision surgeries were revision to silicone implant (22%), arthrodesis (14%), revision with or without cement to original implant (11%), explantation of the implant (10%), amputation (4%), and other procedures (39%).

COMPARISON WITH OTHER JOINTS

Surgical revision rates after PIP implant arthroplasty ranged from 6% to 37% at the mean

Table 2
Summary of extension lag from published articles

Implant Type and Approach	Number of Fingers	Mean Follow-up Period, mo	Mean Postoperative Extension Lag, degree
Silicone volar	168	49	5
Silicone lateral	51	36	12
Silicone dorsal	479	60	8
Surface replacement volar	12	80	17
Surface replacement dorsal	446	56	14

Table 3
Summary of complication rate from published articles

Implant Type and Approach	Number of Fingers	Mean Follow-up Period, mo	Number of Surgical Revisions (%)
Silicone volar	235	41	13 (6)
Silicone lateral	115	37	12 (10)
Silicone dorsal	955	17	107 (11)
Surface replacement volar	27	77	10 (37)
Surface replacement dorsal	907	51	164 (18)

follow-up period, ranging from 17 to 77 months. These results were inferior to arthroplasties at other parts of body, including hip, knee, ankle, and shoulder.[43–49] Revision rates of total hip and knee replacement were reported at approximately 6% after 5 years and 12% after 10 years using cumulative results from worldwide joint register datasets.[45] Using the same datasets, means of 3.29, 1.39, and 5.08 revisions per 100 observed component years were seen after ankle, shoulder, and elbow replacement, respectively.[45] Although the mean revision rate after shoulder replacement (8% at the mean follow-up period 5.8 years) was comparable to those of hip and knee replacement, the highest revision rates for all implants were seen after elbow replacement (20% after 4 years).[45] We found that the revision rate of surface replacements of finger PIP with a dorsal approach (18% at the mean follow-up period 51 months) is comparable with total elbow replacement. Surgical revision rate after silicone implant with a volar approach (6% at the mean follow-up period 41 months) is comparable to total hip and knee replacement (6% after 5 years). However, we need to take into consideration the cases with silicone fracture but no revision surgery.

SUMMARY

We reported the difference of outcomes by exposure and implant designs. According to our literature review, silicone implants using a volar approach showed the best gain in AOM, least extension lag, and fewest complications after surgery among all surgical exposure and implant designs. On the other hand, surface replacement arthroplasty with a volar approach showed the worst gain in AOM, most extension lag, and most complications after surgery. However, there was still significant pain relief and higher satisfaction even after surface replacement arthroplasty, regardless of the considerable complications. These findings define the needs of implant arthroplasty for PIP OA.

Silicone implantation using a volar approach is the preferred technique adopted by the senior author. We had used PyroCarbon arthroplasty for PIP OA, but we changed to silicone implant with a volar approach because of its lower revision rate, ease of revision if necessary, minimal extension lag, and best AOM. A Level 1 study using prospective, randomized, controlled trials are necessary to collect higher evidence for the superiority of any single implant or approach over others. Most importantly, development of an improved implant is needed to ameliorate the outcomes of PIP implant arthroplasty. As silicone implants have shown the best results, we do not think that anatomic implants are always necessary for PIP joint OA. Currently, we can use artificial intelligence to simulate the development of prostheses with better results by modeling for factors that influence results, such as implant materials including surface modification, prosthesis design, surgical approach, and preoperative and postoperative management. After appropriate in vivo studies, we will be able to create an improved implant for the PIP joint in the near future.

ACKNOWLEDGMENTS

We thank Sterbenz Jennifer, BS, a research assistant in the section of Plastic Surgery, Department of Surgery, University of Michigan Health System, Ann Arbor, MI, for her editing of this article.

REFERENCES

1. Haugen IK, Englund M, Aliabadi P, et al. Prevalence, incidence and progression of hand osteoarthritis in the general population: the Framingham Osteoarthritis Study. Ann Rheum Dis 2011;70:1581–6.
2. Brannon EW, Klein G. Experiences with a finger-joint prosthesis. J Bone Joint Surg Am 1959;41:87–102.
3. Flatt A. Reclamation of the rheumatoid hand. Lancet 1961;277:1136–8.
4. Flatt AE, Ellison MR. Restoration of rheumatoid finger joint function. 3. A follow-up note after fourteen years of experience with a metallic-hinge prosthesis. J Bone Joint Surg Am 1972;54:1317–22.

5. Gulke J, Mentzel M, Dornacher D, et al. Linked prosthesis for the proximal interphalangeal joint: 17-year long-term results. Handchir Mikrochir Plast Chir 2016;48:273–80.

6. Swanson AB, Maupin BK, Gajjar NV, et al. Flexible implant arthroplasty in the proximal interphalangeal joint of the hand. J Hand Surg Am 1985;10:796–805.

7. Pellegrini VD Jr, Burton RI. Osteoarthritis of the proximal interphalangeal joint of the hand: arthroplasty or fusion? J Hand Surg Am 1990;15:194–209.

8. Mathoulin C, Gilbert A. Arthroplasty of the proximal interphalangeal joint using the Sutter implant for traumatic joint destruction. J Hand Surg Br 1999; 24:565–9.

9. Silva JB, Schwanke RL, Vicente MG, et al. Arthroplasty with silicone implant in post traumatic lesions of the proximal interphalangeal joint. Rev Bras Ortop 1998;33:79–82.

10. Cesari B, Alnot JY. Proximal interphalangeal joint implant arthroplasty for degenerative or post-traumatic arthritis. Main 1997;2:85–96.

11. Schneider LH. Proximal interphalangeal joint arthroplasty: the volar approach. Semin Arthroplasty 1991; 2:139–47.

12. Lautenbach M, Kim S, Berndsen M, et al. The palmar approach for PIP-arthroplasty according to Simmen: results after 8 years follow-up. J Orthop Sci 2014;19:722–8.

13. Herren DB, Simmen BR. Palmar approach in flexible implant arthroplasty of the proximal interphalangeal joint. Clin Orthop Relat Res 2000;(371):131–5.

14. Merle M, Villani F, Lallemand B, et al. Proximal interphalangeal joint arthroplasty with silicone implants (NeuFlex) by a lateral approach: a series of 51 cases. J Hand Surg Eur Vol 2012;37: 50–5.

15. Stahlenbrecher A, Hoch J. Proximal interphalangeal joint silicone arthroplasty–comparison of Swanson and NeuFlex implants using a new evaluation score. Handchir Mikrochir Plast Chir 2009; 41:156–65.

16. Hage JJ, Yoe EP, Zevering JP, et al. Proximal interphalangeal joint silicone arthroplasty for posttraumatic arthritis. J Hand Surg Am 1999;24:73–7.

17. Minamikawa Y, Imaeda T, Amadio PC, et al. Lateral stability of proximal interphalangeal joint replacement. J Hand Surg Am 1994;19:1050–4.

18. Swanson AB. Lateral stability of proximal interphalangeal joint replacement. J Hand Surg Am 1995; 20:701–2.

19. Daecke W, Kaszap B, Martini AK, et al. A prospective, randomized comparison of 3 types of proximal interphalangeal joint arthroplasty. J Hand Surg Am 2012;37:1770–9.e1-3.

20. Namdari S, Weiss AP. Anatomically neutral silicone small joint arthroplasty for osteoarthritis. J Hand Surg Am 2009;34:292–300.

21. Joyce T, Unsworth A. NeuFlex metacarpophalangeal prostheses tested in vitro. Proc Inst Mech Eng H 2005;219:105–10.

22. Bouacida S, Lazerges C, Coulet B, et al. Proximal interphalangeal joint arthroplasty with Neuflex(R) implants: relevance of the volar approach and early rehabilitation. Chir Main 2014;33:350–5.

23. Foliart DE. Swanson silicone finger joint implants: a review of the literature regarding long-term complications. J Hand Surg Am 1995;20:445–9.

24. Proubasta IR, Lamas CG, Natera L, et al. Silicone proximal interphalangeal joint arthroplasty for primary osteoarthritis using a volar approach. J Hand Surg Am 2014;39:1075–81.

25. Linscheid RL, Dobyns JH, Beckenbaugh RD, et al. Proximal interphalangeal joint arthroplasty with a total joint design. Mayo Clin Proc 1979;54:227–40.

26. Linscheid RL, Murray PM, Vidal MA, et al. Development of a surface replacement arthroplasty for proximal interphalangeal joints. J Hand Surg Am 1997; 22:286–98.

27. Murray PM, Linscheid RL, Cooney WP 3rd, et al. Long-term outcomes of proximal interphalangeal joint surface replacement arthroplasty. J Bone Joint Surg Am 2012;94:1120–8.

28. Cook SD, Beckenbaugh RD, Redondo J, et al. Long-term follow-up of pyrolytic carbon metacarpophalangeal implants. J Bone Joint Surg Am 1999;81: 635–48.

29. Slaughter MS, Pederson B, Graham JD, et al. Evaluation of new Forcefield technology: reducing platelet adhesion and cell coverage of pyrolytic carbon surfaces. J Thorac Cardiovasc Surg 2011;142:921–5.

30. Tuttle HG, Stern PJ. Pyrolytic carbon proximal interphalangeal joint resurfacing arthroplasty. J Hand Surg Am 2006;31:930–9.

31. Sweets TM, Stern PJ. Pyrolytic carbon resurfacing arthroplasty for osteoarthritis of the proximal interphalangeal joint of the finger. J Bone Joint Surg Am 2011;93:1417–25.

32. Ono S, Shauver MJ, Chang KW, et al. Outcomes of pyrolytic carbon arthroplasty for the proximal interphalangeal joint at 44 months' mean follow-up. Plast Reconstr Surg 2012;129:1139–50.

33. Daecke W, Veyel K, Wieloch P, et al. Osseointegration and mechanical stability of pyrocarbon and titanium hand implants in a load-bearing in vivo model for small joint arthroplasty. J Hand Surg Am 2006;31:90–7.

34. Duncan SF, Merritt MV, Kakinoki R. The volar approach to proximal interphalangeal joint arthroplasty. Tech Hand Up Extrem Surg 2009;13: 47–53.

35. Dickson DR, Nuttall D, Watts AC, et al. Pyrocarbon proximal interphalangeal joint arthroplasty: minimum five-year follow-up. J Hand Surg Am 2015; 40:2142–8.e4.

36. Storey PA, Goddard M, Clegg C, et al. Pyrocarbon proximal interphalangeal joint arthroplasty: a medium to long term follow-up of a single surgeon series. J Hand Surg Eur Vol 2015;40:952–6.

37. Pettersson K, Wagnsjo P, Hulin E. Replacement of proximal interphalangeal joints with new ceramic arthroplasty: a prospective series of 20 proximal interphalangeal joint replacements. Scand J Plast Reconstr Surg Hand Surg 2006;40:291–6.

38. Wesemann A, Flügel M, Mamarvar M. Moje prosthesis for the proximal interphalangeal joint. Handchir Mikrochir Plast Chir 2008;40:189–96.

39. Schindele SF, Hensler S, Audigé L, et al. A modular surface gliding implant (CapFlex-PIP) for proximal interphalangeal joint osteoarthritis: a prospective case series. J Hand Surg Am 2015;40:334–40.

40. Flannery O, Harley O, Badge R, et al. MatOrtho proximal interphalangeal joint arthroplasty: minimum 2-year follow-up. J Hand Surg Eur Vol 2016;41:910–6.

41. Athlani L, Gaisne E, Bellemere P. Arthroplasty of the proximal interphalangeal joint with the TACTYS(R) prosthesis: preliminary results after a minimum follow-up of 2 years. Hand Surg Rehabil 2016;35:168–78.

42. Shirakawa K, Shirota M. Post-operative contracture of the proximal interphalangeal joint after surface replacement arthroplasty using a volar approach. J Hand Surg Asian Pac Vol 2016;21:345–51.

43. Canadian Arthroplasty Society. The Canadian Arthroplasty Society's experience with hip resurfacing arthroplasty. An analysis of 2773 hips. Bone Joint J 2013;95:1045–51.

44. Pabinger C, Berghold A, Boehler N, et al. Revision rates after knee replacement. Cumulative results from worldwide clinical studies versus joint registers. Osteoarthritis Cartilage 2013;21:263–8.

45. Labek G, Thaler M, Janda W, et al. Revision rates after total joint replacement: cumulative results from worldwide joint register datasets. J Bone Joint Surg Br 2011;93:293–7.

46. Kasten P, Pape G, Raiss P, et al. Mid-term survivorship analysis of a shoulder replacement with a keeled glenoid and a modern cementing technique. J Bone Joint Surg Br 2010;92:387–92.

47. Young A, Walch G, Boileau P, et al. A multicentre study of the long-term results of using a flat-back polyethylene glenoid component in shoulder replacement for primary osteoarthritis. J Bone Joint Surg Br 2011;93:210–6.

48. Plaschke HC, Thillemann TM, Brorson S, et al. Implant survival after total elbow arthroplasty: a retrospective study of 324 procedures performed from 1980 to 2008. J Shoulder Elbow Surg 2014;23:829–36.

49. Zaidi R, Cro S, Gurusamy K, et al. The outcome of total ankle replacement: a systematic review and meta-analysis. Bone Joint J 2013;95:1500–7.

Microvascular Toe Joint for Proximal Interphalangeal Joint Replacement
Indications, Technique, and Outcomes

Ryan D. Katz, MD, James P. Higgins, MD*

KEYWORDS

- Free joint transfer • Joint replacement • Toe to hand • Indications • Technique • Outcomes

KEY POINTS

- The joint should be harvested with a skin island for microvascular monitoring as well as ease of soft tissue closure.
- Osteosynthesis should be achieved with rigid constructs (multi-planar interosseous wires or plating) if possible to facilitate early motion.
- The long toe extensor is often deficient in allowing full proximal interphalangeal joint (PIPJ) extension; an extensor lag is, therefore, expected.
- The dysfunctional digit PIPJ should be resected generously to position the osteosynthesis sites at high-quality phalangeal bone proximally and distally.
- Positioning the new joint line more proximally than the original joint position can optimize the finger arc of motion by taking full advantage of the concept of angular motion.

INTRODUCTION: NATURE OF THE PROBLEM

The proximal interphalangeal joint (PIPJ) is a bicondylar hinge joint with a normal arc of motion approximating 110°. In its uninjured state, the PIPJ has the greatest contribution to the total arc of digital motion. Loss of motion at the PIPJ, therefore, has considerable impact on digital motion and grip strength.

The complex anatomy of the joint, including its soft tissue and ligamentous attachments, frequently responds unfavorably to trauma and degenerative pathologic conditions. Patients should be counseled to expect limitations in PIPJ motion after any injury or surgery involving the PIPJ or periarticular structures.

In some clinical scenarios, the PIPJ may be deemed unsalvageable. These scenarios include advanced arthritic destruction, posttraumatic joint destruction, avascular necrosis (as can be encountered with condylar fractures of the proximal phalanx), chronic infection/osteolysis, hyperstability (stiffness), or chronic instability. When the native joint is dysfunctional, hampering hand use and quality of life, and cannot be improved on with conventional surgical intervention, treatment options may be motion eliminating (arthrodesis) or motion preserving (fascial arthroplasty, implant arthroplasty, osteochondral grafting, or vascularized toe joint transfer).[1–6]

INDICATIONS

Microvascular toe joint transfer imparts specific benefits not afforded by an alloplastic implant.

Disclosure Statement: The authors have nothing to disclose.
Care of Anne Mattson, The Curtis National Hand Center, MedStar Union Memorial Hospital, 3333 North Calvert Street, #200 JPB, Baltimore, MD 21218, USA
* Corresponding author.
E-mail address: anne.mattson@medstar.net

Hand Clin 34 (2018) 207–216
https://doi.org/10.1016/j.hcl.2017.12.010
0749-0712/18/© 2018 Elsevier Inc. All rights reserved.

hand.theclinics.com

These benefits should be taken into consideration when selecting this technique (**Table 1**):

- The transfer of a microvascular toe joint provides lifelong durability. This durability makes the toe transfer an appealing option in the younger patient population whose decades of stable joint survival are required. Unlike alloplastic implants, the transferred joint
  - Should not lose structural stability over time
  - Should not be subject to adjacent bone cavitation/lysis
  - Will not be subject to implant degradation, fragmentation, or potential host allergy, rejection, or humeral responses
  - Will be as resistant to dislocation as a native interphalangeal joint (IPJ)
- Microvascular toe joint transfer imparts immediate and reliable coronal plane stability through the function of the uninjured collateral ligaments. Unlike alloplastic implants, a free toe joint transfer does not require the presence or reconstruction of native PIPJ collateral ligaments for stability. This advantage makes the free joint transfer an appealing option when patients demonstrate a chronically unstable PIPJ with coronal angulation and/or inadequate collateral ligament integrity.
- As a vascularized flap, the free toe joint is infection resistant and, therefore, may confer an advantage over alloplastic implants when PIPJ dysfunction is caused by chronic infection or osteomyelitis. In such a clinical scenario, the surgeon can confidently resect back to healthy bone and replace the dysfunctional joint with one less likely to fail as a result of prior or long-standing infection.

The joint also brings skin to the recipient site and can be used to reconstruct a dysfunctional PIPJ even in the setting of a compromised soft tissue envelope.

- Microvascular toe joint transfer provides the potential for longitudinal growth in skeletally immature patients. The transferred joint includes the middle phalangeal physis, enabling continued growth after microvascular transfer. Thus, in children for whom other methods of joint reconstruction (arthrodesis, fascial arthroplasty, alloplastic implant) would not provide the potential of continued digital growth, a free microvascular toe PIPJ transfer with physis is the only current method that can achieve the reconstructive goal of replacing like with like.

CONTRAINDICATIONS

Microvascular toe joint transfer has specific disadvantages and should be selected as the method of reconstruction on a case-by-case basis and only after careful consideration of other reconstructive options (see **Table 1**):

- Compared with other forms of joint reconstruction, microsurgical toe joint transfer is also the most technically complex. The indications are infrequent; thus, experience is difficult to amass outside of larger tertiary referral centers. The resources and experience of the operative team may be an additional consideration when selecting the appropriate treatment of a dysfunctional PIPJ.
- Despite being anatomically analogous to the native finger PIPJ, the toe IPJ is not an

Table 1
Indications and contraindications of microvascular toe joint transfer

Indications	Contraindications
Posttraumatic PIPJ dysfunction with pain and limited motion	Absent microvascular surgical resources
Dysfunctional PIPJ with compromised soft tissue	Medical comorbidities contributing to high anesthetic risk
Dysfunctional PIPJ with chronic instability	Patient with prior foot trauma disrupting normal foot vasculature
Dysfunctional PIPJ with chronic infection or osteomyelitis	Patient unwillingness to delete a toe
Dysfunctional PIPJ with need for longitudinal growth	Advanced peripheral vascular disease compromising foot vasculature or requiring prior vascular surgery
Dysfunctional PIPJ that has failed or is not a good candidate for alloplastic reconstruction	Patients with wound healing or connective tissue disorders

identical replacement and has the known and well-described disadvantage of an intrinsic arc of motion less than that of the native finger. Thus, the digital motion achieved with this method of reconstruction will always be less than the normal (uninjured) finger. The reported outcomes of vascularized joint transfer should be reviewed with patients, particularly if their primary goal is achieving near-normal range of motion[1–6]:

- o The transferred joint has 2 primary limitations: an intrinsic extensor lag and ultimate range of motion less than the native finger IPJ.[7,8]
- o The ultimate PIPJ range of motion after a free toe joint has been reported to be comparable with that of a silicone arthroplasty.[1] In one of the largest series reported, a free toe joint for PIPJ reconstruction only achieves an average flexion arc of 42°.[5] In another series of 11 second toe to PIPJ transfers, the investigators found an average range of motion of 47° with 41° of extensor lag at a mean follow-up of 15 years.[6]
- o If the surgeon makes no modifications to the toe joint or no modifications to its inset, the very best range of motion patients can expect is inherently limited. In a clenched-fist position, this provides the hand with a digit that will fail to contact the palm and will protrude beyond the silhouette of the other digits on profile. This limitation may serve as an obstacle to dexterous hand use.
- In comparison with the other options for PIPJ reconstruction, the microvascular toe joint transfer imparts the greatest perioperative burden on patients and has, by necessity, the highest morbidity. The operative time, hospital stay, and donor site requirements are considerable:
  - o Patients should be carefully counseled on these requirements and provided images to review of the typical results on the foot and hand.
  - o Patients often benefit from contacting other patients who have experienced free joint transfer to discuss the realities of their treatment course, therapy requirements, and realistic outcomes.
- Many methods have been described to preserve the donor toe using structural bone grafting, skin grafting, and fusion. However, the most common technique (used by the authors) is deletion of the second toe after toe joint harvest. The loss of the second toe and resultant ray amputation closure of the

second web space is well tolerated, and patients return to normal foot function. Despite this, patients may find the loss of the second toe too great a cost for digit reconstruction.

- In addition to the aforementioned considerations, contraindications for vascularized toe joint transfer include peripheral vascular disease, prior donor site trauma, or factors that may delay or compromise donor site healing (use of chronic immunosuppressive medications, tobacco abuse, connective tissue disorders).

SURGICAL TECHNIQUE/PROCEDURE

1. A clinical examination of the donor and recipient sites to assess vascular adequacy begins with palpation of potential sources of inflow and outflow. If foot pulses cannot be palpated, if patients have a history of prior foot trauma, or if there are scars in potential operative sites on the selected donor foot, an angiogram (either conventional or computed tomography [CT] angiogram) should be considered to ensure the feasibility of the harvest.
2. Patients are positioned supine with the desired upper and lower extremity prepped in the field. The dissection is performed under tourniquet control. The toe can be harvested from either the ipsilateral or contralateral foot. The surgeon selects the donor foot (ipsilateral vs contralateral) with consideration given to the orientation of the pedicle as it relates to the recipient vessels. The vascular pedicle for the second toe PIPJ will typically be the first dorsal metatarsal vessels or plantar vessels in the first intermetatarsal space. When transferred to the hand, these vessels will drape on the radial side of the recipient digit when harvested from the ipsilateral foot; they will drape on the ulnar side of the digit when harvested from the contralateral foot. The laterality of the donor site will, thus, be influenced by the recipient artery in the hand.
3. Vessel orientation is often planned with palmar arterial inflow and dorsal venous outflow. Thus, either a proper digital artery to the involved finger or a common digital artery to an adjacent web space should be considered for inflow. If the selected vessel is the common digital artery, the surgeon must be certain that the uninjured adjacent digit can tolerate the loss of its proper digital artery. Dorsal digital veins, dorsal hand veins, or the cephalic vein may be used for outflow according to the available reach of the harvested venous pedicle to the toe joint.

4. The foot is exsanguinated with gravity before tourniquet inflation to preserve some venous turgor, thus, facilitating venous dissection. A longitudinally oriented elliptical skin island is designed over the dorsal tibial aspect of the toe IPJ with a proximal incision sweeping toward the first web space between the great and second toe. The incision then extends proximally over the dorsal foot in line with the space between the first and second metatarsals (**Fig. 1**). Dissection is begun in the first web space allowing for identification of the proper digital artery to the second toe and early recognition of either a dorsal-dominant or plantar-dominant system. The proper digital branch to the great toe is ligated. Dissection then proceeds distally, following the digital artery distally until branches can be seen splitting off toward the IPJ. Great care is taken to protect these small branches by preserving a cuff of subcutaneous fat over the medial aspect of the digit and around the digital artery. Dermal level veins are not used. The more sizable subcutaneous dorsal veins coursing toward the medial foot are preserved as they coalesce into the saphenous vein.

5. The extensor digitorum communis longus (EDCL) to the second toe is harvested with length. The extensor digitorum brevis (EDB) is often transected, as it has not been definitively shown to significantly improve on IPJ extension.[7,8] If the central slip mechanism is markedly deficient, methods of improving on the expected lag have been described (pinning the IPJ, centralization of the lateral bands, performing a tight extensor repair, or reconstructing the central slip mechanism).[7–10] *Note: As an alternative to EDB transection, if intraoperative testing reveals improved IPJ extension with simultaneous pull on the EDB and EDCL, the EDB can be harvested with length and sutured to the recipient finger EDC along with the EDCL.*

6. The flexor digitorum longus (FDL) and flexor digitorum brevis (FDB) are typically excised and not used in the reconstruction. The latter, however, may be harvested with the flap if the recipient site is flexor tendon deficient.

7. A sagittal saw is used to create transverse osteotomies of the proximal and middle phalanx taking great care to protect the vascular pedicle entering the medial (tibial) side of flap. Any remaining soft tissue attachments are sharply released, thus, isolating the flap on its arterial and venous pedicle.

8. If desired, the leg tourniquet can be released at this point to assess the perfusion of the flap. Perfusion is assessed by identifying punctate bleeding from the cut dermal edge of the skin paddle. The artery is then ligated, followed by the vein, and the flap is brought up to the hand. The amputation of the second toe is then completed. This amputation can be done at either the metatarsophalangeal joint or the metatarsal shaft level to ensure a tension-free closure. The skin is closed over a small closed suction drain.

9. At the hand, the recipient site is prepared under tourniquet control with full exsanguination. A sweeping dorsal skin incision is preferred for access to the extensor mechanism and dorsal veins. This incision also provides access to dorsal arteries (radial artery at the snuff box, princeps pollicis, or dorsal arch) if this is the surgeon's preference. A counter incision in the digit or palm will provide access to palmar arteries if this source of inflow is desired.

10. The native extensor mechanism is elevated from the underlying bone allowing exposure of the PIPJ. Transverse osteotomies are then made through the proximal and middle phalanges extracting the dysfunctional joint. The osteotomies should be taken back to healthy bone proximally and distally and should protect the underlying flexor tendons. In most cases, this will require disinsertion of the flexor digitorum superficialis tendon. The

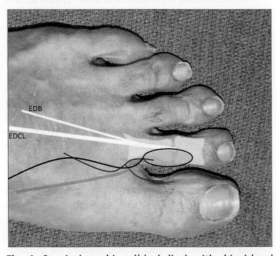

Fig. 1. Surgical marking (*black line*) with skin island (*black oval*) designed over the tibial aspect of the joint so as to optimize periarticular and skin perfusion. White lines indicate extensor tendons. Red line indicates arterial supply to first web space with tibial contribution to second toe. Blue line indicates dorsal venous system draining second toe. EDB, extensor digitorum brevis; EDCL, extensor digitorum communis longus.

flexor digitorum superficialis tendon can be permitted to retract while relying on the flexor digitorum profundus tendon as the sole remaining digital flexor.

11. The proximal phalanx of the free toe joint flap is then shortened to allow provisional insertion into the space created by excision of the dysfunctional native joint. Manual pressure or small-gauge Kirschner wires can be placed to allow provisional fixation and assessment of joint positioning, rotation, angulation, and total range of motion. If full passive range of motion does not allow the digit to touch the palm passively, the gap distance between the fingertip and palm should be determined and recorded. This gap distance equals the amount of proximal phalanx shortening needed to place the joint in a position more favorable to achieving fingertip-to-palm

contact (**Fig. 2**).[11] In this special circumstance, shortening may be performed preferably at the proximal phalanx of the digit rather than the transferred toe proximal phalanx. This location is preferred so that the vascular pedicle is not placed at risk and the osteosynthesis site approaches the more favorable metadiaphysis of the finger proximal phalanx. The total length of the new hybrid proximal phalanx, from base to head, should be the original phalanx length less the gap distance. Care should be taken to place the joint proximally without excessively shortening the finger. This placement can be accomplished by shortening the phalanx in a serial fashion and liberally testing the range of motion after each resection.

12. Once the desired position has been determined, definitive skeletal stabilization is

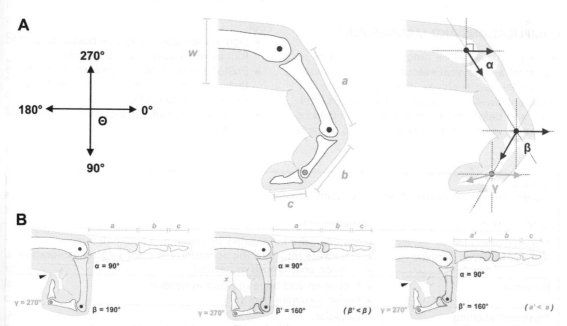

Fig. 2. (*A*) The variables associated with the length of each phalanx and the angles of flexion at each phalangeal joint. *Arrows* reflect the angles relative to the horizontal plane of MCP joint flexion (α) and PIP joint flexion (β) as defined in the legend. (*B*) The schematic at the top demonstrates the normal state. An individual with full range of motion (ROM) of all of the phalangeal joints can achieve touchdown of the digit to the palm. The schematic in the middle demonstrates the situation when toe joint transfer is performed without proximalization. The PIPJ ROM (β') is reduced secondary to stiffness and is less than the normal state. The phalangeal lengths are unchanged. In this case, an individual will most likely not be able to achieve touchdown. In the last schematic, the toe joint transfer is proximalized, and the length of proximal phalanx (A') is less than the normal state. Despite stiffness and reduced PIPJ ROM (β'), the patient is able to achieve touchdown. a, length of proximal phalanx; α, angle of metacarpophalangeal joint flexion relative to the horizontal plane; b, length of middle phalanx; β, angle of proximal IPJ flexion relative to the horizontal plane; c, length of distal phalanx; γ, angle of distal IPJ flexion relative to the horizontal plane; W, width of palm. (*From* Mohan R, Wong VW, Higgins JP, et al. Proximalization of the vascularized toe joint in finger proximal interphalangeal joint reconstruction: a technique to derive optimal flexion from a joint with expected limited motion. J Hand Surg Am 2017;42(2):e127; with permission.)

achieved with Kirschner wires, interosseous 24-gauge wire, or both. These modalities are preferred to plates so that soft tissue stripping may be minimized.

13. With the metacarpophalangeal and IPJs held fully passively flexed, the EDCL is then woven and sutured to the recipient extensor mechanism under maximum tension. This step ensures near full passive flexion will be possible. Any mechanism designed to improve on the expected extensor lag would be used at this point.[7–10] The authors prefer a tight EDCL repair and generally do not pin the IPJ or primarily reconstruct the central slip.

14. Skin is then closed loosely by incorporating the dorsal skin island from the donor toe. A protective splint with bulky soft dressing is applied. A window is created in the dressing to permit visible assessment of the dorsal skin island and the fingertip to ensure viability during the postoperative course.

COMPLICATIONS AND MANAGEMENT

Managing expectations preoperatively is likely as important as technical execution intraoperatively. Complications, such as flap loss, nonunion, persistent swelling, wound healing issues, stiffness, and deformity, are possible and should be discussed in detail with patients. Photos of these (or similar) complications, shown to patients, will aid in their decision-making. It is helpful to arrange contact of candidate patients with previous patients who have undergone toe joint transfer so they may gain insight into the postoperative course and outcomes.

Wound breakdown and delayed wound healing at the donor site is not uncommon. This risk can be minimized by judicious soft tissue handling, meticulous hemostasis, closure over a closed suction drain, light compression, and minimizing dependent positioning of the leg for approximately 3 weeks.

The possibility of complete flap loss, resulting in amputation of a toe with no surgical benefit, is a serious complication. Although this risk cannot be completely eliminated, it can likely be mitigated at a microvascular and hand surgery specialty center (**Table 2**).

POSTOPERATIVE CARE

Foot
- Light compressive wrap or stocking applied to foot as often as possible for 3 weeks
- Postoperative walking minimized to those tasks deemed necessary (eg, bed to bathroom, couch to kitchen)
- Strict elevation of extremity when not in use for 3 weeks

| **Table 2** | |
| **Complications and management of toe joint transfer** | |
Complication	**Management**
Flap microvascular thrombosis/compromise	• Postoperative monitoring to permit immediate detection • Immediate return to the operating room for surgical exploration • Revision anastomosis as needed
Nonunion	• Takedown and bone grafting as needed • Revise hardware construct
Persistent swelling (donor or recipient site)	• Elevation • Minimize unaided walking until foot swelling resolves • Light compression of the foot

Wound breakdown (donor site)	• Dressing changes
	• Elevation
	• Minimize unaided walking until foot swelling resolves
	• Enzymatic or surgical debridement as needed
	• Minimize occurrence by
	  ○ Meticulous hemostasis
	  ○ Closure over a drain
	  ○ Minimize skin flap elevation on foot during harvest to preserve skin perfusion

Stiffness	• A stable osteosynthesis construct should allow early postoperative range-of-motion exercises
Angular/rotational deformity	• May require a postoperative corrective osteotomy

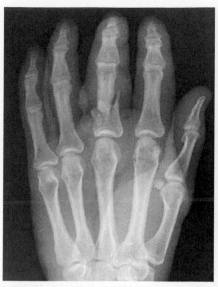
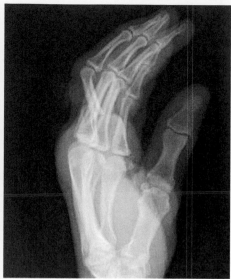

Fig. 3. Radiograph of initial fracture. (*From* Mohan R, Wong VW, Higgins JP, et al. Proximalization of the vascularized toe joint in finger PIPJ reconstruction: a technique to derive optimal flexion from a joint with expected limited motion. J Hand Surg Am 2017;42(2):e128; with permission.)

- Walking short distances in a walking boot from postoperative week 3 to week 6
- Use of a loose-fitting shoe for walking longer distances after postoperative week 6; no walking distances that cause pain or promote swelling
- Unrestricted walking in any shoe once pain and swelling completely resolve (usually around postoperative weeks 10–12)

Hand
- The postoperative splint and dressing are worn full time for the first postoperative week.
- Postoperative day 7: Dressings are removed and the patient is fitted for a custom dorsal blocking splint. Therapy is initiated for light, active range-of-motion exercises.
- A splint is worn at all times between exercises and after hand washing.

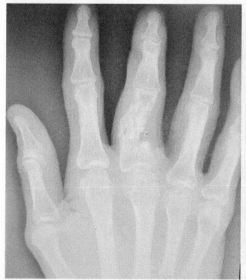
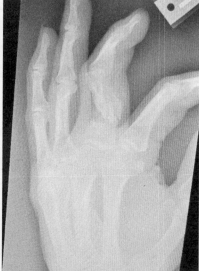

Fig. 4. Radiograph of nonunion. (*From* Mohan R, Wong VW, Higgins JP, et al. Proximalization of the vascularized toe joint in finger PIPJ reconstruction: a technique to derive optimal flexion from a joint with expected limited motion. J Hand Surg Am 2017;42(2):e129; with permission.)

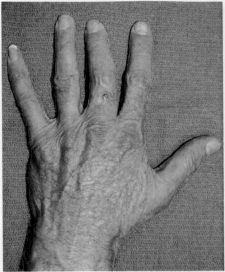
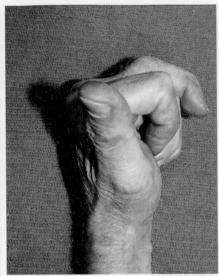

Fig. 5. Demonstration of clinical deformity, sinus tract, and stiffness. (*From* Mohan R, Wong VW, Higgins JP, et al. Proximalization of the vascularized toe joint in finger PIPJ reconstruction: a technique to derive optimal flexion from a joint with expected limited motion. J Hand Surg Am 2017;42(2):e129; with permission.)

- Postoperative week 6: If pain at the osteosynthesis site is minimal and the construct feels stable, patients can transition out of the splint. If external Kirschner wires were used, they are usually removed at this time.
- Postoperative week 8: Consider radiographs to assess the osseous union. Begin strengthening *if* patients are pain free *and* there is evidence of union on radiographs.

- Postoperative week 10: There are no therapy restrictions if patients are pain free.

OUTCOMES

Reports on outcomes for vascularized joint transfers are few. One study compared the different types of joint transfer performed in 26 patients. These types included hetero-digital

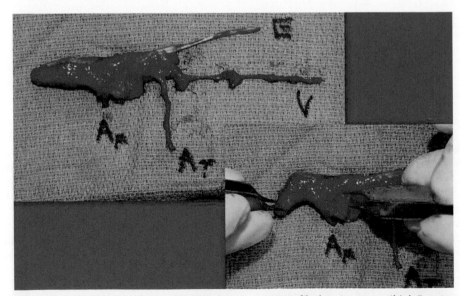

Fig. 6. Intraoperative view of limited native toe IPJ motion. A$_F$, artery fibular; A$_T$, artery tibial; E, extensor; V, vein. (*From* Mohan R, Wong VW, Higgins JP, et al. Proximalization of the vascularized toe joint in finger PIPJ reconstruction: a technique to derive optimal flexion from a joint with expected limited motion. J Hand Surg Am 2017;42(2):e130; with permission.)

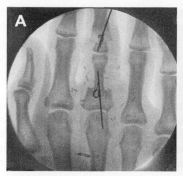
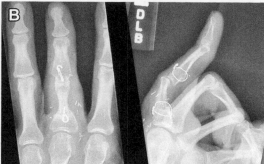

Fig. 7. (A, B) Radiographs of joint inset in a proximalized position. (*From* Mohan R, Wong VW, Higgins JP, et al. Proximalization of the vascularized toe joint in finger PIPJ reconstruction: a technique to derive optimal flexion from a joint with expected limited motion. J Hand Surg Am 2017;42(2):e131; with permission.)

island, homo-digital island, free hetero-digital, and second toe transfers. The mean active range of motion was 33° in the second toe joint transfers included in the study. All had significant extension lag ranging from a mean of 21° to 39°.[10] In a series of 11 second toe to PIPJ transfers, the investigators found an average range of motion of 47° with 41° of extensor lag at a mean follow-up of 15 years.[6] Lam and colleagues[8] reported their results of 9 patients who underwent free joint transfers with most (67%) receiving a modification to address the expected extensor lag. They reported an average total flexion of 72.2° and a persistent extensor lag measuring 18.3° at an average follow-up of 23.4 months.[8] In one of the largest series reported, a free toe joint for PIPJ reconstruction only achieved an average flexion arc of 42°.[5] Indeed, the ultimate PIPJ range of motion after a free toe joint currently seems comparable with that of a silicone arthroplasty.[1] Thus, if the surgeon makes no modifications to the toe joint or no modifications to its inset, the very best range of motion patients can expect is inherently limited. By placing the toe joint more proximally on inset as discussed earlier, some of this known limitation can be mitigated.[11]

Other indicators of success/failure of vascularized joint transfer have not yet been reported in detail. Known benefits inherent to a vascularized and structurally intact ginglymus joint, such as coronal plane stability, lifelong durability, and low infection risk, as well as the potential for continued growth in skeletally immature patients are additional important outcome measures of success that have merit in particular clinical scenarios.

CLINICAL CASE

See **Figs. 3–8**.

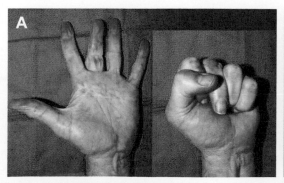
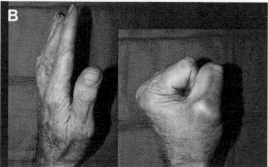

Fig. 8. (A, B) Clinical photographs demonstrating near palm touchdown achieved by joint proximalization despite inherent limitations in joint range of motion. (*From* Mohan R, Wong VW, Higgins JP, et al. Proximalization of the vascularized toe joint in finger PIPJ reconstruction: a technique to derive optimal flexion from a joint with expected limited motion. J Hand Surg Am 2017;42(2):e131; with permission.)

SUMMARY

Vascularized toe joint transfer reconstruction of the dysfunctional finger PIPJ is a valuable tool that should be considered in well-selected patients. The surgeon must weigh the benefits and limitations of this technique as described herein when considering this option.

REFERENCES

1. Squitieri L, Chung KC. A systematic review of outcomes and complications of vascularized toe joint transfer, silicone arthroplasty, and PyroCarbon arthroplasty for posttraumatic joint reconstruction of the finger. Plast Reconstr Surg 2008;121(5): 1697–707.

2. Lin YT, Kao DS, Wan DC, et al. Simultaneous reconstruction of extensor mechanism in the free transfer of vascularized proximal interphalangeal joint. Tech Hand Up Extrem Surg 2013;17(1):20–4.

3. Kimori K, Ikuta Y, Ishida O, et al. Free vascularized toe joint transfer to the hand. A technique for simultaneous reconstruction of the soft tissue. J Hand Surg Br 2001;26(4):314–20.

4. Chen SH, Wei FC, Chen HC, et al. Vascularized toe joint transfer to the hand. Plast Reconstr Surg 1996; 98(7):1275–84.

5. Dautel G, Gouzou S, Vialaneix J, et al. PIP reconstruction with vascularized PIP joint from the second toe: minimizing the morbidity with the "dorsal approach and short-pedicle technique". Tech Hand Up Extrem Surg 2004;8(3):173–80.

6. Tsubokawa N, Yoshizu T, Maki Y. Long-term results of free vascularized second toe joint transfers to finger proximal interphalangeal joints. J Hand Surg Am 2003;28(3):443–7.

7. Waughlock N, Hsu CC, Lam WL, et al. Improving the extensor lag and range of motion following free vascularized joint transfer to the proximal interphalangeal joint: part 1. An observational and cadaveric study. Plast Reconstr Surg 2013;132(2):263e–70e.

8. Lam WL, Waughlock N, Hsu CC, et al. Improving the extensor lag and range of motion following free vascularized joint transfer to the proximal interphalangeal joint: part 2. A clinical series. Plast Reconstr Surg 2013;132(2):271e–80e.

9. Hierner R, Berger AK. Long-term results after vascularised joint transfer for finger joint reconstruction. J Plast Reconstr Aesthet Surg 2008;61(11):1338–46.

10. Foucher G, Lenoble E, Smith D. Free and island vascularized joint transfer for proximal interphalangeal reconstruction: a series of 27 cases. J Hand Surg Am 1994;19(1):8–16.

11. Mohan R, Wong VW, Higgins JP, et al. Proximalization of the vascularized toe joint in finger proximal interphalangeal joint reconstruction: a technique to derive optimal flexion from a joint with expected limited motion. J Hand Surg Am 2017;42(2): e125–32.

Salvaging a Failed Proximal Interphalangeal Joint Implant

Francis J. Aversano, MD, Ryan P. Calfee, MD, MSc*

KEYWORDS

- Salvage • Interphalangeal • Implant • Arthroplasty • Arthrodesis

KEY POINTS

- Revision implant arthroplasty at the PIP joint is feasible with both silicone and resurfacing implants.
- Despite reasonable implant survival data, revision PIP implant arthroplasty is associated with a substantial number of complications and reoperations.
- Risk factors for failure of revision PIP implants include postoperative dislocation, the use of pyrocarbon implants, and the need for bone grafting during the revision surgery.
- Ultimate salvage for the failed PIP joint arthroplasty may require arthrodesis or even amputation.

INTRODUCTION: NATURE OF THE PROBLEM

When treating end-stage arthritic degeneration of the proximal interphalangeal joint (PIP), surgeons can now choose between silicone spacers and surface replacement arthroplasties (pyrocarbon and metallic). Although largely successful in maintaining range of motion and alleviating pain, the outcomes after implant arthroplasty at the PIP joint are imperfect. Reoperations are common, with the incidence of reoperation ranging from 6% to 58%.[1–6] Although less frequently performed, revisions for failed primary implants are also frequent, with an incidence estimated between 8% and 26%.[3,7,8]

At the time of implant salvage, surgeons face a choice of revision arthroplasty, arthrodesis, or amputation. This article details the use of each of these options and discusses the outcomes following these procedures.

INDICATIONS/CONTRAINDICATIONS
Revision Implant Arthroplasty

Revision after implant arthroplasty of the PIP joint is most commonly indicated for pain, restricted motion, and coronal plane deviation (**Boxes 1 and 2**).[9] Although most silicone arthroplasties will eventually fracture by 10 to 15 years,[10,11] the average time between primary implant and revision primary for pain or restricted active motion was only 4 years in a series of 27 patients.[9] Notably, silicone implant breakage is not always symptomatic.

Secondary Arthrodesis

Arthrodesis is an alternative salvage for the failed PIP arthroplasty. A failed PIP implant arthroplasty of the index finger is a relative indication for arthrodesis as the primary revision option.[9] A second relative indication favoring arthrodesis over revision implant arthroplasty is ulnar deviation through the failed PIP joint implant, because this deformity is not reliably corrected with revision implant[9] (**Box 3**).

Amputation is a second salvage that we find most useful when the patient expresses the desire to move on in life without the symptomatic finger and asks that it be removed. There are no absolute

Disclosure Statement: Neither author has a conflict related to the topic of this article.
Department of Orthopedic Surgery, Washington University School of Medicine, 660 South Euclid Avenue, Campus Box 8233, St Louis, MO 63110, USA
* Corresponding author.
E-mail address: calfeer@wudosis.wustl.edu

Hand Clin 34 (2018) 217–227
https://doi.org/10.1016/j.hcl.2017.12.011

Box 1
Indications for revision implant arthroplasty

Recurrent dislocation after PIP implant arthroplasty

Hyperextension or contracture of PIP after implant arthroplasty

Malaligned implant arthroplasty

Symptomatic fractured silicone implant

Symptomatic loose resurfacing implant

Box 3
Indications for secondary arthrodesis

Recurrent dislocation after PIP implant arthroplasty

Hyperextension or contracture of PIP after implant arthroplasty

Symptomatic fractured silicone implant

Symptomatic loose resurfacing implant

Failed arthroplasty of index PIP joint

---

contraindications to amputation, as it can be used to treat recalcitrant infection and the level of amputation can be chosen to ensure adequate soft tissue closure (**Box 4**). As the technical aspects of digit amputations are similar for failed arthroplasty and other diagnoses, the details of performing amputations are not included in the techniques to follow.

SURGICAL TECHNIQUE/PROCEDURE
Preoperative Planning

When planning a revision surgery for any PIP arthroplasty, equal consideration is required for both the technical planning and setting appropriate patient expectations. A detailed preoperative conversation with the patient should discuss the ultimate goals for the digit and expectations for the surgery. The surgeon should openly discuss the risks of surgery, acknowledging that these patients have already failed one attempt at arthroplasty. At times, surgical consent may need to include multiple possibilities, such as revision implant arthroplasty versus arthrodesis, depending on intraoperative evaluation of the bone and soft tissues.

Technical planning requires consideration of the soft tissue envelope around the PIP joint, the status of the extensor apparatus, the location of prior incisions, and the remaining bone stock to support the revision arthroplasty. As part of the preoperative assessment, the surgeon should carefully examine for any clinical evidence of infection complicating the failed PIP arthroplasty.

Box 2
Contraindications for revision implant arthroplasty

Active infection

Inadequate soft tissue coverage for joint

Incompetent or nonrepairable collateral ligaments (for resurfacing implants)

Lack of flexor tendon function

Preparation and Patient Positioning

Revision surgery for a failed PIP implant arthroplasty is expected to be outpatient surgery with preparation and patient positioning similar to most elective hand surgeries. Either a high arm or forearm tourniquet is used at the surgeon's discretion. A regional nerve block anesthesia may be sufficient for patient comfort. This may be supplemented with sedation as needed. Typically, the patient remains supine on an operative stretcher with the shoulder abducted and hand resting on an arm table. A mini C-arm should be available.

Surgical Approach

The surgical approach for salvage of the failed PIP implant arthroplasty is often dictated by the prior incision and quality of the soft tissue envelope. Similar to Satteson and colleagues,[12] we prefer to use the existing incision from the primary surgery. Most commonly, this results in a dorsal approach and requires dissection through the extensor tendon, which introduces the risk of extensor tendon dysfunction, including adhesion formation, incompetence, and imbalance.[3,4,13–16] When the extensor apparatus is insufficient or damaged, the dorsal approach provides access for reconstruction of the extensor apparatus during the surgery.[17]

Although less commonly performed, the volar approach to the PIP joint offers the advantages of allowing any necessary flexor tenolysis and immediate postoperative motion, as the extensor apparatus is not violated.[18,19] However, this approach risks flexor tendon bowstringing, swan-neck deformity, heterotopic ossification, and an increased risk of implant failure.[4,13,20] For

---

Box 4
Contraindications for secondary arthrodesis

Active infection

Inadequate soft tissue coverage for joint

a volar approach, a wide V-shaped incision is made, with the apex at the radial or ulnar border of the PIP flexion crease. The skin and subcutaneous fat are dissected off the flexor pulley sheath while preserving both digital neurovascular bundles. The flexor tendon sheath is opened with a window between the A2 and A4 pulleys. The flexor tendons are retracted, and the volar plate is released along its medial and lateral border as well as either proximal or distal to expose the PIP joint. The collateral ligaments are then recessed off of the proximal phalanx allowing the PIP joint to be hyperextended or "shotgunned" for visualization of the complete articular surfaces of both the proximal and middle phalanx.

When implanting silicone implants, a lateral approach also may be considered.[21,22] This requires release and subsequent repair of the collateral ligament, but preserves the extensor and flexor tendons. For this approach, a mid-axial incision places the operative exposure dorsal to the digital neurovascular bundle. The transverse retinacular ligament of the extensor apparatus is incised and the collateral ligament is released from the head of the proximal phalanx and the volar plate. The joint can then be deviated coronally for access to the articular surface of the proximal and middle phalanx.

Surgical Procedure

Revising a silicone implant arthroplasty to a silicone arthroplasty

When revising a PIP implant arthroplasty, we will most commonly approach the joint dorsally (**Figs. 1–8**). Adherent scar between the skin and extensor apparatus is released sharply. Then, we access the PIP joint with a Chamay exposure to raise a distally based flap of the central slip for wide exposure of the PIP joint. Alternatively, the extensor mechanism can be split longitudinally, with elevation to either side of the proximal and

middle phalanx. This longitudinal incision divides the central slip insertion and requires subsequent repair through small bone tunnels. After dissecting through the extensor apparatus, the existing implant needing revision is removed. When removing silicone implants, explantation is readily accomplished and often requires removal of fractured implant fragments. At this point, the bone quality, collateral ligaments, and extensor mechanism are assessed to determine if revision implant arthroplasty is feasible. When replacing a silicone implant with a new silicone implant, the proximal and distal bone tunnels are freshened gently with the broach, and the trial implant is placed. In all cases, trial implants are placed checking for appropriate tension and alignment relative to other digits. After the implants are placed, the extensor mechanism is repaired with a 3 to 0 or 4 to 0 nonabsorbable suture. If collateral ligaments have been compromised during the procedure, they are repaired through bone tunnels (made with 0.035-inch Kirschner wires) with sutures (3–0 or 4–0 nonabsorbable) passed before final implant placement. We prefer to deflate the tourniquet before skin closure to ensure hemostasis. The skin is closed with 4 to 0 nylon suture and a short-arm plaster splint is applied to support the finger and the adjacent digits.

Revising a resurfacing implant arthroplasty to a silicone arthroplasty

For primary resurfacing implants, revision is typically performed because of loosening or migration, which also results in the implants being removed without undue difficulty. If the primary arthroplasty was cemented, the surgeon faces the challenge of removing the remaining cement during revision. Well-fixed implants may require drilling around the implant components to break the cement-implant interface. Subsequently, the cement may be removed with careful use of a bur and osteotomes. When placing a silicone implant after

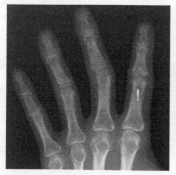 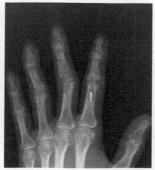 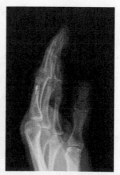

Fig. 1. Preoperative radiographs of a 53-year-old patient with pain and deformity in the index and long finger PIP joints after silicone arthroplasties of the index, long, and ring fingers. (*Courtesy of* M. Rizzo, MD, Rochester, MN.)

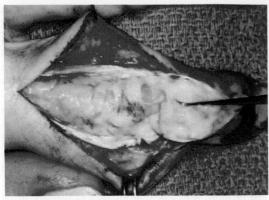

Fig. 2. Wide exposure of PIP joint of index finger after Chamay approach. (*Courtesy of* M. Rizzo, MD, Rochester, MN.)

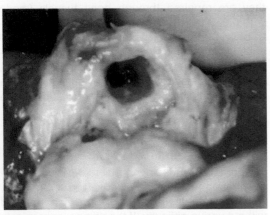

Fig. 3. Intraoperative view of irregular but contained canal of index finger after implant removal. (*Courtesy of* M. Rizzo, MD, Rochester, MN.)

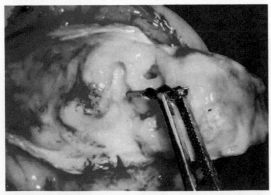

Fig. 4. Broken bur retrieved from index finger proximal phalanx. (*Courtesy of* M. Rizzo, MD, Rochester, MN.)

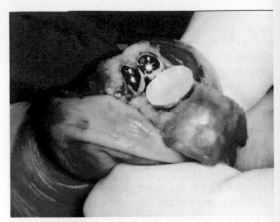

Fig. 5. Revision resurfacing implant placed for index finger PIP joint. (*Courtesy of* M. Rizzo, MD, Rochester, MN.)

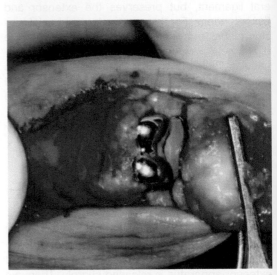

Fig. 6. Reduction of revision resurfacing implant for index finger PIP joint. (*Courtesy of* M. Rizzo, MD, Rochester, MN.)

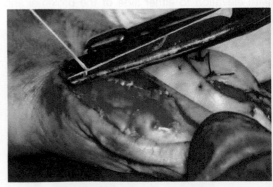

Fig. 7. Closure of Chamay exposure with multiple interrupted sutures in extensor mechanism. (*Courtesy of* M. Rizzo, MD, Rochester, MN.)

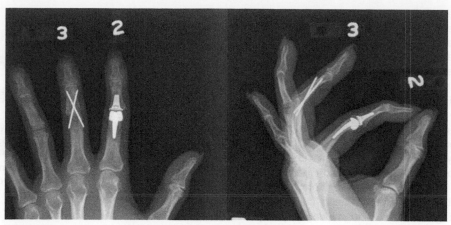

Fig. 8. Final radiographs after revision arthroplasty of index finger and arthrodesis of long finger PIP joint. (*Courtesy of* M. Rizzo, MD, Rochester, MN.)

removing a resurfacing implant, broaching and sizing will be necessary, and it is necessary to have removed any old cement within the canals.

Revising a silicone or resurfacing implant arthroplasty to a resurfacing arthroplasty

If placing a revision resurfacing implant, care must be taken to ensure proper placement along the long axis of the proximal and middle phalanx and new bony cuts may be necessary according to manufacturer specifications. For pyrocarbon press-fit implants, bone grafting may be necessary based on the amount of bone loss or expansion of the canal space as a result of previous implant migration. As a result, when revising a PIP implant arthroplasty with a pyrocarbon resurfacing implant, the proximal and distal components are often up-sized or down-sized relative to each other.[13]

If placing a metallic resurfacing implant, the new implant is cemented as opposed to being press-fit. This is often necessary in revision cases because of the size mismatch between appropriate-sized implants and the expanded canal space with associated poor bone stock.

Revision surgery for swan-neck deformity

Although soft tissue imbalance resulting in joint instability or abnormal motion may prompt implant revision, those digits complicated by swan-neck deformity may be salvaged while maintaining the implant arthroplasty. Froelich and Rizzo[23] published the technique of performing a slip of flexor digitorum superficialis as a hemi-tenodesis combined with VY lengthening of the extensor apparatus for those implants complicated by swan-neck deformity. These patients typically present for further treatment to correct functional limitations attributed to stiff swan-neck deformities, as opposed to pain. Through a volar approach, one slip of the flexor digitorum superficialis (FDS) is identified and cut proximal to A2, preserving its distal insertion on the middle phalanx. That slip of FDS is then routed from deep to superficial through a transverse opening in the A2 pulley. The PIP is flexed 25° and the FDS is tensioned before being sutured to the superficial surface of A2 to create the static volar restraint to PIP hyperextension. If the PIP cannot passively flex, a dorsal incision is made, and the extensor mechanism is incised as in a Chamay approach, preserving the distal insertion of the central slip. The FDS tenodesis is then secured after restoration of passive flexion. The extensor apparatus is closed in a V to Y fashion to lengthen the extensor sufficiently to preserve the gained PIP flexion. Postoperatively, the PIP is splinted in slight flexion for 4 to 6 weeks to allow soft tissue healing. The advantage of this approach is that the implant can be maintained and motion preserved. In a series of 12 patients with 14 fingers affected, the posture of the PIP joint was satisfactorily improved. At final the follow-up visit, patients averaged a 38° arc of PIP motion.

Secondary arthrodesis

When performing a secondary arthrodesis after PIP implant arthroplasty, we perform a dorsal approach with sharp dissection from the skin to the bone. Elevating the extensor apparatus directly off the bone with the surrounding soft tissue sleeve may prevent compromise of thin skin flaps. Next, the failed implant and any associated cement is removed. Removing cement is always challenging. We recommend working carefully with a bur, as well as rongeurs and osteotomes to remove the cement. To achieve bony apposition between the proximal and middle phalanx after the previous bony resections, one must either substantially shorten the finger or preferably place interposition bone graft to more closely replicate native anatomy.[24] We prefer autograft harvested from the distal radius or alternatively from the iliac crest. Bone graft is placed with the goal of restoring overall finger length as judged relative to adjacent digits. Most commonly, this is accomplished with Kirschner wires supplemented with tension band fixation or small plate and screw fixation constructs. Once stabilized, we recommend carefully reassessing finger rotation and making any adjustments before placing all hardware. If possible, any periosteum and the extensor mechanism should be closed over hardware. This reduces the chance of symptomatic hardware requiring later removal. The skin is closed in routine fashion and a plaster splint is placed on the finger before leaving the operating room (see **Figs. 1** and **8**; **Figs. 9–12**).

COMPLICATIONS AND MANAGEMENT

Complications are frequent after salvage procedures for the failed PIP implant arthroplasty. Common complications and potential approaches for treatment are detailed as follows. Depending on patient preference and the number of surgeries that have been performed on the digit, secondary arthrodesis or amputation of the affected digit remain ultimate salvage options for all of the complications listed.

Revision Implant Arthroplasty

- Extensor tendon adhesions limiting flexion
  - Tenolysis or tendon lengthening
- Flexion contracture with extensor tendon disruption

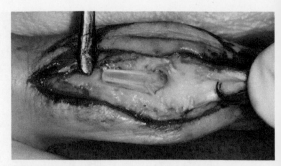

Fig. 10. Confirmed complete loss of proximal phalanx dorsal bone making revision arthroplasty not possible. (*Courtesy of* M. Rizzo, MD, Rochester, MN.)

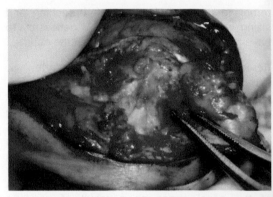

Fig. 11. Bone grafting to fill defect at PIP joint for long finger. Cancellous bone harvested from distal radius. (*Courtesy of* M. Rizzo, MD, Rochester, MN.)

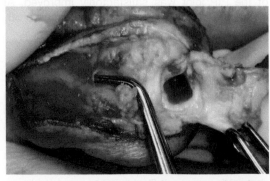

Fig. 9. Exposure of failed long finger PIP arthroplasty noting implant extruded from proximal phalanx dorsal cortex. (*Courtesy of* M. Rizzo, MD, Rochester, MN.)

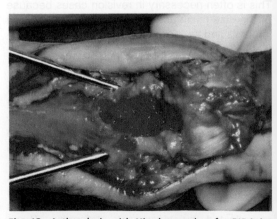

Fig. 12. Arthrodesis with Kirschner wires for PIP joint of long finger. (*Courtesy of* M. Rizzo, MD, Rochester, MN.)

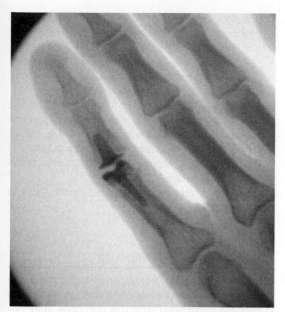

Fig. 13. Surface replacement arthroplasty for post-traumatic arthritis of index PIP joint that developed radial collateral ligament instability. (*Courtesy of* M. Rizzo, MD, Rochester, MN.)

○ Manipulation with soft tissue reconstruction of the extensor apparatus
• PIP joint instability
○ Suture repair of the collateral ligaments (**Figs. 13–15**)
○ FDS hemi-tenodesis for hyperextension (**Figs. 16–19**)
• PIP joint dislocation
○ Potential implant revision with altered component positioning or sizing or bone grafting to support implants

○ Conversion of surface replacement implant to silicone implant
• Infection
○ Surgical debridement with intravenous anti-biotics and implant removal based on severity of infection

Secondary Arthrodesis

The primary complications after secondary arthrodesis of the PIP joint are nonunion and symptomatic hardware. Nonunion is addressed with revision arthrodesis using autograft, whereas symptomatic hardware may require removal of that hardware after union is achieved.

POSTOPERATIVE CARE
Revision Implant Arthroplasty

• Postoperative splint maintained for 10 to 14 days
• Sutures removed at 10 to 14 days and custom orthosis fashioned to support PIP joint in extension
○ Orthosis may be static and removed or un-strapped for exercises; alternatively, a day-time dynamic extension orthosis may be applied to allow active flexion with assisted extension
• At time of suture removal, active range of motion of the finger is initiated and elastic wrap used to minimize edema
○ If the extensor apparatus was divided and repaired, initial active motion recommended through limited arc with gradual advancement to full flexion only after 6 weeks

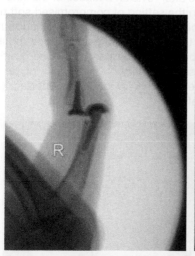
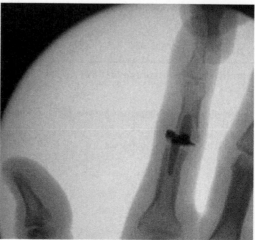

Fig. 14. Several months after radial collateral ligament repair, index PIP joint returns now with recurrent instability and dislocation. (*Courtesy of* M. Rizzo, MD, Rochester, MN.)

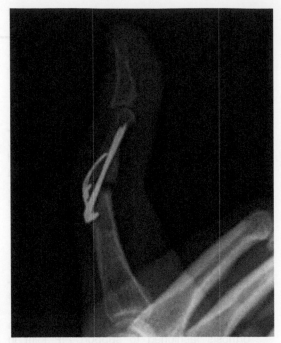

Fig. 15. Ultimate salvage for index PIP joint instability now with arthrodesis. Current radiograph at 3 months without union, although delayed union eventually occurred.

- Any coronal plane deviation treated with buddy strapping to adjacent finger during first 6 weeks postoperatively
- At 6 weeks:
  ○ Grip strengthening initiated
  ○ Daytime orthosis discontinued
  ○ Allowed to perform basic activities of daily living
- At 3 months:
  ○ Night orthosis discontinued
  ○ Unrestricted activity allowed
- Elastic wrapping continued until edema resolved

Secondary Arthrodesis

- Postoperative splint maintained for 10 to 14 days

- Sutures removed at 10 to 14 days and custom orthosis fashioned to support PIP joint in position of arthrodesis
  ○ Orthosis may be finger based with buddy strap or hand based depending on patient comfort and compliance
- At time of suture removal, active range of motion of the distal interphalangeal and metacarpophalangeal finger is initiated, and elastic wrap used to minimize edema
- No lifting or gripping until radiographic union (no sooner than 6 weeks)
- Elastic wrapping continued until edema resolved

OUTCOMES
Revision Implant Arthroplasty

Similar to most revision surgeries in the hand, the average outcome of revision implant arthroplasty is modest compared with the outcome after primary implant arthroplasty. Among 75 consecutive revision PIP joint arthroplasties, 25% of fingers required additional revision surgery over a 14-year period.[13] Overall survival for the revision implants was 70% at 5 and 10 years. Indications for subsequent revision surgery included dislocation, limited motion, component loosening or fracture, and infection, with additional reoperations for either limited range of motion or PIP instability. In that series, most implants placed were pyrocarbon but the use of silicone implants or metal on polyethylene implants for the revision were associated with fewer postoperative complications. Those investigators suggested that the constrained design of silicone implants may reduce the incidence of complications after revision because of the inherent stability in the setting of compromised soft tissue joint stabilizers. Other predictors of poor outcome after the revision surgery include postoperative dislocation or the need for bone grafting during revision surgery.[13] However, at a mean of 5 years, 98% of patients reported good pain relief.

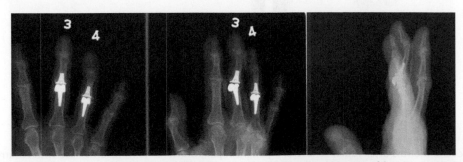

Fig. 16. Surface replacement arthroplasties of PIP joints complicated by development of fixed swan-neck deformity.

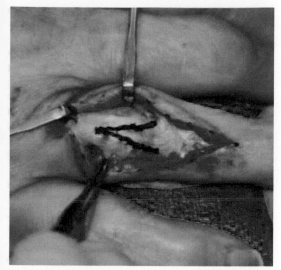

Fig. 17. Chamay exposure for V to Y lengthening of extensor apparatus.

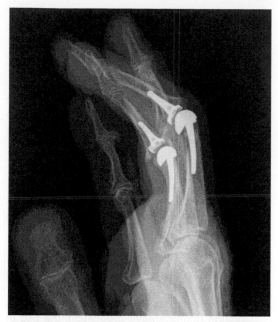

Fig. 19. Final resting radiographs demonstrating correction of swan-neck deformities.

After revision silicone arthroplasty, 12% of digits required a second revision with all performed for painful implant breakage.[9] In addition, correction of substantial coronal plane deformity with revision silicone arthroplasty has proven difficult.[9] Following revision surgery, PIP motion was largely unchanged from preoperative measurements; however, when revisions were performed for severely restricted active range of motion, then revision was able to substantially improve flexion.[9]

Secondary Arthrodesis and Amputation

Reporting on revision surgery after 294 nonconstrained PIP implants, Pritsch and Rizzo[14] noted that 6 fingers were eventually amputated, 9 underwent PIP arthrodesis, and 2 required resection arthroplasty. The likelihood of arthrodesis or amputation increased as the number of operations on the finger increased. As such, arthrodesis was the first reoperation in only 1 of 76 fingers, but

was performed in 5 of 12 third operations on affected fingers.[14]

Primary arthrodesis of the PIP joint has a high rate of union with successful fusion achieved and more than 95% of cases.[25–27] Arthrodesis of the PIP joint after implant arthroplasty is associated with a higher rate of nonunion. Jones and colleagues[28] reported nonunion in 39% of 13 arthrodeses following arthroplasty. In that series, 7 of 8 fingers treated with Kirschner wire and tension band constructs successfully fused. All but one of these patients required bone grafting. Notably, nonunion was only associated with subtle differences in patient-reported outcomes. Eight of 13 digits required subsequent removal of painful hardware with 1 patient's hardware eroding through the skin. Three patients healed with residual deformity present.

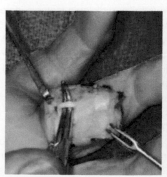
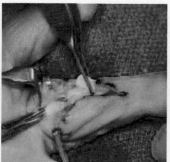
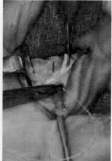

Fig. 18. FDS tenodesis to A2 to prevent PIP hyperextension.

Amputation of a persistently painful, unstable, or infected digit following PIP arthroplasty remains the ultimate salvage.[24] Patients can expect reliable pain relief but may face functional challenges adapting to the removal of a digit. Typically, preoperative conversations with the patient can determine the optimal level of amputation and dictate whether to preserve some digit length versus considering a more aesthetic final appearance with a ray resection.

SUMMARY

- Revision implant arthroplasty at the PIP joint is feasible with both silicone and resurfacing implants.
- Despite reasonable survival of revision PIP implants, this procedure is associated with a substantial number of complications and reoperations.
- Risk factors for failure of revision PIP implants include postoperative dislocation, the use of pyrocarbon implants, and the need for bone grafting.
- Ultimate salvage for the failed PIP joint arthroplasty may require arthrodesis or even amputation.

REFERENCES

1. Wijk U, Wollmark M, Kopylov P, et al. Outcomes of proximal interphalangeal joint pyrocarbon implants. J Hand Surg Am 2010;35(1):38–43.
2. Meier R, Schulz M, Krimmer H, et al. Proximal interphalangeal joint replacement with pyrolytic carbon prostheses. Oper Orthop Traumatol 2007; 19(1):1–15.
3. Bravo CJ, Rizzo M, Hormel KB, et al. Pyrolytic carbon proximal interphalangeal joint arthroplasty: results with minimum two-year follow-up evaluation. J Hand Surg Am 2007;32(1):1–11.
4. Luther C, Germann G, Sauerbier M. Proximal interphalangeal joint replacement with surface replacement arthroplasty (SR-PIP): functional results and complications. Hand (NY) 2010;5(3):233–40.
5. Herren DB, Schindele S, Goldhahn J, et al. Problematic bone fixation with pyrocarbon implants in proximal interphalangeal joint replacement: short-term results. J Hand Surg Br 2006;31(6): 643–51.
6. Chung KC, Ram AN, Shauver MJ. Outcomes of pyrolytic carbon arthroplasty for the proximal interphalangeal joint. Plast Reconstr Surg 2009;123(5): 1521–32.
7. Jennings CD, Livingstone DP. Surface replacement arthroplasty of the proximal interphalangeal joint using the PIP-SRA implant: results, complications,

and revisions. J Hand Surg Am 2008;33(9):1565. e1–11.
8. Johnstone BR, Fitzgerald M, Smith KR, et al. Cemented versus uncemented surface replacement arthroplasty of the proximal interphalangeal joint with a mean 5-year follow-up. J Hand Surg Am 2008;33(5):726–32.
9. Herren DB, Keuchel T, Marks M, et al. Revision arthroplasty for failed silicone proximal interphalangeal joint arthroplasty: indications and 8-year results. J Hand Surg Am 2014;39(3):462–6.
10. Takigawa S, Meletiou S, Sauerbier M, et al. Longterm assessment of Swanson implant arthroplasty in the proximal interphalangeal joint of the hand. J Hand Surg Am 2004;29(5):785–95.
11. Bales JG, Wall LB, Stern PJ. Long-term results of Swanson silicone arthroplasty for proximal interphalangeal joint osteoarthritis. J Hand Surg Am 2014; 39(3):455–61.
12. Satteson ES, Langford MA, Li Z. The management of complications of small joint arthrodesis and arthroplasty. Hand Clin 2015;31(2):243–66.
13. Wagner ER, Luo TD, Houdek MT, et al. Revision proximal interphalangeal arthroplasty: an outcome analysis of 75 consecutive cases. J Hand Surg Am 2015;40(10):1949–55.e1.
14. Pritsch T, Rizzo M. Reoperations following proximal interphalangeal joint nonconstrained arthroplasties. J Hand Surg Am 2011;36(9):1460–6.
15. Nunley RM, Boyer MI, Goldfarb CA. Pyrolytic carbon arthroplasty for posttraumatic arthritis of the proximal interphalangeal joint. J Hand Surg Am 2006; 31(9):1468–74.
16. Linscheid RL, Murray PM, Vidal MA, et al. Development of a surface replacement arthroplasty for proximal interphalangeal joints. J Hand Surg Am 1997; 22(2):286–98.
17. Iselin F, Pradet G, Gouet O. Conversion to arthroplasty from proximal interphalangeal joint arthrodesis. Ann Chir Main 1988;7(2):115–9.
18. Kobayashi KT. A proximal interphalangeal joint arthroplasty of the hand. J Am Soc Surg Hand 2003; 3(4):219–26.
19. Schneider HJ, Weiss MA, Stern PJ. Silicone-induced erosive arthritis: radiologic features in seven cases. AJR Am J Roentgenol 1987;148(5):923–5.
20. Murray PM, Linscheid RL, Cooney WP 3rd, et al. Long-term outcomes of proximal interphalangeal joint surface replacement arthroplasty. J Bone Joint Surg Am 2012;94(12):1120–8.
21. Segalman KA. Lateral approach to proximal interphalangeal joint implant arthroplasty. J Hand Surg Am 2007;32(6):905–8.
22. Merle M, Villani F, Lallemand B, et al. Proximal interphalangeal joint arthroplasty with silicone implants (NeuFlex) by a lateral approach: a series of 51 cases. J Hand Surg Eur Vol 2012;37(1):50–5.

23. Froelich JM, Rizzo M. Reconstruction of swan neck deformities after proximal interphalangeal joint arthroplasty. Hand (NY) 2014;9(1):93–8.
24. Sauerbier M, Cooney WP, Linscheid RL. Operative technique of surface replacement arthroplasty of the proximal interphalangeal joint. Tech Hand Up Extrem Surg 2001;5(3):141–7.
25. Stern PJ, Gates NT, Jones TB. Tension band arthrodesis of small joints in the hand. J Hand Surg Am 1993;18(2):194–7.
26. Ayres JR, Goldstrohm GL, Miller GJ, et al. Proximal interphalangeal joint arthrodesis with the Herbert screw. J Hand Surg Am 1988;13(4):600–3.
27. Stahl S, Rozen N. Tension-band arthrodesis of the small joints of the hand. Orthopedics 2001;24(10): 981–3.
28. Jones DB Jr, Ackerman DB, Sammer DM, et al. Arthrodesis as a salvage for failed proximal interphalangeal joint arthroplasty. J Hand Surg Am 2011;36(2):259–64.

Treatment of Proximal Interphalangeal Joint Contracture

Sami H. Tuffaha, MD, W.P. Andrew Lee, MD*

KEYWORDS

- Proximal interphalangeal joint • Contracture • Contracture release • Trauma • Dynamic splinting
- Serial splinting

KEY POINTS

- Proximal interphalangeal joint contracture can involve many structures, including the accessory collateral ligaments, volar plate, checkrein ligaments, retinacular ligaments, flexor and extensor tendons, and articular surfaces.
- Results with treatment are unpredictable and often modest.
- Treatment typically begins with conservative modalities, including dynamic splinting and serial casting.
- Surgery typically requires stepwise release of affected structures, with extent of release determined intraoperatively, under local anesthesia, with patient participation.

INTRODUCTION

Proximal interphalangeal joint (PIPJ) flexion contracture is a challenging and often frustrating problem commonly faced by patients, hand surgeons, and therapists. With a wide arc of motion, the PIPJ is responsible for 85% of total finger motion.[1] As such, patients with PIPJ contracture often experience significant functional impairment.[2] Normal PIPJ function depends upon adequate bony support, intact articular surfaces, and competent periarticular stabilizers. Damage to any of these critical structures resulting from trauma or other disease processes can lead to diminished joint motion and fixed contracture. Several conservative and surgical approaches are available to treat PIPJ contracture, the choice of which depends upon the severity and etiology of the contracture. The multiple described treatment options for PIPJ contracture and lack of consensus regarding the optimal approach speak to the unpredictable and often unsatisfactory outcomes that are achieved, regardless of which treatment approach is chosen. This article briefly reviews the pertinent anatomy and pathologic processes that can result in PIPJ contracture and then describes the various treatment options that can be used to address this difficult problem.

ANATOMY

The PIPJ is a hinge joint with a flexion/extension arc of 90° to 100° and minimal motion in the coronal plane.[3] The articulation of the intercondylar eminence of the middle phalanx within the intercondylar sulcus of the proximal phalanx provides some lateral stability in full extension. However, joint stability and integrity, particularly during flexion, depend heavily upon the periarticular capsuloligamentous and tendinous structures, including the volar plate, collateral and checkrein ligaments, flexor tendons, and extensor hood. The fibrocartilaginous volar plate is the primary

Department of Plastic and Reconstructive Surgery, Johns Hopkins School of Medicine, Baltimore, MD, USA
* Corresponding author. 601 North Caroline Street, Suite 8152F, Baltimore, MD 21287.
E-mail address: wpal@jhmi.edu

Hand Clin 34 (2018) 229–235
https://doi.org/10.1016/j.hcl.2017.12.012
0749-0712/18/© 2018 Elsevier Inc. All rights reserved.

hand.theclinics.com

restraint against hyperextension and glides across the bony surfaces with flexion and extension.[4,5] The checkrein ligaments extend from the proximal volar plate and anchor it to the proximal phalanx, also serving to prevent hyperextension. Bony adhesions of the volar plate or contracture of the checkrein ligaments can result in diminished range of motion and flexion contracture. The collateral ligaments are primarily responsible for radial and ulnar stability. The proper collateral ligaments originate from the head of the proximal phalanx and insert into the middle phalanx, whereas the accessory collateral ligaments also arise from the proximal phalanx and insert onto the volar plate and flexor sheath. Because the accessory collateral ligaments do not insert into the middle phalanx, they remain lax in full flexion, rendering them susceptible to fibrosis and contracture if immobilized for a prolonged period of time in this position.[2] The relatively weaker dorsal stabilizers of the PIPJ include the thin dorsal capsule and overlying central slip, lateral bands, and transverse retinacular ligaments of the extensor hood. Disruption of any of these delicate structures can result in joint imbalance and contracture.[6] See **Fig. 1** for illustrations of pertinent PIPJ anatomy.

PATHOGENESIS

Traumatic PIPJ contracture can occur as a result of lacerations, fractures, dislocations, stress injuries, burns, traumatic nerve palsies, and ischemic insult. PIPJ contracture following trauma typically develops in a delayed fashion as a

sequela of the physiologic injury response and prolonged joint immobilization owing to the injury itself or treatment of the injury. Soon after injury occurs, edema fluid and blood tend to accumulate within and around the tendons, ligaments, sheaths, and articular space of the joint, resulting in swelling of the digits and hand that mechanically limits joint motion.[7,8] The swollen, injured hand tends to assume a characteristic posture, with the metacarpophalangeal joint (MPJ) extended and the interphalangeal joints (IPJ) flexed 30° to 40°, serving to maximize joint space and reduce pressure and discomfort.[9–11] Prolonged immobilization of the PIPJ in a flexed posture, whether because of swelling and discomfort or as part of injury management, can cause contracture. The mechanisms by which this occurs include secondary contracture of the skin envelope, joint capsule, collateral and checkrein ligaments, tendon sheath, and superficial fascia, as well as adherence of the retinacular ligaments and volar plate to the proximal phalanx and collateral ligaments.[12] Contractures following proximal phalangeal fracture are most likely to occur initially as a result of flexor tendon adhesions, which typically occur at the site of the fracture but can also extend proximally and distally.[13,14] Following fractures involving the articular surfaces, exostoses, arthrosis, and bony block can also cause joint contracture.[15] Regardless of injury mechanism, the final common pathway for most PIPJ contractures involves contraction and fibrosis of the volar plate-checkrein ligament complex.[16,17] It should also be noted that there are many nontraumatic causes

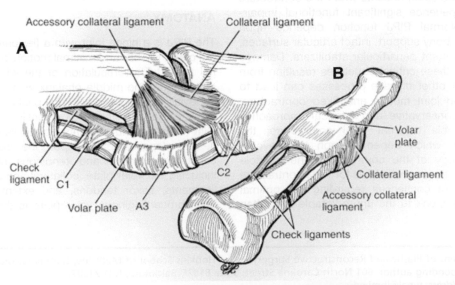

Fig. 1. Illustration of PIP joint anatomy. (*A*) Lateral view. (*B*) Volar view. (*Courtesy of* Elizabeth Martin MA, FAMI, Waynesville, NC; with permission from Green's Operative Hand Surgery, 7th edition.)

of PIPJ contracture, including Dupuytren disease,[18] rheumatoid arthritis,[19,20] gout,[21] and diabetes mellitus.[22,23]

TREATMENT
Evaluation

Given the many potential causes of PIPJ contracture, a systematic approach should be used to determine the most likely etiology and optimal treatment plan. When examining the stiff joint, it is important to differentiate between limitations in active and passive range of motion and to be cognizant of the relative position of the adjacent joints during each maneuver. When active range of motion is more limited than passive range of motion, musculotendinous problems or adhesions are more likely.[17] In contrast, equal limitation of active and passive range of motion suggests intraarticular block or capsuloligamentous contracture. Following fracture, if there is evidence of arthritis or articular misalignment on imaging, contracture release surgery should be avoided. In such cases, silicone joint replacement can be considered, with favorable results reported using a volar approach.[24,25] A contracture of greater than 70° may cause attenuation of the extensor mechanism requiring correction during surgery.[10] Intrinsic and extrinsic tightness should be specifically assessed. When assessing extrinsic tightness, diminished passive PIP flexion with the MP held in flexion suggests extensor tightness or adhesion, whereas diminished passive PIP extension with the MP held in extension suggests flexor tightness or adhesion. The Bunnell intrinsic tightness test is considered positive when there is less PIP flexion noted with the MP held in extension than when the MP is held in flexion. It should be noted that the etiology of PIPJ contracture at times cannot be determined during the preoperative examination.

Prevention

Before discussing treatment, it should be emphasized that PIPJ contracture is much easier to prevent than to treat after it has occurred. Prevention strategies center on the principle of early mobilization. When necessary, the PIPJ should be immobilized in full extension for no longer than 3 weeks.[14] Allowing even minimal glide of as little as 5 mm can translate to 40° gain in PIPJ motion by preventing adhesions.[11] Treatment approaches that allow for early motion include buddy taping to adjacent fingers for collateral ligament injury, extension block splinting for fracture-dislocations, and achieving optimal bony fixation and ligamentous/tendinous repair at the time of injury.[14] Effective strategies for pain and edema control, including compressive wraps and distal to proximal massage, should not be overlooked.[14]

Nonsurgical Treatment

Conservative management of PIPJ contractures can be effective[26] and should be attempted before considering surgical interventions.[17,27,28] Conservative measures include joint mobilization, encouraging functional use in daily activities, exercises that incorporate steady and prolonged loading, compression, massage, splinting, and casting.

Splinting and casting protocols are the mainstay of conservative treatment, with the goal of applying constant, distributed extension force perpendicular to the flexed middle phalanx so as to gradually lengthen the contracted periarticular capsuloligamentous structures that limit joint motion.[29] These techniques are typically considered first-line for contractures less than 45° but should be used with caution for more severe contractures given the risk of skin breakdown.[2,30] Splinting can be classified as static, serial static, static progressive, or dynamic.[23] Dynamic splints make use of mechanical energy or elastics to apply steady extension force that is maintained as the contracture is gradually released. The efficacy of this approach is dependent on patient compliance, as outcomes tend to improve with greater duration and frequency of use.[23,31–34] Regarding optimal daily splint use, a prospective study by Glasgow and colleagues[34] demonstrated improved outcomes with 6 to 12 hours of use per day compared with less than 6 hours of daily use, and greater than 12 hours of use being poorly tolerated by patients.[35] Several studies have demonstrated a direct relationship between degree of correction and longitudinal duration of therapy,[32,33,36] leading to a general consensus that therapy should continue for as long as improvement is being achieved. The amplitude of applied force is another important variable that must be considered. Although enough force should be applied to provide adequate correction, excessive force can cause severe pain, inflammation, swelling, and skin tears.[23,37] Dynamic splints are typically avoided when the patient is sleeping, as pressure sores can develop. However, nighttime static splinting can be used in conjunction with dynamic splinting to maintain gains and prevent relapse during sleep.[17,38]

Static progressive splints and serial casting can be used as alternatives to dynamic splinting. These approaches may have an advantage over dynamic splinting with more severe contractures that are greater than 45° and lack a springy endpoint.[14] However, dynamic splinting has the advantages of promoting active and passive range of motion and easier hygiene.[14] Furthermore, static progressive splints require constant adjustment to maintain adequate force as correction of the contracture is achieved, and serial casting requires application of the cast multiple times per week for the same reason.

External fixation is another approach used to correct of PIPJ contracture that has been gaining favor.[39] External fixators can be used in 1 of 2 ways, to either extend or distract the joint. Extension correction is achieved with a unilateral hinged external fixator that is placed under radiologic guidance and is slowly activated by the patient in increments of 3° to 5° per day.[2,40] Distraction correction involves use of a monolateral external fixator that is gradually activated by the patient until 5 to 8 mm of joint distraction are achieved.[2] Although not widely used, distraction correction has been shown to be more effective than extension correction,[41] perhaps because distraction allows for elongation of all of the periarticular structures, whereas extension correction only stretches the volar structures. Although favorable results can be achieved with external fixation, application of the device can be cumbersome and requires precise placement and adjustment to achieve the desired effect. Furthermore, because the device prevents joint flexion, gain in extension can come at the expense of loss of flexion motion.[42]

Surgical Treatment

PIPJ contracture release can be carried out using either a midlateral or a volar approach. Although a volar approach using a Bruner incision may provide easier exposure, most surgeons tend to prefer the midlateral approach.[5,10,12,14,16,17,43–45] Bruser and colleagues[43] reviewed a series of 42 patients with PIPJ contracture treated with either a midlateral or a volar approach and noted greater improvement in joint motion with the midlateral approach. They concluded that the advantage of midlateral incisions was likely due the ability to begin early mobilization and dynamic splinting before wound healing is complete, whereas the volar approach places the volar flap under tension after the joint is extended, which requires the skin flap to heal sufficiently before starting motion.

Although there are differences of opinion regarding which anatomic structures are most critical to address, a stepwise approach under local anesthesia is typically recommended, with sequential releases of structures from proximal to distal and extra-articular to intra-articular.[2,14,17,45,46] Use of local anesthesia encourages patient participation after each structure is released to determine the need to proceed with subsequent releases.

Outcomes following surgical contracture release are unpredictable and often less than desired. In some of the earliest work on open PIPJ contracture release, Curtis performed sequential capsulectomy, checkrein ligament resection, and collateral ligament excision.[12] He reported modest gains with this technique, noting that the degree of improvement with release diminished as the number of affected structures requiring release increased. Sprague came to similar conclusions using this technique, noting poor outcomes in patients who underwent capsulotomy and excision of collateral ligaments, volar plate, and extensor tendon.[6] Regardless of which technique is used, most authors report less than full range of motion following release, typically in the range of 25° to 30°.[14] Use of postoperative dynamic splinting and other mobilization techniques is likely helpful in improving outcomes, and may obviate the need for extensor tendon shortening.[47]

The authors' preferred stepwise approach to surgical contracture release is as follows:

- Single midlateral incision is made under local anesthesia (**Fig. 2**)
- Visualize neurovascular bundle and retract volarly (**Fig. 3**)
- Incise lateral flexor sheath at A3 pulley and transverse retinacular ligament and retract flexor tendons volarly (**Fig. 4**)
- Release checkrein ligaments and accessory collateral ligaments (**Fig. 5**)
- Assess active extension and proceed if needed
- Elevate volar plate subperiosteally and excise proximal portion (**Fig. 6**)
- Assess active extension and proceed if needed (**Fig. 7**)

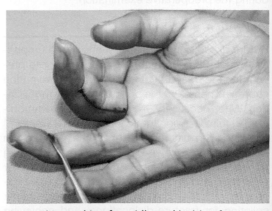

Fig. 2. Skin marking for midlateral incision from proximal aspect of proximal phalanx to distal aspect of middle phalanx. (*Courtesy of* KC Chung, MD, MS, Ann Arbor, MI.)

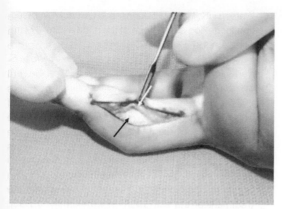

Fig. 3. Neurovascular bundle (*white arrow*) is retracted volarly, exposing flexor sheath (*black arrow*). (*Courtesy of* KC Chung, MD, MS, Ann Arbor, MI.)

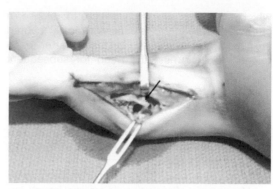

Fig. 6. Volar plate (*black arrow*) is elevated subperiosteally and released proximally from proximal phalanx. (*Courtesy of* KC Chung, MD, MS, Ann Arbor, MI.)

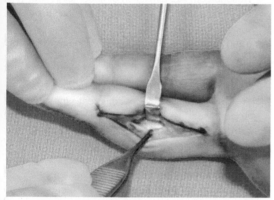

Fig. 4. Flexor sheath A3 pulley and transverse retinacular ligament and incised and flexor tendons retracted volarly, exposing volar plate. (*Courtesy of* KC Chung, MD, MS, Ann Arbor, MI.)

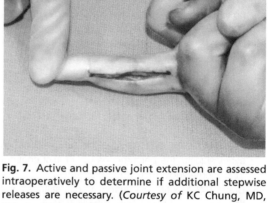

Fig. 7. Active and passive joint extension are assessed intraoperatively to determine if additional stepwise releases are necessary. (*Courtesy of* KC Chung, MD, MS, Ann Arbor, MI.)

- Dorsal exposure for extensor tenolysis and central slip repair if needed
- Aggressive mobilization begins 2 to 3 days after surgery

SUMMARY

Treatment of PIPJ contracture should begin with conservative measures that include dynamic or serial splinting or casting, particularly for contractures less than 45°. With good compliance and prolonged use, favorable results can be achieved using these modalities. For contractures that fail to respond to conservative treatment, surgical intervention can be considered. The affected structures that can be released during surgery include the accessory collateral ligaments, volar plate, checkrein ligaments, retinacular ligaments, and the flexor and extensor tendons. Although there is disagreement about

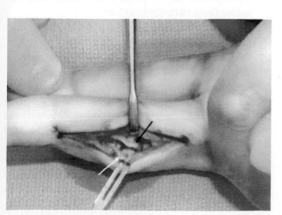

Fig. 5. Accessory collateral ligament (*white arrow*) released from volar plate (*black arrow*). (*Courtesy of* KC Chung, MD, MS, Ann Arbor, MI.)

which structures are most critical to release, a stepwise approach to release is typically favored in which active motion is tested after each release to determine the need for subsequent releases.

REFERENCES

1. Leibovic SJ, Bowers WH. Anatomy of the proximal interphalangeal joint. Hand Clin 1994;10(2): 169–78.

2. Houshian S, Jing SS, Chikkamuniyappa C, et al. Management of posttraumatic proximal interphalangeal joint contracture. J Hand Surg Am 2013;38(8): 1651–8.

3. Bailie DS, Benson LS, Marymont JV. Proximal interphalangeal joint injuries of the hand. Part I: anatomy and diagnosis. Am J Orthop (Belle Mead NJ) 1996; 25(7):474–7.

4. Bain GI, Mehta JA, Heptinstall RJ, et al. Dynamic external fixation for injuries of the proximal interphalangeal joint. J Bone Joint Surg Br 1998; 80(6):1014–9.

5. Mansat MF. Volar aspect of the proximal interphalangeal joint. An anatomical study and pathological correlations. Bull Hosp Jt Dis Orthop Inst 1984;44(2): 309–17.

6. Sprague BL. Proximal interphalangeal joint injuries and their initial treatment. J Trauma 1975;15(5): 380–5.

7. Akeson WH, Amiel D, Woo SL. Immobility effects on synovial joints the pathomechanics of joint contracture. Biorheology 1980;17(1–2):95–110.

8. Brand PW. Mechanical factors in joint stiffness and tissue growth. J Hand Ther 1995;8(2):91–6.

9. Watson HK. Treatment of the stiff finger and hand. In: Green DP HR, Pederson WC, editors. Green's operative hand surgery. Philadelphia: Churchill Livingstone; 1999. p. 552–62.

10. Allieu Y, Ould Ouali A, Gomis R, et al. Simple arthrolysis for flexor rigidity of the proximal interphalangeal joint. Ann Chir Main 1983;2(4):330–5.

11. Freeland AE, Hardy MA, Singletary S. Rehabilitation for proximal phalangeal fractures. J Hand Ther 2003;16(2):129–42.

12. Curtis RM. Capsulectomy of the interphalangeal joints of the fingers. J Bone Joint Surg Am 1954; 36-A(6):1219–32.

13. Schneider LH. Tenolysis and capsulectomy after hand fractures. Clin Orthop Relat Res 1996;(327): 72–8.

14. Hogan CJ, Nunley JA. Posttraumatic proximal interphalangeal joint flexion contractures. J Am Acad Orthop Surg 2006;14(9):524–33.

15. Chinchalkar SJ, Gan BS. Management of proximal interphalangeal joint fractures and dislocations. J Hand Ther 2003;16(2):117–28.

16. Watson HK, Light TR, Johnson TR. Checkrein resection for flexion contracture of the middle joint. J Hand Surg Am 1979;4(1):67–71.

17. Hotchkiss R. Treatment of the stiff finger. In: Wolfe S, Pederson WC, Hotchkiss RN, et al, editors. Green's operative hand surgery, vol. 7. Philadelphia: Elsevier; 2017. p. 338–44.

18. Shaw RB Jr, Chong AK, Zhang A, et al. Dupuytren's disease: history, diagnosis, and treatment. Plast Reconstr Surg 2007;120(3):44e–54e.

19. Rizio L, Belsky MR. Finger deformities in rheumatoid arthritis. Hand Clin 1996;12(3):531–40.

20. Scott FA, Boswick JA Jr. Palmar arthroplasty for the treatment of the stiff swan-neck deformity. J Hand Surg Am 1983;8(3):267–72.

21. Hernandez-Cortes P, Caba M, Gomez-Sanchez R, et al. Digital flexion contracture and severe carpal tunnel syndrome due to tophaceus infiltration of wrist flexor tendon: first manifestation of gout. Orthopedics 2011;34(11):e797–9.

22. Rosenbloom AL. Limitation of finger joint mobility in diabetes mellitus. J Diabet Complications 1989; 3(2):77–87.

23. Yang G, McGlinn EP, Chung KC. Management of the stiff finger: evidence and outcomes. Clin Plast Surg 2014;41(3):501–12.

24. Yamamoto M, Malay S, Fujihara Y, et al. A systematic review of different implants and approaches for proximal interphalangeal joint arthroplasty. Plast Reconstr Surg 2017;139(5): 1139e–51e.

25. Stoecklein HH, Garg R, Wolfe SW. Surface replacement arthroplasty of the proximal interphalangeal joint using a volar approach: case series. J Hand Surg Am 2011;36(6):1015–21.

26. Weeks PM, Wray RC Jr, Kuxhaus M. The results of non-operative management of stiff joints in the hand. Plast Reconstr Surg 1978;61(1):58–63.

27. Young VL, Wray RC Jr, Weeks PM. The surgical management of stiff joints in the hand. Plast Reconstr Surg 1978;62(6):835–41.

28. Curtis RM. Management of the stiff proximal interphalangeal joint. Hand 1969;1:32–7.

29. Flowers KR. Reflections on mobilizing the stiff hand. J Hand Ther 2010;23(4):402–3.

30. Fess EE. Splints: mechanics versus convention. J Hand Ther 1995;8(2):124–30.

31. Hunter E, Laverty J, Pollock R, et al. Nonoperative treatment of fixed flexion deformity of the proximal interphalangeal joint. J Hand Surg Br 1999;24(3): 281–3.

32. Flowers KR, LaStayo P. Effect of total end range time on improving passive range of motion. J Hand Ther 1994;7(3):150–7.

33. Prosser R. Splinting in the management of proximal interphalangeal joint flexion contracture. J Hand Ther 1996;9(4):378–86.

34. Glasgow C, Wilton J, Tooth L. Optimal daily total end range time for contracture: resolution in hand splinting. J Hand Ther 2003;16(3):207–18.

35. Glasgow C, Fleming J, Tooth LR, et al. Randomized controlled trial of daily total end range time (TERT) for Capener splinting of the stiff proximal interphalangeal joint. Am J Occup Ther 2012;66(2):243–8.

36. Glasgow C, Fleming J, Tooth LR, et al. The Long-term relationship between duration of treatment and contracture resolution using dynamic orthotic devices for the stiff proximal interphalangeal joint: a prospective cohort study. J Hand Ther 2012; 25(1):38–46 [quiz: 47].

37. Flowers KR. A proposed decision hierarchy for splinting the stiff joint, with an emphasis on force application parameters. J Hand Ther 2002;15(2): 158–62.

38. Cantero-Tellez R, Cuesta-Vargas AI, Cuadros-Romero M. Treatment of proximal interphalangeal joint flexion contracture: combined static and dynamic orthotic intervention compared with other therapy intervention: a randomized controlled trial. J Hand Surg Am 2015;40(5):951–5.

39. Schenck RR. Dynamic traction and early passive movement for fractures of the proximal interphalangeal joint. J Hand Surg Am 1986;11(6):850–8.

40. Houshian S, Gynning B, Schroder HA. Chronic flexion contracture of proximal interphalangeal joint treated with the compass hinge external fixator. A consecutive series of 27 cases. J Hand Surg Br 2002;27(4):356–8.

41. Houshian S, Jing SS, Kazemian GH, et al. Distraction for proximal interphalangeal joint contractures: long-term results. J Hand Surg Am 2013;38(10): 1951–6.

42. Kasabian A, McCarthy J, Karp N. Use of a multiplanar distracter for the correction of a proximal interphalangeal joint contracture. Ann Plast Surg 1998; 40(4):378–81.

43. Bruser P, Poss T, Larkin G. Results of proximal interphalangeal joint release for flexion contractures: midlateral versus palmar incision. J Hand Surg Am 1999;24(2):288–94.

44. Pittet-Cuenod B, della Santa D, Chamay A. Total anterior tenoarthrolysis to treat inveterate flexion contraction of the fingers: a series of 16 patients. Ann Plast Surg 1991;26(4):358–64.

45. Abbiati G, Delaria G, Saporiti E, et al. The treatment of chronic flexion contractures of the proximal interphalangeal joint. J Hand Surg Br 1995; 20(3):385–9.

46. Mansat M, Delprat J. Contractures of the proximal interphalangeal joint. Hand Clin 1992;8(4):777–86.

47. Diao E, Eaton RG. Total collateral ligament excision for contractures of the proximal interphalangeal joint. J Hand Surg Am 1993;18(3):395–402.

Treating Congenital Proximal Interphalangeal Joint Contracture

Sarah M. Yannascoli, MD, Charles A. Goldfarb, MD*

KEYWORDS

- Proximal interphalangeal joint • Contracture • Camptodactyly • Congenital

KEY POINTS

- Congenital proximal interphalangeal (PIP) joint contracture, also known as camptodactyly, is a nontraumatic PIP joint flexion deformity most commonly affecting 1 or both small fingers, sometimes involving other fingers in isolation or in conjunction with a small finger deformity, and presenting in a bimodal age distribution during periods of rapid growth (<2 years old and >10 years old).
- There is no unified consensus on the cause of camptodactyly; however, the comprehensive theory of an imbalance between the flexor and extensor mechanisms acting across the PIP joint is well accepted.
- Early, diligent passive stretching, extensor strengthening, and splinting regimens are often successful and sufficient, leading therapy to be the mainstay of treatment. These protocols must be altered based on patient age and activity level.
- Surgical treatment should proceed in a stepwise manner addressing the skin, underlying fascial structures, intrinsic muscles, lateral bands, flexor digitorum superficialis tendon, intrinsic PIP joint disorder, and secondary distal interphalangeal joint deformity.
- Patient expectations must be managed preoperatively, compliance is a requirement, and the goals of surgery should be to place the digit in a more functional and extended position, while maintaining finger flexion.

CURRENT DEFINITION

Congenital proximal interphalangeal (PIP) joint contracture is often referred to as camptodactyly. The term camptodactyly stems from a Greek word translated as bent finger.[1] Its first description was likely by Tamplin in 1846, whose *Lectures on the Nature and Treatment of Deformities* described a congenital flexion contracture.[1] Still, the term camptodactyly was not applied until 1906, when Landouzy used it to describe young girls with fixed flexion deformities of the PIP joint.[2]

The current accepted definition of camptodactyly is a nontraumatic finger PIP joint flexion deformity, often occurring bilaterally. Patients present in a bimodal age distribution during periods of rapid growth. Younger patients, less than 2 years old, are classified as having infantile camptodactyly, whereas patients greater than 10 years old are classed as having

Disclosure: The authors have no disclosures of any relationship with a commercial company that has a direct financial interest in subject matter or materials discussed in this article or with a company making a competing product.

Department of Orthopedic Surgery, Washington University School of Medicine, 660 South Euclid Avenue, Campus Box 8233, St Louis, MO 63110, USA

* Corresponding author.

E-mail address: goldfarbc@wustl.edu

Hand Clin 34 (2018) 237–249
https://doi.org/10.1016/j.hcl.2017.12.013

adolescent camptodactyly. Camptodactyly has been described in conjunction with numerous other congenital anomalies. Difficulty in identifying a unifying cause and treatment recommendation has left the full characterization of the condition controversial.

CAUSE

Despite the vast array of descriptions, theories, and pathologic structures implicated in campto-dactyly, the exact cause remains debatable. Some of the earliest reports on the condition by Landouzy in 1906 identified tuberculosis and rheumatic disorders to be the underlying cause of this disorder.[3] In 1954, Oldfield[2] attributed his findings to sluggish peripheral circulation found predominantly in young women. By the late 1960s, Courtemanche[3] and Smith and Kaplan[4] described a nontraumatic flexion defor-mity of the PIP joint without evidence of circula-tory compromise. Courtemanche[3] additionally noted volar skin tightness with passive exten-sion, as well as abnormal insertion of the fourth lumbrical in 2 of 3 cases.[3] McFarlane and colleagues[5] found similar abnormalities in the insertion of the fourth lumbrical in 21 consecu-tive cases with absence or diminished appear-ance of the palmar interossei in a small subset of patients. In a later study, he had accumulated a total of 74 consecutive cases, all with fourth lumbrical anomalies or complete absence (4%).[6] Siegert and colleagues[7] identified only 2 lumbrical abnormalities in 17 cases, suggesting that the inability of the volar skin to stretch during rapid growth was the primary pathologic cause of the deformity. Ogino and Kato[8] described a hypoplastic flexor digitorum superfi-cialis (FDS) tendon with no continuity of the distal end with the proximal muscle in 5 of 6 pa-tients, with others identifying tightness or slow retraction of the FDS tendon to be the cause.[4] In addition to implicating many of these struc-tures, Smith and Grobbelaar[9] further identified adherence of the lateral bands to the proximal phalanx as a cause of loss of extension force. Congenital absence of the extensor mechanism or central slip have been described,[10] and extensor mechanism anomalies were implicated as the primary cause of camptodactyly by Koman and colleagues.[11] Smith and Kaplan[4] succinctly summarized that nearly every anatomic structure at the base of the finger has been implicated as the deforming disorder in camptodactyly.

Later publications acknowledged the hetero-geneous causes, unifying the description as an imbalance in the flexion and extension forces acting on the PIP joint. Although it is possible that a single structure may be the primary cause for the development of this condition, at presentation there are often multiple structures involved in the pathogenesis of the disease, given that these abnormal forces lead to secondary changes and deformities. Thus, when considering surgical intervention, many have advocated a stepwise assessment of all potentially involved structures (skin, fascia, the FDS tendon, lumbricals, interossei, lateral bands, volar plate, accessory collateral ligaments, joint surfaces, and central slip insertion).[9,12,13]

CLINICAL PRESENTATION

The true incidence of congenital PIP joint contracture is unknown, but it has been reported to occur in less than 1% of the popula-tion.[1,4,9,14–16] It has been noted to affect male and female patients equally[3,9,11,17] but in other studies has been found to affect female patients more commonly.[1,5–8,18,19] Patients present in a bimodal age distribution, with early or infantile presentation occurring before the age of 2 years (**Fig. 1**A, B), and late or adolescent presentation occurring after 10 years of age (**Fig. 1**C, D). Engber and Flatt[1] found patient presentation to occur within the first year of life in 84%, more than the age of 10 years in 13%, with only 3% (2 patients) presenting between the ages of 1 and 10 years. Progression of the PIP joint deformity has been noted until 20 years of age[1]; however, conventional theory describes halting of progression once skeletal growth has ceased.[7] The deformity is painless, and many patients present with a concern over appearance and functional limitations such as difficulty typing, playing a musical instrument, participating in sporting activities, or wearing gloves.

The characteristic presentation is a flexion deformity of the PIP joint. However, many have noted compensatory intrinsic minus posturing of the hand with metacarpophalangeal (MCP) joint hyperextension,[1,3,5] as well as a secondary boutonnière deformity with distal interphalangeal (DIP) joint hyperextension.[12,13] The PIP joint flexion deformity may be fixed or correctable, but there is no natural history evidence that the deformity progresses from a correctable form to a fixed contracture.[6,7,9,16] Likewise, it has not been shown that a fixed deformity represents the end stage of disease. The deformity classi-cally involves the small finger, sometimes

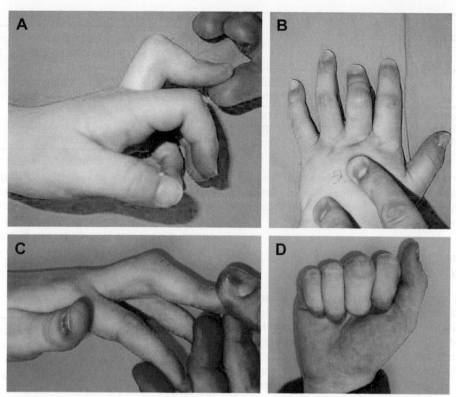

Fig. 1. The clinical presentation of camptodactyly. (*A*, *B*) Infantile presentation with isolated long finger involvement. (*C*) Adolescent presentation with more mild deformity. (*D*) Note that full finger flexion is maintained.

involving multiple digits, and is often bilateral and asymmetric. Many clinicians think that the ulnar aspect of the hand is more frequently involved; however, Rhee and colleagues[17] found that the long finger was most commonly affected in a cohort of children less than 3 years old (22 patients, 61 fingers). Koman and colleagues[11] found equal prevalence of long finger, ring finger, and small finger involvement, with the index finger being the rarest presentation. In a series of 142 patients, Miura and colleagues[19] identified 44% of patients with isolated small finger presentation, 11% with small finger and other digits involved, and 29% with no small finger involvement. This finding was mirrored by Evans and colleagues,[15] who identified 55% of cases to involve the small finger.

CLASSIFICATION

Multiple classification systems have been described for camptodactyly, all of which are descriptive. Initial classification of camptodactyly used the bimodal age presentation to describe congenital and acquired types. The congenital type was described as affecting boys and girls

equally and was isolated to small finger involvement. The acquired variant was noted in adolescents and more commonly identified in girls.[3] Similarly, the terminology of early and delayed was used according to age of onset. Courtemanche[3] disliked this terminology given that it did not have relevance to the severity, cause, or management of the condition. He preferred to classify the condition based on the number of involved digits. He thought that multiple-digit involvement showed volar skin shortage only, whereas single-digit involvement isolated to the small finger was representative of abnormal lumbrical insertion.[3] Siegert and colleagues[7] separated patients into simple and complex types, with the latter having additional finger anomalies in addition to a PIP joint contracture. Benson and colleagues[14] were the first to divide camptodactyly into types, describing type I as an isolated, infantile presentation, type II as a deformity occurring during adolescence, and type III as a deformity presenting in conjunction with other congenital anomalies (**Table 1**). Foucher and colleagues[16] described a classification system based on whether the PIP joint was fixed or correctable. However, despite this differentiation, they did not

Table 1
Classification of camptodactyly

Type I	Infantile
Type II	Adolescent
Type III	Syndromic

From Benson LS, Waters PM, Kamil NI, et al. Camptodactyly: classification and results of nonoperative treatment. J Pediatr Orthop 1994;14(6):814–9; with permission.

find a consistent association between a fixed or correctable deformity and age of presentation, finger involved, family history, or associated syndromes.

INHERITANCE AND ASSOCIATED CONDITIONS

The most common presentation of camptodactyly is sporadic occurrence without a family history.[1] The familial variant shows an autosomal dominant pattern of inheritance with variable penetrance.[1] Flexion contractures associated with clinodactyly, syndactyly, polydactyly, brachydactyly, or longitudinal ray defects represent a different form of camptodactyly,[1] and have been classified as complex camptodactyly by Siegert and colleagues.[7] In addition, camptodactyly has been associated with several syndromes, including arthrogryposis, mucopolysaccharidoses, Marfan syndrome, trisomy 13 and other chromosomal trisomy disorders, oculodentaldigital dysplasia, Freeman-Sheldon syndrome, windblown hand, and camptomelic dysplasia.[1,19,20]

DIFFERENTIAL DIAGNOSIS

Accurate diagnosis can be deduced from a thorough history and clinical examination. First, an appropriate history specifically assessing for traumatic injuries, family history, and other congenital anomalies must be obtained.

Traumatic Boutonniere Deformity

Any history of trauma, swelling, pain, and/or DIP joint hyperextension should alert the examiner to a traumatic boutonnière deformity.

Dupuytren Contracture

Dupuytren contracture may have a family history; however, this rarely presents in younger patients and MCP contracture, palpable cords, skin dimpling, and nodules are typically present on physical examination.

Trigger Finger

Trigger finger in pediatric patients can similarly present with a fixed flexion contracture, frank triggering, or decreased range of motion.[21] Careful examination to evaluate for a palpable mass over the MCP joint reveals nodularity of the flexor tendons.

Extensor Mechanism Absence

The patient's ability to actively extend the finger should be carefully evaluated, allowing the provider to distinguish between a contracture and possible absence of the extensor mechanism.[10] Weakness of the extensor mechanism can be a contributing factor in a diagnosis of camptodactyly; therefore, carefully assessing finger extension (discussed later) is important for guiding both nonoperative and operative treatment.

Arthrogryposis

The diagnosis of arthrogryposis is given when 2 or more body areas have congenital joint contractures. Distal arthrogryposis refers to a subset of these patients in whom the proximal, larger joints are spared, and contractures are isolated to the hands and feet. Although these patients may also present with PIP joint contractures mimicking camptodactyly, the MCP joints are often involved with a flexion and ulnar deviation deformity. In addition, the thumb and first web space may be involved, distinguishing it from classic camptodactyly (**Fig. 2**).[22]

PHYSICAL EXAMINATION

Once the diagnosis of camptodactyly has been made, there are several specific examination maneuvers that assist in the understanding and ultimate management of the condition. Given the lack of a singular pathologic entity, the integration of the clinical examination with surgical technique is essential to achieving an effective solution. Should surgical management be pursued, each physical examination maneuver should guide surgeons with their intraoperative decision making[9,12,16]:

1. The skin should be assessed for tightness and presence of a pterygium.
   - Treatment requires Z-plasties, a rotational flap, and possible need for full-thickness skin grafting.
2. The degree of PIP joint contracture should be noted with the wrist and MCP joint flexed.
   - Wrist and MCP joint flexion takes tension off the FDS tendon, allowing assessment of the volar plate and intrinsic joint structures.[1,4,12]

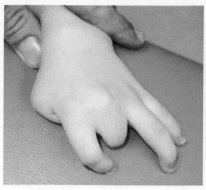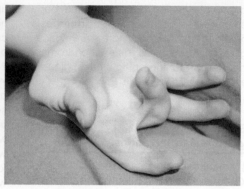

Fig. 2. A patient with distal arthrogryposis with associated camptodactyly, type III. Note the slight MCP flexion and ulnar deviation of the fingers, as well as involvement of the thumb.

3. The degree of PIP joint passive extension should be tested with the wrist and MCP joint maximally extended.
   - Loss of passive PIP joint extension indicates tightness in the flexor tendons.[16]
4. Evaluation of active PIP joint extension with the MCP joint flexed (Bouvier maneuver).
   - This maneuver identifies attenuation of the central slip, which can be corrected with postoperative splinting, PIP joint pinning, or tendon transfer at the time of surgery.
5. Assessment of DIP joint hyperextension indicating a boutonnière deformity.
   - Rarely, a terminal tenotomy may be indicated for correction of a fixed, secondary deformity at the DIP joint.[12]
6. Assessment of flexor digitorum profundus (FDP) strength.
   - If planning to transect the FDS tendon, adequate FDP strength must be maintained to preserve finger flexion.
7. If the small finger is involved, examination for independent small finger FDS function is important if considering surgical intervention, particularly a tendon transfer.[6,16]
   - The small finger FDS tendon should be isolated by maintaining the index finger, long finger, and ring finger PIP joints in extension while the patient attempts to flex the small finger.
   - If the small finger FDS is unable to fire, allow the ring finger to flex with the small finger to identify a tendon that is functional but not independent from the ring finger FDS.

RADIOGRAPHIC FINDINGS

Radiographic changes are frequently noted and radiograph examination may be helpful during the initial visit. The head of the proximal phalanx is examined for evidence of degeneration and joint congruency. Camptodactyly produces flattening and beaking of the proximal phalangeal head.[13] As beaking of the proximal phalangeal head increases, the middle phalanx subluxates volarly. This volar translation can cause the volar lip of the middle phalangeal base to create an indentation in the volar neck of the proximal phalanx.[13] The angulation of the phalangeal condyles in relation to the phalangeal shaft has also been noted to be increased (**Fig. 3**).[1] In a series of 155 fingers by Foucher and colleagues,[16] they identified 29% to have radiographic phalangeal bony changes, with findings increased to 58% if the PIP joint had a fixed contracture. Ogino and Kato[8] identified radiographic abnormalities in 63% of 35 patients with small finger camptodactyly. Remodeling of the PIP joint radiographic abnormalities after correction by nonoperative or operative means has been reported[18,20] and recently was studied by Netscher and colleagues,[13] who followed serial radiographs of surgical patients who underwent soft tissue correction and documented radiographic remodeling 9 months after surgery in 15 of 16 children. In older patients with significant PIP joint degeneration, soft tissue surgery is

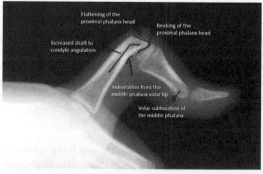

Fig. 3. Radiographic changes noted in association with camptodactyly.

unlikely to provide lasting correction, and bony procedures such as osteotomy or arthrodesis were recommended.[1,9] Furthermore, rare space-occupying lesions, such as osteochondromas, have been noted on radiographic examination as the cause of camptodactylylike PIP joint flexion deformity.

TREATMENT
Managing Patient Expectations

Managing patient expectations is the most important aspect of treatment in patients with campto-dactyly. The complex nature of the condition should be explained, emphasizing that diligent adherence to passive stretching and splinting protocols is often sufficient and can achieve an acceptable result. It is important that families understand that the deformity worsens during periods of rapid growth. A therapy protocol to which the family subscribes is especially important during these periods. Patients should be counseled to accept mild deformity and be discouraged from early operative intervention. Patients with more severe contracture should be encouraged to comply with nonoperative regimens, because increased severity of the joint contracture has not been correlated with worse outcomes or end-stage disease.[6,7,9,16] Patients should be aware that surgery has not yielded consistent results in any case series, and unrealistic expectations of a normal finger are not the goal of surgical correction. Evans and colleagues[15] recently showed that surgical correction did not improve overall arc of motion but placed the existing arc of motion in a more functional, hygienic position for improved large-object grasp. These goals should be discussed with the patient at length before surgery.

Nonoperative Treatment

Passive stretching protocols and splinting regimens are the mainstay of treatment of camptodac-tyly. In order to properly institute these regimens, many clinicians have emphasized the need for strict compliance and frequent initial visits to reinforce teaching points.[7,17–19] A lack of motivation from the patient or family to comply with these regimens excludes the patient as a surgical candidate. Only patients who show no improvement or progression despite compliance for at least 3 months are offered surgery.[15]

Outcomes

Results of conservative treatment have generally been encouraging compared with the unpredictable results associated with surgical intervention. Engber and Flatt[1] followed 14 patients who underwent passive stretching and splinting, and noted improvement in 43%, compared with surgical treatment, which yielded improved results in only 19%. Hori and colleagues[18] used a strict 24-hour-per-day Cabener-type coil splint, noting improvement in 22 of 24 patients and a residual posttreatment contracture of 10°. Recurrence several years after splint discontinuation was noted. Siegert and colleagues[7] noted that patients with mild deformity (contracture <30°) who underwent conservative treatment attained good results (correction to within 20° of full PIP joint extension), whereas mild camptodactyly treated surgically produced a near doubling of the flexion deformity postoperatively (19°–39°). Moderate deformities (30°–60°) additionally had overall greater improvement with conservative management compared with surgically treated patients, leading the investigators to recommend surgical intervention only for severe contractures of greater than 60°.[7] Miura and colleagues[19] instituted a dynamic splint for 12 h/d in children less than 6 years old, and 24 h/d in those who were greater than 6 years old. Only 3.5% (5 patients of 142 cases) failed conservative treatment. Those who failed conservative therapy went on to surgical intervention, during which an abnormal structure was noted to be anchored to the proximal phalanx in all cases.[19] Rhee and colleagues[17] showed that a regimen consisting of passive stretching only in children less than 3 years old could attain significant improvement without loss of flexion in 20 of 22 patients. The average time to full extension or plateau was 5 months (mild, <30° contracture), 10 months (moderate, 30°–60°), and 13 months (severe, >60°). They emphasized frequent visits during initial treatment to ensure the parents were performing the stretch properly with the wrist and MCP joint extended. In a small series of 8 children with multidigit involvement (27 digits), Koman and colleagues[11] found that although stretching and splinting prevented progression, it did not produce significant improvement.

Recommended protocol
There are 4 components to our nonoperative treatment.

Passive stretching First, and depending on patient age, our protocol includes passive stretching at least 4 times each day for 5 minutes. Patients are counseled generally on isolated PIP joint stretching, placing a finger on the dorsum of the proximal phalanx, and using the thumb to apply force to the volar aspect of the middle phalanx. In young patients, parents are counseled to stretch with each diaper change, whereas, in adolescents, success depends on patient and family engagement.

Active extensor strengthening Second, many patients present with weakness in the extensor mechanism. The authors therefore supplement passive stretching of the volar structures with active extension exercises. Initial repetitions of PIP joint extension with MCP joint flexion can later be supplemented with resistance either by using a rubber band wrapped around the hand and involved finger (**Fig. 4**), or by extending the finger into putty.

Nighttime static, progressive splint Third, a nighttime static extension splint can be effective and is usually well tolerated and can be worn during naptime and bedtime. These splints are fashioned by our therapist in a position of maximal extension. The splint can be modified at each subsequent therapy visit as extension improves. For children less than 8 years old, a forearm-based splint is required to maintain the splint in place. Children and adolescents more than 8 years old generally do well with hand-based splints. Standard Velcro is placed over the hand to secure the splint, and elastic strap is placed over the dorsum of the PIP joint to provide an additional, constant stretch (**Fig. 5**).

Dynamic finger extension splint In addition, and again depending on patient age, a dynamic splint can be used during selected waking hours for a more intense stretch. The authors have found adolescents who are very active during the day and unable to comply with stretching and active extensor strengthening protocols to benefit the most from this splint. It is generally recommended only for flexion contractures less than 45°.

Operative Treatment

Described surgical procedures

The variety of anatomic structures associated with camptodactyly has led to several surgical techniques to address the pathologic cause. Almost all surgical procedures report addressing volar skin tightness with Z-plasties, rotational flaps, full-thickness skin grafting, or cross-finger flaps. Several have implicated an abnormal lumbrical insertion as the cause of camptodactyly, leading to excision of abnormal insertions[1,5] or reinsertion of the lumbrical to the lateral bands.[3] Smith and Kaplan[4] were proponents of FDS sectioning, finding that the location of sectioning (finger, palm, or wrist) was unimportant.[4] FDS sectioning with subsequent transfer to the extensor mechanism has been advocated in the setting of weak PIP joint extension[1,6]; however, this has been discouraged by some clinicians because of its restriction on immediate postoperative range of motion.[7] Some have proposed transfer of the ring finger FDS to the extensor mechanism of the involved small finger in patients who lack an independent small finger FDS tendon.[5] The Zancolli lasso procedure has been used in patients who have active, full PIP joint extension with MCP joint flexion (positive Bouvier maneuver).[6,16,23] Patients with an intrinsic PIP joint contracture often undergo release of the volar plate and collateral ligaments.[6,8] PIP joint pinning has been used to augment joint release, repairs, or transfers for the immediate postoperative period.[1,6,8,15] Most protocols institute some measure of postoperative splinting to mediate extensor tendon attenuation rather than directly addressing the extensor surface through surgical means.[12,20] One group did advocate using a dorsal approach to allow lateral band relocation and release of the transverse retinacular ligament.[11]

Indications

Surgical treatment is reserved for patients who have failed aggressive splinting and stretching regimens.[7,14,19] Lack of compliance with these regimens should alert the surgeon that postoperative compliance may also be compromised. Patients who show failure to improve with

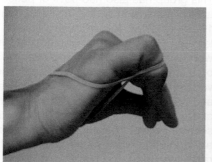
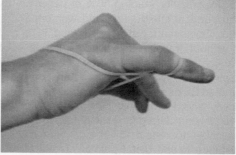

Fig. 4. Active extensor strengthening against resistance using a rubber band wrapped around the hand and the involved finger middle phalanx.

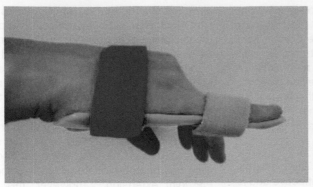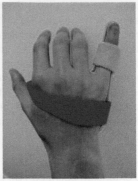

Fig. 5. A typical hand-based, nighttime static splint, which can be remolded for maximal PIP joint extension at each therapy visit. Note the elastic strap placed over the dorsal aspect of the PIP joint to provide additional stretch.

adherence to a stretching and splinting regimen for more than 3 months[15] and have progressive, severe deformity with functional limitations are generally the best candidates for surgery. Some clinicians have advocated that contractures greater than 30° warranted intervention,[5,6,13] but lack of convincing improvement has led many to less aggressive indications, offering surgery for patients with a contracture greater than 60°[7,9,15] or 70°.[11]

Outcomes

Surgical results of camptodactyly correction have been generally discouraging. In addition to less-than-optimal results, variations in surgical techniques have increased uncertainty for the most effective surgical intervention. Engber and Flatt[1] identified 18 patients who underwent 20 corrective operations and showed improvement in 35%, no difference in 30%, and worse results in 35%. Worse results were associated with phalangeal joint recontouring and decompression. In 1990, Siegert and colleagues[7] described a classification system for results, labeling outcomes as excellent, good, fair, or poor based on the degree of residual contracture and loss of flexion. In their cohort, surgical intervention yielded 0 excellent, 7 good, 6 fair, and 25 poor results, leading 50% of patients to state that surgical intervention had worsened the problem. Ogino and Kato[8] performed FDS sectioning without transfer and found improvements in active extension but noted a loss of flexion postoperatively. McFarlane and colleagues[6] treated 35 cases of isolated small finger camptodactyly and found only 50% to have a less than 15° flexion deformity at final follow-up, with 33% unable to regain full flexion with an average distance to the distal palmar crease of 1.8 cm. Koman and colleagues[11] performed FDS sectioning in 8 digits and found no improvement

but had 10 good and 2 fair results when the extensor mechanism was realigned. These studies represent a heterogeneous group with regard to camptodactyly type, treatment approach, and surgical technique. In addition, they are limited by their small cohorts in many subgroups, varied and often short-term follow-up, and retrospective nature. Nonetheless, although moderate successes had been shown, overall outcomes were severely short of optimal.

Once the understanding that all structures in and around the PIP joint may be involved, either primarily or by secondary compensation, surgeons began to address all potential deforming forces intraoperatively. This development led many to proceed with a stepwise surgical approach to manage the deformity and produced improved surgical outcomes.[9,12,13,15] Smith and Grobbelaar[9] had 83% good to excellent results using a stepwise approach, noting only 1 poor result in a patient who had degeneration of the PIP joint before surgery. Netscher and colleagues[13] used a stepwise approach to show improvement in radiographic PIP joint deformity in 15 of 16 patients, noting a decrease in the average contracture from 62° preoperatively to 4° postoperatively. This group has also had 83% of patients with full active extension with no recurrences after 11 months of follow-up.[12] Foucher and colleagues[16] compared their outcomes in patients who were treated before and after the institution of a stepwise surgical approach, finding 55% versus 86% improvement, respectively. Evans and colleagues[15] noted no improvement in either active or passive PIP joint range of motion in their series; however, they found that the postoperative arc of motion was in a more extended, and thus more functional and hygienic, position. These results, although only modestly improved, have been encouraging to surgeons who treat this complex deformity. This stepwise approach integrates the preoperative examination with the intraoperative findings to bring some consistency to a procedure that has historically been unsystematic.

Recommended protocol

Preoperative planning Some clinicians have argued to delay surgical intervention until the patient has reached maturity and the growth plates of the finger have closed.[18] Others have noted that radiographic remodeling may still be possible while the physes remain open, thus advocating early surgical intervention in patients with impending radiographic joint destruction to improve skeletal alignment of the PIP joint.[13] Because of the skeletal alignment, as well as increased plasticity of the tissues in younger patients, the authors prefer to intervene once it is clear that conservative treatment is not effective, compliance has been established, and the patient and family have realistic expectations. On deciding to proceed with surgery, a detailed preoperative examination helps guide surgical techniques (discussed earlier). Radiographic changes showing articular degeneration in older patients warrant salvage operations with either a PIP joint arthrodesis or a proximal phalanx osteotomy.[1]

Operative technique Our approach[12] is a summary of published techniques with acceptable success and personal experience. Steps 1 to 4 and 9 are always performed, whereas steps 5 to 8 depend on the preoperative examination and intraoperative findings:

- Step 1: skin
  - Planning for adequate soft tissue coverage after correction is essential. Z-plasties, rotational flaps, full-thickness skin grafting, and cross-finger flaps have been reported. In most patients with a camptodactyly of at least 60°, the authors have found Z-plasties insufficient and prefer a random pattern rotational flap for exposure and coverage of the volar defect (**Fig. 6**).
- Step 2: subcutaneous tissues and fascia
  - Release of the subcutaneous fibrous tissue allows both exposure and occasionally minor deformity correction.
- Step 3: assessment of lumbrical and FDS anatomy
  - The lumbricals must be identified and their insertions traced distally. Any anomalous insertions are removed (**Fig. 7**). The lumbrical insertion and lateral bands are inspected from the volar aspect of the finger and any adhesions to the proximal phalanx are released using a tenotomy scissor or Freer.
- Step 4: FDS tenotomy

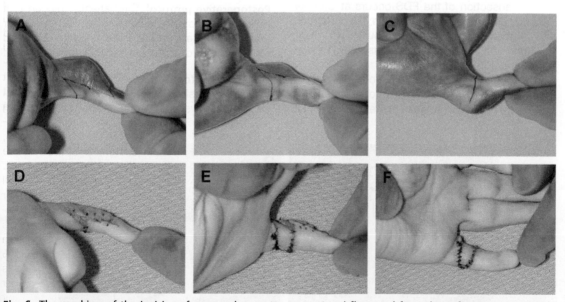

Fig. 6. The marking of the incisions for a random pattern rotational flap used for volar soft tissue coverage in camptodactyly. (*A*) The flap is drawn over the dorsal aspect of the finger with the distal tip reaching to the level of the DIP joint. (*B*) The volar, proximal incision is curvilinear starting from the palmodigital crease and carried over the middle of the proximal phalanx. (*C*) This incision is carried to the other side of the finger to approximately the level of the midaxial line. (*D–F*) After insetting and closure of the flap allowing correction of the deformity.

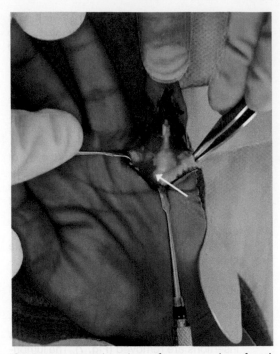

Fig. 7. Intraoperative view of an anomalous fourth lumbrical insertion into the flexor tendon sheath (*white arrow*).

○ Assuming adequate FDP strength on preoperative examination, the authors include FDS transection as a part of our approach. Transection of the FDS occurs at Camper chiasm after entry into the flexor tendon sheath proximal to the A3 pulley.

• Step 5: release of intrinsic PIP joint contracture
  ○ If on preoperative examination flexion of the wrist and MCP joint does not allow full PIP joint extension, release of the proximal volar

plate and accessory collateral ligaments is performed.

• Step 6: correction of PIP joint extension lag
  ○ If preoperative Bouvier maneuver shows a mild extension lag (<60°), the patient receives a postoperative splint for 4 weeks.
  ○ If the preoperative Bouvier maneuver shows a severe extension lag (>70°), a tendon transfer using the released FDS to the extensor mechanism is performed.

• Step 7: PIP joint pinning
  ○ Once surgical correction is obtained, tension is required to maintain this correction, and the PIP joint is pinned using a Kirschner wire appropriately sized according to the age and size of the patient. The pin is left in place for 7 to 10 days before initiation of postoperative therapy (discussed later).

• Step 8: terminal tenotomy
  ○ Rarely, a hyperextended DIP joint warrants release of the terminal tendon.

• Step 9: release of the tourniquet
  ○ It is of critical importance to release the tourniquet before termination of the procedure to assess digit perfusion in full extension. Should the neurovascular bundles limit full correction, the PIP joint should be placed in the appropriate degree of flexion to maximize correction and permit perfusion (**Fig. 8**).

Postoperative protocol The patient is placed in a bulky, soft postoperative dressing with the finger maximally extended, and the fingertip exposed for monitoring of perfusion and fingertip sensation.

Ten days postoperative
Patients are asked to return to the office approximately 10 days after surgery. The surgical team

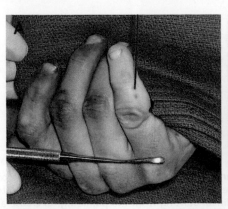
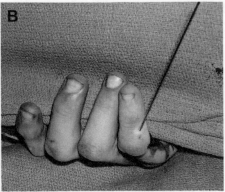

Fig. 8. (*A*) Release of the tourniquet at the end of the procedure shows an avascular, white fingertip. (*B*) Removal of the pin, allowing the PIP joint to flex, restores perfusion. The finger is pinned in slight flexion in order to avoid digital ischemia.

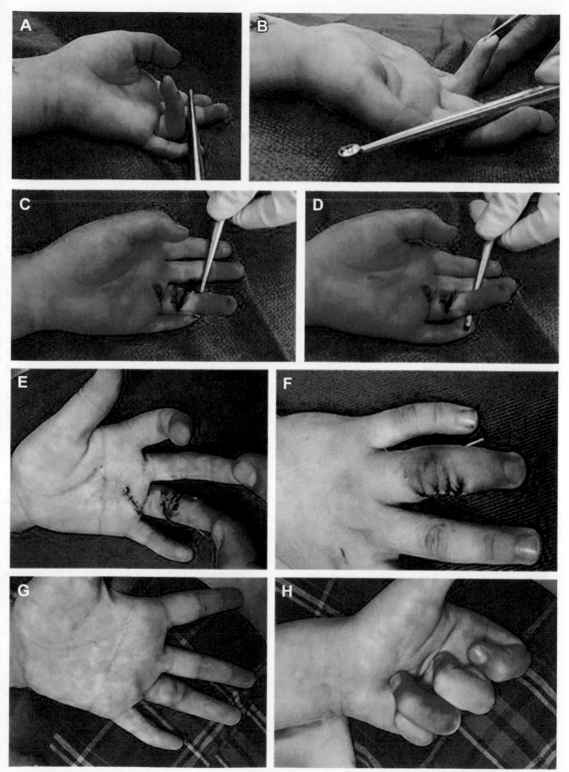

Fig. 9. Clinical example of surgical treatment of camptodactyly of the ring finger. (*A*) Preoperative flexion contracture. (*B*) Passive extension shows persistent, significant deformity. (*C*, *D*) After operative correction and PIP joint pinning. Note the use of a random pattern rotational flap for volar skin coverage. An additional proximal incision allows inspection of the lumbricals and proximal FDS tendon. (*E*, *F*) At the 2-week postoperative visit. (*G*, *H*) Clinical views at final follow-up showing full active extension without loss of full finger flexion.

removes the initial dressing to assess the incision and remove the PIP joint pin if placed intraoperatively. Therapy is asked to initiate scar management and edema control, as well as fashion a forearm-based or hand-based finger extension splint depending on the age and maturity of the child. The splint is worn at all times but removed hourly for the following therapy exercises:

- The authors initiate active and passive MCP joint range of motion.
- Active PIP joint extension with MCP held in flexion is taught.
- Ranges of motion for the PIP joint and DIP joint are initiated via proximal and middle phalanx blocking exercises, respectively.
- Passive PIP joint flexion is avoided if an extension transfer has been performed.

Four weeks postoperative

The patient returns at 4 weeks postoperatively and may occasionally remove the splint for light activity and continuation of the exercises discussed earlier.

Six weeks postoperative

At 6 weeks postoperatively, passive flexion of the PIP joint may begin for patients who underwent a tendon transfer. If a flexion contracture of the PIP joint has recurred, a dynamic finger extension splint may be initiated. The static extension splint is now worn only at night.

Twelve weeks postoperative

By 12 weeks postoperatively the nighttime splint is discontinued, unless there is a residual PIP joint extension lag. Progressive strengthening is initiated.

Final assessment

A final assessment makes specific note of active and passive range of motion, sensation, ability to perform activities of daily living, a functional assessment, and grip strength (**Fig. 9**).

SUMMARY

Congenital PIP joint contracture-camptodactyly is a nontraumatic PIP joint flexion deformity caused by an imbalance between the flexion and extension forces that act across the joint. Managing patient expectations is the cornerstone of successful outcomes. All deformities are initially treated with a passive stretching protocol and splinting regimen, often showing sufficient correction and allowing the patient to show motivation and compliance. Surgery is only considered for contracture greater than 60°, failed conservative measures, and persistent limitations in function. The preoperative

physical examination and radiographs help guide surgical treatment, which should proceed in a stepwise manner addressing all potentially involved structures. To date, the efficacy of surgical outcomes remains modest and continued efforts to improve on current techniques are necessary.

REFERENCES

1. Engber WD, Flatt AE. Camptodactyly: an analysis of sixty-six patients and twenty-four operations. J Hand Surg Am 1977;2(3):216–24.
2. Oldfield MC. Campylodactyly: flexor contracture of the fingers in young girls. Br J Plast Surg 1956; 8(4):312–7.
3. Courtemanche AD. Campylodactyly: etiology and management. Plast Reconstr Surg 1969;44(5):451–4.
4. Smith RJ, Kaplan EB. Camptodactyly and similar atraumatic flexion deformities of the proximal interphalangeal joints of the fingers. A study of thirty-one cases. J Bone Joint Surg Am 1968;50(6): 1187–203.
5. McFarlane RM, Curry GI, Evans HB. Anomalies of the intrinsic muscles in camptodactyly. J Hand Surg Am 1983;8(5 Pt 1):531–44.
6. McFarlane RM, Classen DA, Porte AM, et al. The anatomy and treatment of camptodactyly of the small finger. J Hand Surg Am 1992;17(1):35–44.
7. Siegert JJ, Cooney WP, Dobyns JH. Management of simple camptodactyly. J Hand Surg Br 1990;15(2): 181–9.
8. Ogino T, Kato H. Operative findings in camptodactyly of the little finger. J Hand Surg Br 1992;17(6): 661–4.
9. Smith PJ, Grobbelaar AO. Camptodactyly: a unifying theory and approach to surgical treatment. J Hand Surg Am 1998;23(1):14–9.
10. Carneiro RS. Congenital attenuation of the extensor tendon central slip. J Hand Surg Am 1993;18(6): 1004–7.
11. Koman LA, Toby EB, Poehling GG. Congenital flexion deformities of the proximal interphalangeal joint in children: a subgroup of camptodactyly. J Hand Surg Am 1990;15(4):582–6.
12. Hamilton KL, Netscher DT. Evaluation of a stepwise surgical approach to camptodactyly. Plast Reconstr Surg 2015;135(3):568e–76e.
13. Netscher DT, Hamilton KL, Paz L. Soft-tissue surgery for camptodactyly corrects skeletal changes. Plast Reconstr Surg 2015;136(5):1028–35.
14. Benson LS, Waters PM, Kamil NI, et al. Camptodactyly: classification and results of nonoperative treatment. J Pediatr Orthop 1994;14(6):814–9.
15. Evans BT, Waters PM, Bae DS. Early results of surgical management of camptodactyly. J Pediatr Orthop 2017;37(5):e317–20.

16. Foucher G, Lorea P, Khouri RK, et al. Campto-dactyly as a spectrum of congenital deficiencies: a treatment algorithm based on clinical examination. Plast Reconstr Surg 2006;117(6): 1897–905.

17. Rhee SH, Oh WS, Lee HJ, et al. Effect of passive stretching on simple camptodactyly in children younger than three years of age. J Hand Surg Am 2010;35(11):1768–73.

18. Hori M, Nakamura R, Inoue G, et al. Nonoperative treatment of camptodactyly. J Hand Surg Am 1987;12(6):1061–5.

19. Miura T, Nakamura R, Tamura Y. Long-standing extended dynamic splintage and release of an abnormal restraining structure in camptodactyly. J Hand Surg Br 1992;17(6):665–72.

20. Hamilton KL, Netscher DT. Multidigit camptodactyly of the hands and feet: a case study. Hand (N Y) 2013;8(3):324–9.

21. Shah AS, Bae DS. Management of pediatric trigger thumb and trigger finger. J Am Acad Orthop Surg 2012;20(4):206–13.

22. Beals RK. The distal arthrogryposes: a new classification of peripheral contractures. Clin Orthop Relat Res 2005;(435):203–10.

23. Almeida SF, Monteiro AV, Lanes RC. Evaluation of treatment for camptodactyly: retrospective analysis on 40 fingers. Rev Bras Ortop 2014;49(2):134–9.

Management of Flexor Pulley Injuries with Proximal Interphalangeal Joint Contracture

Elizabeth Inkellis, MD*, Emily Altman, DPT, CHT, Scott Wolfe, MD

KEYWORDS

- Flexor pulley injuries • Flexor tendon bowstringing • PIP contractures

KEY POINTS

- Injuries to the flexor pulley system cause bowstringing and increase work of flexion.
- Neglected flexor pulley injuries with proximal interphalangeal (PIP) joint contracture are a difficult challenge.
- This article describes a technique for managing patients with delayed presentation of pulley rupture and fixed PIP flexion contracture with Digit Widget® application followed by splinting without pulley reconstruction.
- This technique allows for correction of the flexion contracture and high patient satisfaction without invasive open surgery.

INTRODUCTION

The flexor pulley system is an elegant, efficient system that converts tendon excursion to angular motion at the joints of the fingers. Injuries to the flexor pulleys cause volar displacement of the flexor tendons by disrupting the balance of the system. Closed pulley injuries may occur from an extension forced applied over a short period of time to a flexed digit, notably in rock climbers.[1] Pulley injuries may also occur postoperatively, most commonly after tendon repairs or exuberant trigger finger releases.[2] Acute, single-pulley ruptures typically are treated conservatively.[3] A statewide database review in New York State found the incidence of operative pulley reconstruction to be 0.27 per 100,000 persons, with an annual frequency of 52 procedures state wide.[4]

Anatomy

The flexor pulley system consists of 5 annual pulleys, 3 cruciate pulleys, and the palmar aponeurosis pulley.[5] The A1, A3, and A5 pulleys are located over the metacarpophalangeal (MP), proximal interphalangeal (PIP), and distal interphalangeal (DIP) joints, respectively. The critical pulleys are the A2 and A4 pulleys, which overly the proximal and middle phalanges.

Function and Biomechanics

The purpose of the pulley system is to convert the longitudinal motion of tendon excursion into angular motion across the interphalangeal joints. The pulleys maintain close contact between the flexor tendons and the phalanges, ensuring a short moment arm.[6] The system permits a 3-cm flexor

Hospital for Special Surgery, Hand and Upper Extremity Service, 535 East 70th Street, New York, NY 10021, USA
* Corresponding author.
E-mail address: liz.inkellis@gmail.com

Hand Clin 34 (2018) 251–266
https://doi.org/10.1016/j.hcl.2017.12.001
0749-0712/18/© 2018 Elsevier Inc. All rights reserved.

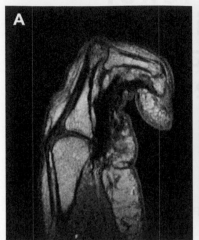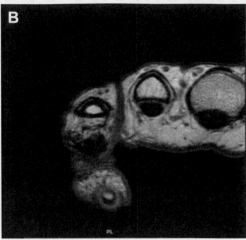

Fig. 1. (*A*) Sagittal and (*B*) Axial MRI demonstrating bowstringing in the small finger of Patient 3. Note the distance of the flexor tendon away from the volar surface of the proximal phalanx as well as the PIP flexion contracture. (*Courtesy of* S. Wolfe, MD, New York, NY.)

tendon excursion to produce a digital arc of motion of 260°.[7] With injury to the A2 pulley, the flexor tendons bowstring and translate palmarward, increasing the moment arm on the interphalangeal joints (**Fig. 1**). The inability of the relatively weak intrinsic extensor to compensate for the increased moment arm of PIP flexion leads to a flexion contracture.[7,8] The change in excursion of the flexor muscle-tendon unit that results in an effective lengthening of the tendon leads to a loss of active flexion.[1] It is widely held that the integrity of the A2 and A4 pulleys are the most important for preventing bowstringing.[9] Biomechanical studies have demonstrated that the sectioning of both the A2 and A4 pulleys leads to a 30% increase in tendon excursion and markedly increased work of flexion as well as decreased range of motion.[10]

Management of Pulley Injuries

Patients present clinically with bruising, swelling, and localized tenderness. They may recall a tearing or popping sensation at the time of injury.[11] Patients also may present after prior surgery. Bowstringing may not be present immediately and also may not always occur after isolated pulley ruptures. Although radiographs are the initial imaging modality of choice, MRI and dynamic ultrasound can both be useful in confirming pulley injuries and resultant bowstringing (**Table 1**).[12]

Conservative treatment with a ring splint or taping is recommended for isolated pulley injury.[11] In a study of 21 rock climbers with complete or

partial isolated pulley ruptures of A2, A3, or A4 treated conservatively, all had excellent clinical outcomes and regained their level of climbing within 1 year.[13] Another study examining 47 complete pulley ruptures in 45 rock climbers treated with a pulley-protection thermoplastic splint for 2 months found normalization of tendon-phalanx distance on ultrasound as well as return to climbing at their prior level in 38 of 43 patients at an average of 8.8 months.[14]

Surgical treatment is indicated for patients with multiple pulley ruptures and impairment of function or those with persistent symptoms after nonoperative treatment.[11] Reconstructive techniques are based either on weaving an

Table 1 Management of pulley rupture	
Injury	**Treatment**
Single closed pulley rupture without contracture	Conservative
Multiple pulley ruptures, persistent pain after conservative treatment, good digital range of motion	Pulley reconstruction
Pulley rupture with bowstringing and fixed PIP flexion contracture	Pulley rescue with Digit Widget followed by splinting

autogenous tendon graft through the remaining pulley rim or making a new pulley loop around bone.[2] Biomechanically, techniques incorporating a new loop around the bone are stronger.[15] Kleinert and Bennet[16] adapted the technique of Weilby, weaving a free tendon graft through the fibro-osseous pulley rim. Repairs involving a loop of graft around bone include the belt loop technique,[17] the Lister repair with extensor retinaculum,[18] the single-loop technique of Bunnell, the loop-and-a-half technique,[19] and the triple-loop technique.[20]

All of the surgical treatment modalities, however, are predicated on the absence of digital flexion contractures.[2] In the setting of subacute pulley ruptures with an interphalangeal joint contracture, the contracture must be addressed prior to proceeding with pulley reconstruction.[1] In other settings of PIP joint contracture, such as Dupuytren disease, extension torque transmitted from an external device, such as the Digit Widget (Hand Biomechanics Lab, Sacramento, California), has been used to correct the contracture.[21] The device helps resolve the torque imbalance that drives the PIP contracture. The authors have found this a useful technique to correct the imbalance associated with chronic pulley injuries and one that has the potential to avoid the need for open reconstruction of the pulley system.

Between 2014 and 2017, the authors treated 4 patients with a delayed presentation of pulley rupture and fixed PIP flexion contracture with a technique of Digit Widget application followed by splinting without pulley reconstruction. Each patient presented with a fixed PIP contracture of greater than 45°. The diagnosis of pulley rupture was made based on patient history, clinical examination demonstrating bowstringing, and imaging. MRI or ultrasound confirmed multiple pulley ruptures in each patient.

INDICATIONS

For acute isolated pulley ruptures without contracture, the authors recommend conservative treatment with a ring splint. For patients with multiple closed pulley ruptures or who have failed conservative treatment, any number of reconstructive techniques, discussed previously, can be effective. For patients with pulley ruptures and a fixed digital flexion contracture, the authors recommend a pulley rescue technique of application of the Digit Widget to produce an extension torque, followed by a precise splinting regimen. In 1 of the 4 patients, the pulley loss and bowstringing were accompanied by recurrent Dupuytren disease,

which was not considered a contraindication to this technique.

Contraindications include current or history of infection or the inability to tolerate a digital external fixator.

SURGICAL TECHNIQUE
Preoperative Planning

Prior to surgery, it is important for a to arrange a time when they are able to tolerate up to 3 months of treatment with the external fixator, followed by a prolonged period (3–6 months) of full-time to intermittent splinting. Possible concurrent procedures should also be planned, such as palmar fasciectomy, completed at the same operative setting just prior to external fixator application.

Preparation and Patient Positioning

Patients are placed supine on a standard operating table with a hand table attachment and access for fluoroscopy. An arm tourniquet may be placed but is typically not inflated. At the authors' institution, the anesthesia choice is most commonly regional anesthesia with intravenous sedation. Patients receive a standard weight-based dose of intravenous antibiotics. The arm and forearm are prepped out with chlorhexidine.

Application of External Fixator Device

The procedure is performed percutaneously with the aid of a mini fluoroscopy unit, using the manufacturer's guide for application (https://handbiolab.com/wp-content/uploads/2017/07/320401B_DW-SM-for-web.pdf). Importantly, the pin block is secured 5 mm from the dorsal skin to allow for swelling. The cuff is then attached to the patient's hand and wrist. The connector assembly is attached from the pin block to the wrist cuff. Extension torque is then generated by placing a variable number of rubber bands around the posts on the device (**Fig. 2**).

Posoperative Care

The pins are dressed in the operating room with thin strips of Xeroform gauze and then wrapped with a gauze stretch bandage. Pin site care with hydrogen peroxide with cotton swabs is initiated at 1 week postoperatively. Radiographs are monitored periodically.

Postoperative Therapy

Prior to placement of the Digit Widget, the patient has 1 visit with the hand therapist. During this visit

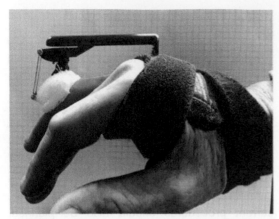

Fig. 2. Assembled Digit Widget. Note the rubber band between the posts as well as the wrist cuff. (*Courtesy of* Hand Biomechanics Lab, Sacramento, CA; and S. Wolfe, MD, New York, NY.)

the therapist explains the role of therapy in the pulley rescue protocol and evaluates the status of the PIP joint contracture, the condition of the soft tissue of the digit, and the overall mechanics of the hand and finger. The therapist preoperatively notes any special considerations, such as a tendency toward hyperextension of the MP joint during active digit extension, severely thickened and contracted tissue volar to the PIP joint, or concomitant DIP joint flexion or extension contracture. The general guideline presented to the patient is as follows:

- Minimum period of 6 weeks to 8 weeks with external fixator in place to extend the PIP joint with rubber band tension.
- Within that period, once the PIP joint has been fully extended for 1 week, testing the joint's response to torque release (removal of rubber bands) can be initiated. It is not unusual to see a surprising return of a flexed posture after a short a time, such as just a few hours. This indicates that the tissue is not ready for Digit Widget removal. If this happens, replace rubber bands and extension returns quickly.
- Once PIP joint extension can be maintained for approximately 3 days with no torque and near full-time extension splinting, Digit Widget removal can be considered. It is easy to fabricate a simple volar finger gutter splint that accommodates the fixator.
- After the Digit Widget is removed, contact with the hand therapist becomes critically important and more frequent. Each PIP joint behaves slightly differently and the patient-surgeon-therapist team needs to respond as it declares itself.

- After Digit Widget removal, the PIP joint is splinted in extension full time for as long as 16 weeks. The patient is encouraged to remove the splint and perform strictly passive digit flexion at least twice daily. Active engagement of the extrinsic finger flexors without a splint on is to be avoided. The splint may be removed for hygiene. Close monitoring of the PIP joint position is critical. If a 20° or greater loss of full PIP joint extension is allowed to re-establish itself, the patient may be on track for an aggressive return of a significant, passively uncorrectable PIP joint flexion contracture. Small PIP joint flexion contractures are relatively easy to reverse with basic splinting and stretching techniques.

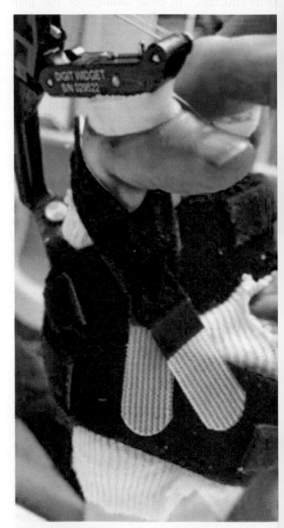

Fig. 3. Short strap holding the MP joint in slight flexion. (*Courtesy of* Hand Biomechanics Lab, Sacramento, CA; and E. Altman, DPT, CHT, New York, NY.)

The authors have found that the role of the hand therapist varies considerably from patient to patient. Some patients require more assistance with the management of the fixator whereas others quickly learn how to handle the device. At the least, 1 immediate postoperative visit is indicated to instruct patients in pin care and management of the fixator (how to remove the connector assemble from the pin block and how to apply and remove rubber bands). Every effort should be made to encourage patient independence and facility with removal of the cuff and connecting rod, changing rubber bands, and cleaning the pins. Patients are instructed to use a light (purple) rubber band and then progress to stronger bands as tolerated. Too much force results in excessive pain and inflammation, which are counterproductive. The rubber bands are removed 3 times per day for the performance of passive digit range-of-motion exercises. Active PIP and DIP blocking exercises can also be performed if the pulley is supported using the contralateral thumb. Some surgeons are comfortable allowing patients to remove the connector assembly for showering. After the initial postoperative a visit, once every

Table 2
Suggestions for managing various scenarios after Digit Widget removal

Excessive active MP joint hyperextension The extended position of the MP joint significantly diminishes the capacity of the intrinsic muscles of the hand to extend the PIP joint and should be mechanically blocked. MP joint hyperextension becomes a learned behavior seen in patients with long standing PIP flexion contractures. It moves the bent finger out of the way during hand use.	• $2\frac{1}{2}$ Buddy Ring (Silver Ring Splint, Charlottesville, VA) with half-ring on top (**Fig. 4**)
	  ○ Recommend 4-mm band width
	  ○ Use depth options according to clinical presentation and judgment
	• Thermoplastic extension block splint (**Fig. 5**)
	• Custom relative motion flexion splint (**Fig. 6**)
	• Buddy Ring (Silver Ring Splint) with offset as needed (**Fig. 7**)

Aggressive tendency of PIP joint to return to flexion	• Windowed extension splint (**Fig. 8**) • Bivalved extension splint (**Fig. 9**) • Dynamic extension splint (**Fig. 10**) • Finger gutter splint (**Fig. 11**) • Cylinder night extension splint (**Fig. 12**) • Intermittent simple extension casting (**Fig. 13**) • Combination MP joint extension block + interphalangeal extension device (**Fig. 14**)

Pulley ring options The use of pulley rings can contribute to increased swelling of the digit (possibly caused by the compromise of lymphatic drainage). This sabotages efforts to extend the PIP joint.	• Pulley Ring (Silver Ring Splint) (**Fig. 15**)
	  ○ One wide band
	  ○ Two narrow bands
	  ○ Hinged version for prominent PIP joint
	• Custom thermoplastic splint with dorsal slit (**Fig. 16**)
	• 0.5-in self-grip straps/cable ties
	  ○ Reinforce volar aspect with thin rigid thermoplastic (**Fig. 17**)

Hand therapy treatment ideas	• Paraffin + polyethylene food handling glove + dynamic extension splint + heat for pretreatment (**Fig. 18**)
	• Gentle traction of the PIP joint using distal radius fracture reduction finger trap + volar glide of proximal phalanx on the middle phalanx at the PIP joint (**Fig. 19**)
	• Focused soft tissue techniques
	  ○ Volar aspect of the PIP joint (volar plate)
	  ○ Lateral band
	  ○ Passive DIP joint flexion with PIP joint held in maximum available extension
	• Active PIP joint extension with MP joint held firmly in flexion (reverse blocking)

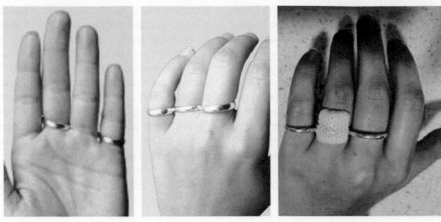

Fig. 4. A 2¹/₂ Buddy Ring (Silver Ring Splint). Half-ring is dorsal. Can be used for border digits. Limits capacity to hyperextend the MP joint of involved digit. Note addition of thermoplastic material dorsally to distribute force distribution. (*Courtesy of* Silver Ring Splint Company, Charlottesville, VA; and E. Altman, DPT, CHT, New York, NY.)

2 weeks for a brief check is usually sufficient. In some cases, the MP joint is pulled into hyperextension by the dynamic fixator mechanism. This too is counterproductive and must be managed by the addition of a small strap to hold the MP joint in slight flexion (**Fig. 3**).

After the Digit Widget has been removed, regular hand therapy visits become more important. The focus of each session is on soft tissue management and adjustments to the splint regimen. In most cases, the finger has been in a flexed position for a prolonged period

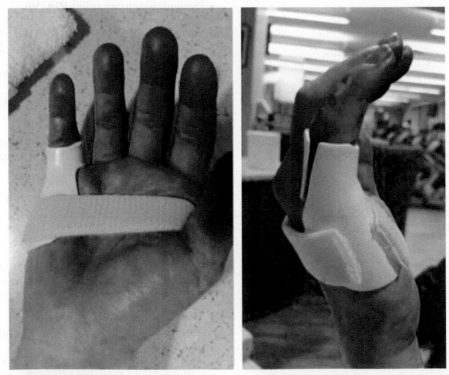

Fig. 5. Simple thermoplastic splint to block MP joint hyperextension. Can be used after the strict extension splinting phase as patient is beginning to use finger actively during the day. (*Courtesy of* E. Altman, DPT, CHT, New York, NY.)

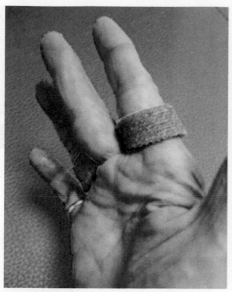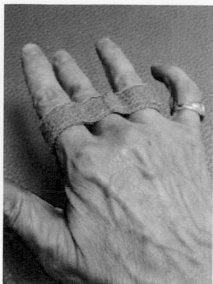

Fig. 6. Relative motion flexion splint used to limit active MP joint hyperextension. Can be fabricated for border and middle digits. (*Courtesy of* E. Altman, DPT, CHT, New York, NY.)

of time. Moist heat followed by appropriate soft tissue techniques and protected passive range-of-motion exercises are performed at each session. Patients can also actively flex the involved PIP joint if a therapist firmly applies pressure to the volar proximal phalanx and holds the MP joint in full extension, blocking bowstringing of the flexor tendons. If patients are capable of correctly performing this carefully protected active motion exercise, they may be permitted to do so at home.

After 16 weeks of strictly protected motion, patients are free to remove the extension splint during the day. Some type of pulley support device is recommended for use during the day. If the digit has a strong tendency to hyperextend

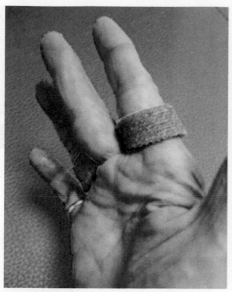

Fig. 7. Buddy Rings (Silver Ring Splint) are effective for limiting less pronounced MP joint hyperextension. (*Courtesy of* Silver Ring Splint Company, Charlottesville, VA; and E. Altman, DPT, CHT, New York, NY.)

at the MP joint with active digit extension, an MP joint extension blocking splint should be considered. Night extension splinting is recommended for up to 9 months, depending on the patient. Lifelong monitoring of the PIP joint and intermittent attention to stretching and splinting may be necessary.

Suggestions for managing various scenarios after Digit Widget removal are found in **Table 2**.

COMPLICATIONS AND MANAGEMENT

A superficial pin site infection developed in 3 of 4 patients. The average time after surgery to the infection was 6 weeks. All infections were successfully treated with a reduction in the rubber band torque across the device, adjustment of the height of the pin block by the surgeon and a 7-day course of oral cephalexin. One patient had a recurrent infection at 2 months after surgery, which was treated with a 5-day course of cephalexin as well as pin removal.

One of the 4 patients, after achieving full extension of the PIP joint, developed a recurrence of her contracture to 30° 4 months after removal of the Digit Widget. The patient was treated with intermittent LMB (DeRoyal LMB splint, Knoxville, TN) splinting and responded to splinting.

OUTCOMES

The clinical data from the authors' series are summarized in **Table 3**. Three patients were male and 1 female. The average age at presentation was 46

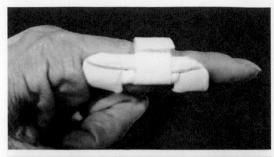

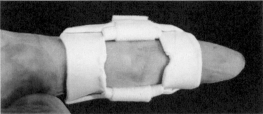

Fig. 8. Volar window, cinch strap at dorsal PIP joint, molded over straight object, such as a highlighter pen barrel. Provides effective extension force. (*Courtesy of* E. Altman, DPT, CHT, New York, NY.)

(range 33–57). Two pulley ruptures occurred with closed trauma, and 2 postoperatively (1 after zone II flexor tendon repair [patient 4] and 1 after Dupuytren excision [patient 3]). Surgery was

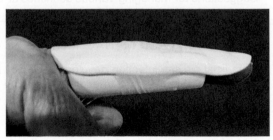

Fig. 9. Bivalve design. Use 1/16-in Polyform splint material. Volar piece is molded first over the barrel of a highlighter to ensure full extension. Distal end is trimmed to allow DIP joint flexion if desired. Side walls only are then resoftened and gently contoured to the patient's finger. Dorsal piece is molded on finger, overlapping existing volar piece. Pieces are snapped apart when hardened. Fabrication pearl: radial and ulnar side walls of volar piece are then shortened by approximately 1/16-in to create a very snug extension force. A piece of foam tape can be added to the inside of the volar piece at the level of the distal end of the middle phalanx to further improve PIP joint extension forces. If patient presents with underlying DIP hyperextension (boutonniere deformity), the distal end of the dorsal piece can be shaped in some flexion. (*Courtesy of* E. Altman, DPT, CHT, New York, NY.)

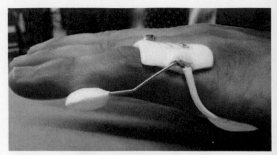

Fig. 10. Dynamic PIP joint extension splint. Many prefabricated options for this are available. (*Courtesy of* E. Altman, DPT, CHT, New York, NY.)

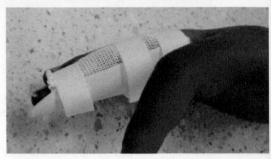

Fig. 11. Simple, low-profile finger gutter, PIP joint extension splint. Mold splint over barrel of highlighter and then resoften radial and ulnar border to conform to patient's finger. (*Courtesy of* E. Altman, DPT, CHT, New York, NY.)

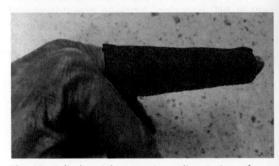

Fig. 12. Cylinder night extension splint. A circumferential cylinder cast can be fabricated with 2-in Orficast Thermoplastic Tape. Easy to take on and off due to gentle flexibility of material. (*Courtesy of* Orfit Industries, Wijnegem, Belgium; and E. Altman, DPT, CHT, New York, NY.)

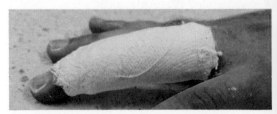

Fig. 13. Intermittent thin (3 layers) plaster cylinder casting is effective in some cases. Cast can be lined with a light coating of paraffin wax, making it removable. (*Courtesy of* E. Altman, DPT, CHT, New York, NY.)

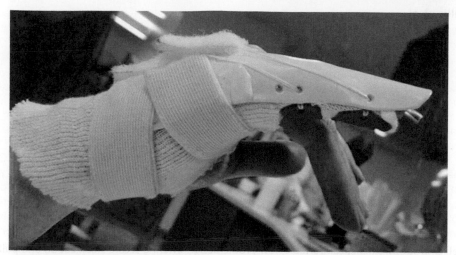

Fig. 14. Combination MP hyperextension block and interphalangeal extension splint providing secure control of PIP extension via adjustable, pull-through cuff design. This splint was used after Digit Widget removal for 1 patient who exhibited extreme MP joint hyperextension. (*Courtesy of* E. Altman, DPT, CHT, New York, NY.)

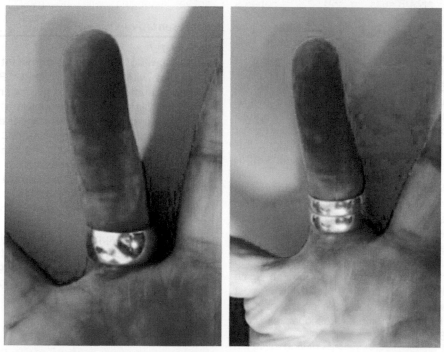

Fig. 15. Pulley Ring (Silver Ring Splint) options. (*Courtesy of* Silver Ring Splint Company, Charlottesville, VA; and E. Altman, DPT, CHT, New York, NY.)

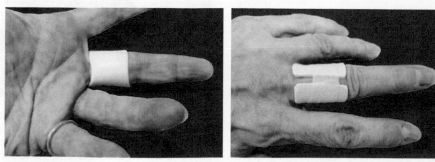

Fig. 16. Custom thermoplastic splint with dorsal slit, which permits secure closure with tape. (*Courtesy of* E. Altman, DPT, CHT, New York, NY.)

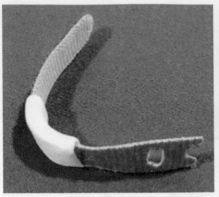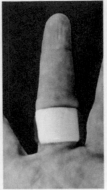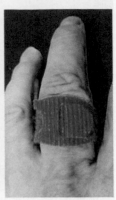

Fig. 17. Self-grip straps. Simple, comfortable, low-profile design offering secure stabilization and pulley protection. Addition of rigid thermoplastic volar piece significantly enhances splint mechanics. Fabrication pearl: flatten middle portion of thermoplastic piece to further enhance pulley support. (*Courtesy of* E. Altman, DPT, CHT, New York, NY.)

performed at an average of 23 months after injury (range 8–60). All patients at presentation had demonstrable bowstringing on physical examination as well as fixed PIP flexion contracture, which averaged 66° (range 45°–90°). All patients had A2 and A3 pulley ruptures demonstrated on MRI or ultrasound; 1 patient (patient 3) also had a rupture of the A4 pulley. The patients spent an average of 12 weeks (range 9–14) in the Digit Widget, followed by splinting for up to 11 months after surgery.

At final follow-up, at mean of 17 months (range 5–33) after Digit Widget removal, all patients had improvement in their PIP contracture. PIP flexion contracture averaged 19° (range 0°–30°). Visual analog scale score for pain averaged 1. Patients were overall satisfied with the procedure, rating their likelihood to undergo the procedure again using a Likert scale from 0 to 5, with 5 the most likely to undergo the procedure again, as 4.75. Michigan Hand Outcomes Questionnaire Score averaged 87.

Representative Cases

Patient 1

A 56-year-old right hand–dominant engineer presented with a right ring finger PIP flexion contracture after an injury to his finger 8 months prior after his finger was caught in a dog collar while breaking up a fight between 2 dogs. Prior to presentation, he had been treated elsewhere with multiple types of splints and hand therapy. His PIP range of motion was 45° to 100°, and he lacked 20° of terminal composite flexion at the DIP joint. MRI demonstrated ruptures of the A2 and A3 pulleys with bowstringing (**Fig. 20**).

He underwent application of the Digit Widget 8 months after his injury. At 10 days after surgery, his flexion contracture was 10° (**Fig. 21**). By 4 weeks postoperatively, his PIP had achieved

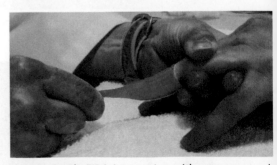

Fig. 18. Dynamic PIP joint extension splint placed over paraffin using a polyethylene food handling glove during pretreatment heat/stretch is effective. (*Courtesy of* E. Altman, DPT, CHT, New York, NY.)

Fig. 19. Gentle PIP joint traction with concurrent volarly directed force at the dorsal distal aspect of the proximal phalanx results in a volar glide of the proximal phalanx on the middle phalanx, increasing PIP joint extension. (*Courtesy of* E. Altman, DPT, CHT, New York, NY.)

Table 3
Summary of clinical data reported from management of pulley ruptures

Patient	Age (y)	Hand/ Finger	Dominant	Pulleys Ruptured	Mechanism	Other Injuries/ Surgeries	Time to Presentation (mo)	Preoperative Proximal Interphalangeal Range of Motion	Postoperative Proximal Interphalangeal Range of Motion	Time in Widget (w)	Follow-up (mo)	Visual Analog Scale Score	Likelihood of Having Surgery Again (0–5 Likert Scale, 5 Most Likely)	Michigan Hand Outcomes Questionnaire Score
1	56	R/ring	Y	A2, A3	Finger stuck in dog collar	None	8	45–100	0–100	13	5	0	5	97
2	57	R/ring	Y	A2, A3	Wrestling case of beer out of son's friend's hand	None	13	60–100	15–85	9	11	1	5	93
3	33	L/small	N	A2, A3, A4	Rock climbing	Dupuytrens/ fasciectomy	60	90–100	30–80	14	18	0	5	97
4	38	R/small	Y	A2, A3	Knife laceration	Zone II FDS/FDP lacerations/ tendon repair	9	70–100	30–80	13	33	2	4	64

Abbreviations: FDP, flexor digitorum profundus; FDS, flexor digitorum superficialis; L, left; N, non, non-dominant hand; R, right; Y, yes, dominant hand.

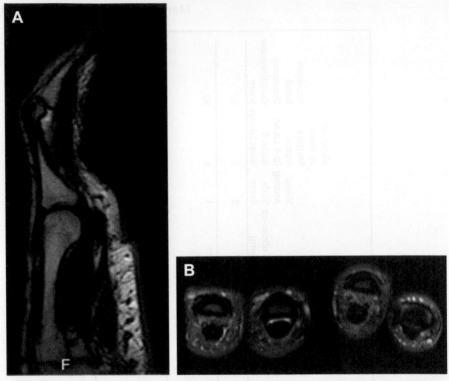

Fig. 20. (*A*) Sagittal and (*B*) Axial MRI of patient 1 with multiple pulley ruptures and bowstringing of the ring finger. (*Courtesy of* S. Wolfe, MD, New York, NY.)

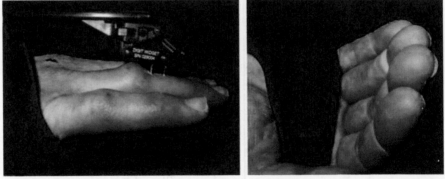

Fig. 21. Patient 1 at 10 days after application of Digit Widget. The flexion contracture at the ring PIP has decreased from 45° to 10°. (*Courtesy of* Hand Biomechanics Lab, Sacramento, CA; and S. Wolfe, MD, New York, NY.)

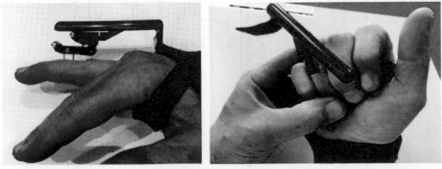

Fig. 22. Two months postoperatively with a mild extensor lag at the DIP. Passive flexion at the PIP to 90°. (*Courtesy of* Hand Biomechanics Lab, Sacramento, CA; and S. Wolfe, MD, New York, NY.)

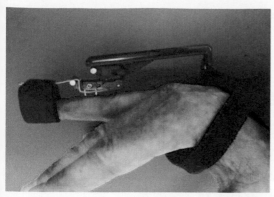

Fig. 23. DIP outrigger. (*Courtesy of* Hand Biomechanics Lab, Sacramento, CA; and S. Wolfe, MD, New York, NY.)

full extension. Flexion, however, was now limited to 45°. At 6 weeks, he developed a superficial pin site infection, which was successfully treated with 10 days of oral cephalexin. At 2 months postoperatively, he had full extension at the PIP, 90° of passive flexion at the PIP, and a slight extensor lag at the DIP (**Fig. 22**). He began wearing an outrigger for the DIP as well as taking the bands off for 5 hours to 6 hours per day with no loss of extension at the PIP (**Fig. 23**). The Digit Widget was removed at 13 weeks. He went into a pulley ring at all times. Three weeks after removal, he started a program of active short arc flexion with the pulley

supported. By 6 weeks after removal, he continued to have full extension and could flex to his palm without bowstringing (**Fig. 24**).

Patient 3
A 33-year-old right hand–dominant male retail manager presented with a left small finger contracture 4 years after a rock climbing injury. After the injury, he rapidly developed Dupuytren contracture. He was initially managed elsewhere and underwent 2 Xiaflex injections but nevertheless had progression of the contracture. He subsequently underwent palmar digital fasciectomy at another facility. The patient was unable to achieve full extension postoperatively and he continued to have a 45° PIP contracture. His operative report noted that the A3 pulley was sacrificed at the time of surgery. The PIP contracture worsened over time and by the time he presented he had a flexion contracture at the PIP of 90°, a DIP contracture of 45°, and an MP contracture of 50° (**Fig. 25**). He had a pretendinous cord on examination and also had evidence of bowstringing. MRI revealed disruptions of A2, A3, and A4 pulleys.

Five years after his initial injury, the authors took him to the operating room for planned Dupuytren fasciectomy followed by Digit Widget application. Intraoperatively, the A2 through A4 pulleys were found disrupted, confirming the MRI findings. After the palmar fasciectomy, the MP contracture was completely corrected, but the PIP was still

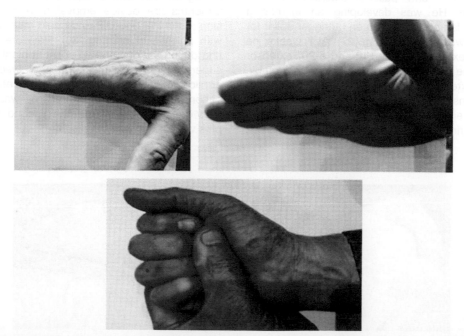

Fig. 24. Six weeks after removal of Digit Widget (Patient 1). (*Courtesy of* S. Wolfe, MD, New York, NY.)

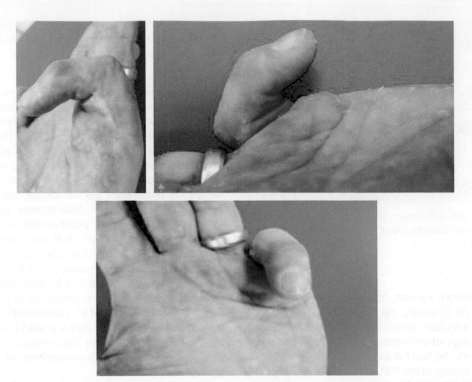

Fig. 25. Patient 3 on presentation. Note the MP, PIP, and DIP contractures. (*Courtesy of* S. Wolfe, MD, New York, NY.)

contracted to 70° and the DIP contracted 20°. The Digit Widget was then applied. By 11 days postoperatively the PIP contracture had improved to 50°. At 4 weeks postoperatively, he had active extension to 25° and passive extension to 15° (**Fig. 26**). He was developing an increasing extensor lag at the DIP, so an outrigger splint for the DIP was fashioned (**Fig. 27**). At 7 weeks, he had full extension at the PIP and a 20° extensor lag at the DIP, which was passively correctable to full extension (**Fig. 28**). By 12 weeks, he had full extension at the PIP and DIP (**Fig. 29**). He started removing the bands during the day and only wearing the Digit Widget at night. At 14 weeks,

the device was removed. He started a program of serial casting, which was removed for passive flexion exercises only; 5 weeks after removal of the Digit Widget, he transitioned to an LMB splint during the day with a night extension splint. At 2 months after device removal, he had full extension at the PIP and DIP and could make a full fist with pulley support (**Fig. 30**). He wore a pulley ring during the day and no splint at night. He had superficial pin site infections at 7 weeks after application of the device and 14 weeks after application of the device. Both times he was treated with oral cephalexin, and the second time his pins were removed as well.

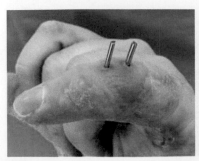
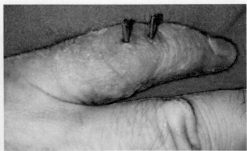

Fig. 26. Patient 3 at 3 weeks postoperatively. (*Courtesy of* S. Wolfe, MD, New York, NY.)

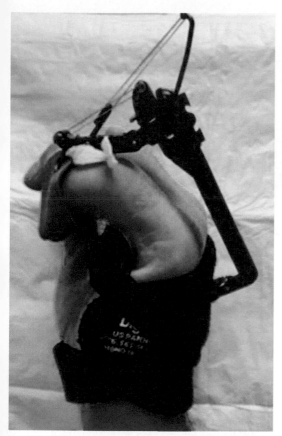

Fig. 27. DIP outrigger attachment to Digit Widget. (*Courtesy of* Hand Biomechanics Lab, Sacramento, CA; and S. Wolfe, MD, New York, NY.)

At final follow-up 18 months after surgery, he was no longer wearing any splints and had returned to all his prior activities. He had a slight recurrence of his PIP contracture with MP range of motion 30° of hyperextension to 80° of flexion, PIP motion of 30° to 80°, and DIP range of motion of 20° to 60°.

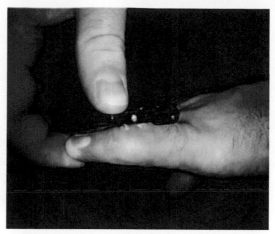

Fig. 28. Patient 3 at 7 weeks postoperatively. (*Courtesy of* S. Wolfe, MD, New York, NY.)

SUMMARY

Delayed flexor pulley rupture with severe PIP flexion contracture presents a challenging problem. There is no recent literature on management of this complex situation. This article presents a technique for the rescue of the delayed presentation of pulley ruptures with fixed flexion contracture with application of a Digit Widget followed by a customized splinting regimen. The authors' technique provides early promising results for closed management of this difficult problem. The authors are not certain why this technique is effective at reducing PIP contractures after pulley injury, because the pulley injury remains. The authors speculate that the technique may help rebalance the forces across the PIP joint by enabling a prolonged period of intrinsic strengthening. The technique facilitates and does not preclude staged tendon graft pulley reconstruction, which may be performed at surgeon discretion.

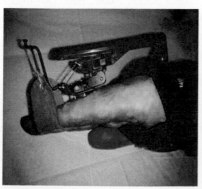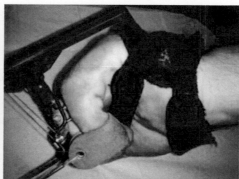

Fig. 29. Patient 3 at 12 weeks postoperatively, prior to removal of the fixator. (*Courtesy of* Hand Biomechanics Lab, Sacramento, CA; and S. Wolfe, MD, New York, NY.)

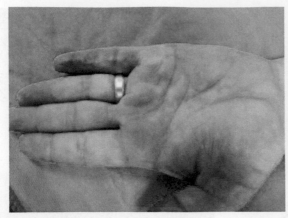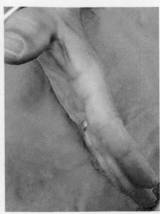

Fig. 30. Twenty-two weeks after application of the Digit Widget and 7 weeks after removal. (*Courtesy of* S. Wolfe, MD, New York, NY.)

ACKNOWLEDGMENTS

The authors would like to acknowledge Schneider Rancy, BA, for his assistance in contacting patients for this article.

REFERENCES

1. Bowers WH, Kuzma GR, Bynum DK. Closed traumatic rupture of finger flexor pulleys. J Hand Surg Am 1994;19(5):782–7.

2. Clark TA, Skeete K, Amadio PC. Flexor tendon pulley reconstruction. J Hand Surg Am 2010;35(10): 1685–9.

3. King EA, Lien JR. Flexor tendon pulley injuries in rock climbers. Hand Clin 2017;33(1):141–8.

4. Dy CJ, Lyman S, Schreiber JJ, et al. The epidemiology of reoperation after flexor pulley reconstruction. J Hand Surg Am 2013;38(9):1705–11.

5. Doyle JR. Anatomy of the finger flexor tendon sheath and pulley system. J Hand Surg Am 1988;13(4): 473–84.

6. Roloff I, Schoffl VR, Vigouroux L, et al. Biomechanical model for the determination of the forces acting on the finger pulley system. J Biomech 2006;39(5): 915–23.

7. Goodman HJ, Choueka J. Biomechanics of the flexor tendons. Hand Clin 2005;21(2):129–49.

8. Doyle JR. Palmar and digital flexor tendon pulleys. Clin Orthop Relat Res 2001;(383):84–96.

9. Mehta V, Phillips CS. Flexor tendon pulley reconstruction. Hand Clin 2005;21(2):245–51.

10. Peterson WW, Manske PR, Bollinger BA, et al. Effect of pulley excision on flexor tendon biomechanics. J Orthop Res 1986;4(1):96–101.

11. Dy CJ, Daluiski A. Flexor pulley reconstruction. Hand Clin 2013;29(2):235–42.

12. Martinoli C, Bianchi S, Cotten A. Imaging of rock climbing injuries. Semin Musculoskelet Radiol 2005;9(4):334–45.

13. Schoffl VR, Einwag F, Strecker W, et al. Strength measurement and clinical outcome after pulley ruptures in climbers. Med Sci Sports Exerc 2006;38(4): 637–43.

14. Schneeberger M, Schweizer A. Pulley ruptures in rock climbers: outcome of conservative treatment with the pulley-protection splint-A series of 47 cases. Wilderness Environ Med 2016;27(2):211–8.

15. Lin GT, Amadio PC, An KN, et al. Biomechanical analysis of finger flexor pulley reconstruction. J Hand Surg Br 1989;14(3):278–82.

16. Kleinert HE, Bennett JB. Digital pulley reconstruction employing the always present rim of the previous pulley. J Hand Surg Am 1978;3(3):297–8.

17. Karev A, Stahl S, Taran A. The mechanical efficiency of the pulley system in normal digits compared with a reconstructed system using the "belt loop" technique. J Hand Surg Am 1987;12(4):596–601.

18. Lister G. Indications and techniques for repair of the flexor tendon sheath. Hand Clin 1985;1(1):85–95.

19. Widstrom CJ, Johnson G, Doyle JR, et al. A mechanical study of six digital pulley reconstruction techniques: part I. Mechanical effectiveness. J Hand Surg Am 1989;14(5):821–5.

20. Okutsu I, Ninomiya S, Hiraki S, et al. Three-loop technique for A2 pulley reconstruction. J Hand Surg Am 1987;12(5 Pt 1):790–4.

21. Agee JM, Goss BC. The use of skeletal extension torque in reversing dupuytren contractures of the proximal interphalangeal joint. J Hand Surg Am 2012;37(7):1467–74.

Complications of Proximal Interphalangeal Joint Injuries: Prevention and Treatment

Sirichai Kamnerdnakta, MD[a,b], Helen E. Huetteman, BS[a],
Kevin C. Chung, MD, MS[c,*]

KEYWORDS

- Proximal interphalangeal joint • Complications • Prevention • Treatment

KEY POINTS

- Proximal interphalangeal (PIP) joint stability is maintained through the congruency of the bony structures and its soft tissue stabilizers.
- Complications regularly arise after PIP joint injuries, yet they can often be prevented through early detection of injury and appropriate initial treatment protocols.
- The main goals of any treatment of a PIP joint complication are maintaining concentric reduction of the joint, restoring joint stability, and facilitating early range-of-motion exercises.

The ability to flex and extend the proximal interphalangeal (PIP) joint is crucial for adequate grip strength. Estimates show that the PIP joint accounts for approximately 85% of the motion required in a functional grip.[1] As a hinge joint, it is extremely stable in the sagittal plane, but has limited tolerance to angular, axial, and rotational stress. Thus, the PIP joint is one of the most susceptible joints to injury. The vulnerability of the PIP joint stems from its unprotected position in the digit and its long moment arm. Of potential injuries to the hand, PIP joint injuries are common among the general population and are especially pronounced in athletes.[2–4]

Because injury type can range from minor sprains to complex intra-articular fractures, classifying PIP joint injuries can be a complex task for therapists and surgeons. PIP joint injuries are often overlooked by patients or even athletic trainers or coaches; thus, improper treatment occurs regularly. Necessary treatment and rehabilitation techniques may be delayed and lead to permanent deformities of the digit. For example, prolonged immobilization of the PIP joint can cause stiffness and may subsequently result in irreversible loss of motion in the digit.[5,6] Given that this joint has a predilection for stiffness, pain, arthritis, and residual deformities caused by soft tissue imbalance or adhesions, timely and accurate diagnosis and appropriate treatment are critical for all PIP joint injuries. Certain complications may be more easily prevented than treated. Therefore, concerted measures promoting prevention of further complications following PIP joint injuries are needed.

Disclosure Statement: This work was supported by a Midcareer Investigator Award in Patient-Oriented Research (2 K24-AR053120-06) to Dr K.C. Chung. The content is solely the responsibility of the authors and does not necessarily represent the official views of the National Institutes of Health.

[a] Department of Surgery, Section of Plastic Surgery, University of Michigan, NCRC, Building 18, G200, 2800 Plymouth Road, Ann Arbor, MI 48109, USA; [b] Division of Plastic Surgery, Department of Surgery, Faculty of Medicine, Siriraj Hospital, Mahidol University, 12th Floor, Siamintr Building, Bangkok-noi, Bangkok 10700, Thailand; [c] Section of Plastic Surgery, University of Michigan, 2130 Taubman Center, SPC 5340, 1500 East Medical Center Drive, Ann Arbor, MI 48109-5340, USA

* Corresponding author.

E-mail address: kecchung@med.umich.edu

RELEVANT ANATOMY

The PIP joint is composed of a delicate balance of bony and soft tissues. The combination of the tongue-in-groove articulation of the intercondylar eminence at the base of the middle phalanx and the bicondylar head of the proximal phalanx permits increased resistance of torque and translational displacements. Although the joint is commonly classified as uniaxial, some lateral movement and rotation may occur during flexion, facilitating rotation of the finger toward the scaphoid tubercle.[1,7,8] This unique property results from slight anatomic differences in the radial and ulnar condyles of the proximal phalanx, as illustrated by the trapezoidal cross-section at the head of proximal phalanx. Moreover, the index and middle fingers display a more prominent ulnar condyle, whereas the ring and little fingers possess a more prominent radial condyle[9] (**Fig. 1**). Further discrepancies exist between the articular surfaces of the proximal and middle phalanxes at the PIP joint. Most notably, the articular facet of the proximal phalanx facilitates 210° of motion, whereas the middle phalangeal side encompasses approximately 110°.[10]

Given the asymmetry among condyles, bony structure alone cannot effectively stabilize the joint during motion, and surrounding soft tissues play an important role in joint stability. A 3-sided box analogy is useful to identify relevant soft tissue structures. The PIP joint is intrinsically supported along the volar, radial, and ulnar side but devoid of a stout dorsal restraint, as if it were surrounded by a 3-sided box (**Fig. 2**). The true and accessory collateral ligaments (ACLs) embrace the radial and ulnar walls of the box and prevent lateral deviation. Along the base, the volar plate functions to limit hyperextension of the joint.[11] In addition to the 3 primary stabilizers, the joint is further supported by the central slip, the lateral bands, and the flexor tendons, collectively referred to as secondary stabilizers. These secondary stabilizers determine the balanced posture and facilitate motion of the joint.[12] Dislocation of the PIP joint requires that the volar plate and at least one of the collateral ligaments be disrupted.[13] However, small disruptions or incongruities to the intricate structure of the joint or its stabilizers may lead to abnormal wear, arthritis, or more extreme complications after injury.[1,14]

CLASSIFICATION OF PROXIMAL INTERPHALANGEAL JOINT INJURIES

Because injuries of the PIP joint can affect many combinations of the bony structures and surrounding soft tissues, various classification systems of PIP joint injuries are available. Individual fracture or dislocation patterns are affected by the characteristics of the specific mechanism of injury. The most common pattern of injury is observed when a force drives proximally along the middle phalanx against the dorsal lip of the head of the proximal phalanx. This mechanism of injury can lead to fracture of the palmar lip of the base of middle phalanx with dorsal subluxation of the PIP joint. The volar plate of the PIP joint may be avulsed (**Fig. 3**). Occasionally, injury mechanisms are substantially more complex, with the direction and magnitude of a force determining a unique fracture location and pattern. To facilitate the best prognosis and treatment option for each injury, it is important to classify PIP joint injuries with a standard system according to the structural involvement, mechanism of injury, and joint stability.[14–16] The classification systems used in this article are described in later discussion.

Collateral Ligament Injuries

Any laterally deviating force to the tip of the finger will affect the distribution of stress over the collateral ligaments. Significant injury may also disrupt the secondary PIP joint stabilizers. With enough force, the true collateral ligament will tear from its origin at the proximal phalanx. The disruption may also progress to the ACL and the attachment of volar plate at the middle phalanx.[11,17] Bowers and colleagues[8] developed the following grading system for classification of collateral ligament injuries:

- Grade 1: Asymmetric swelling and tenderness over the collateral ligament without instability on the lateral stress test.
- Grade 2: Complete disruption of the collateral ligament, but the volar plate remains intact.

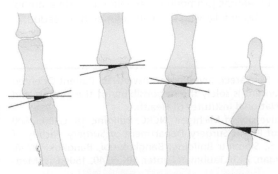

Fig. 1. The dorsal aspect of the right hand demonstrates size discrepancies between the ulnar and radial condyles of the proximal phalanx in the fingers. (*Courtesy of* N. Fujihara, MD, Nagoya, Japan.)

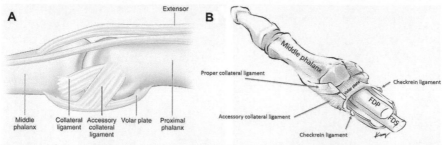

Fig. 2. (*A*) Anatomy of the soft-tissue stabilizers of the PIP joint. (*B*) A 3-sided box analogy is useful to identify volar, radial, and ulnar restraints of the joint. ([*A*] *From* Chung KC, Brown M. Capsulotomy for proximal interphalangeal contracture. In: Chung KC, editor. Operative techniques: hand and wrist surgery. 3rd edition. Philadelphia: Elsevier; 2018. p. 368; with permission; and [*B*] *Courtesy of* C. Hokierti, MD, Bangkok, Thailand.)

Clinical examination displays a stable active arc of motion (AOM) and less than 20° of deviation with a firm end point on the lateral stress test.

- Grade 3: Total collateral ligament disruption and volar plate rupture. Clinical examination depicts evidence of subluxation or dislocation on active extension and greater than 20° of joint laxity on a varus and valgus stress test with a firm end point.

The implications of an open approach for ligament repair must be considered because open repair can aggravate the injury and further induce fibrosis. Furthermore, the collateral ligament may spontaneously heal itself over time and does not always require surgical correction. Eaton and colleagues[18] demonstrated this process through the formation of a "neocollateral" ligament after total ligament excision for treatment of PIP stiffness in 10 PIP joints over a 3-month period. Thus, open ligament repair should be preserved for only grade 3 collateral ligament injuries that require restoration of the volar plate integrity.[5,19]

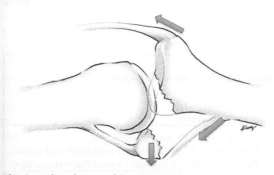

Fig. 3. Volar plate avulsion injury. The dynamic forces across the PIP joint can lead to fracture of palmar lip of the base of middle phalanx with dorsal subluxation of the PIP joint. Arrows indicate the direction of force. (*Courtesy of* C. Hokierti, MD, Bangkok, Thailand.)

Proximal Phalanx Articular Fractures

Condylar fractures of the proximal phalanx result from strong lateral deviation forces or forceful axial loading. They are classified into the following 3 types:

- Type 1: stable fractures without displacement
- Type 2: unicondylar, unstable fractures
- Type 3: bicondylar or comminuted fractures

For lateral deviation injuries of the PIP joint, an applied force may lead to avulsion fracture of the condyle or rupture of the collateral ligament. This injury pattern is particularly relevant for a joint that exhibits slight flexion because joint stability is maintained solely by the soft tissue stabilizers, making the joint vulnerable to stress. Type 1 and 2 injuries are referenced by subtle comminution or displacement. A type 3 injury pattern is usually the result of aggressive force and high-energy axial loading at the fingertips. Such injuries are vastly comminuted and displaced. Most of these fractures, including type 1 nondisplacement fractures, will require fixation. Considering the substantial force and torque exhibited during joint movement and minimal periosteal sleeve surrounding the fracture site, restoration of appropriate bicondylar morphology through adequate fixation is necessary to maintain lateral and rotational stability (**Fig. 4**). Various techniques of fixation have been described, including the use of K-wires, lag screws, or an external fixation device.[20–23]

Base of the Middle Phalanx Fractures

The most common type of PIP joint injury is a volar lip fracture at the base of the middle phalanx with PIP joint dorsal dislocation.[9,24] This type of injury is typically the result of hyperextension or axial loading at the tip of the finger during joint flexion.[25] Classification not only is defined by fracture morphology and stability but also depends on

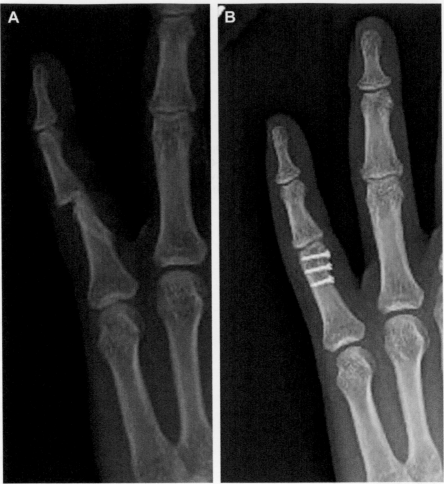

Fig. 4. (A) A unicondylar oblique fracture pattern is seen at the head of the proximal phalanx. (B) After fixation with 3 lag screws, restoration of bicondylar morphologic pattern was achieved to maintain stability.

the involvement of the articular surface of the base of middle phalanx. The amount of articular surface involvement can be used to determine postreduction joint stability (**Table 1**). The main goals of any

treatment plan for fracture-dislocation injuries should focus on maintaining concentric reduction of the subluxated or dislocated joint, restoring stability to achieve a normal AOM, facilitating early

Table 1
Stability-based classification of proximal interphalangeal joint fracture dislocation

Fracture Type	Articular Surface Involvement	Stability	Clinical Stability
Volar lip	<30%	Stable	Stable with full active ROM
	30%–50%	Tenuous	Requires <30° of flexion to maintain reduction
	>50%	Unstable	Requires >30° of flexion to maintain reduction
Dorsal lip	<50%	Stable	Reduced in full extension
	Any percentage	Unstable	Volar subluxation/dislocation in full extension
Pilon	100%	Stable	Stable through full active ROM
	100%	Unstable	Grossly unstable

range of motion (ROM) exercises, and, if feasible, performing an anatomic reduction of the articular surface. Nonetheless, existing evidence shows that imperfections to the joint articular surface are not correlated with clinically relevant posttraumatic arthrosis of the PIP joint and will not worsen clinical outcomes.[26–29] In other words, if a smooth articular surface cannot be obtained technically, the outcomes may not suffer as long as alignment and concentric reduction are achieved.

Available treatment options include immobilization, protected motion, traction, open reduction and internal fixation (ORIF), buttress reconstruction, joint arthroplasty, or arthrodesis.[30–36] By principle, stable PIP joint fracture dislocations can be treated nonsurgically if closed reduction can restore a normal AOM. However, surgical treatment is indicated for injuries that are unable to achieve concentric joint reduction or cannot maintain stability after reduction.[37] Whenever possible, the selected treatment should permit early-protected motion with a stable AOM. Early motion exercises enhance cartilage healing and promote remodeling of the injured articular surface to a great congruency.[38]

COMPLICATIONS OF PROXIMAL INTERPHALANGEAL JOINT INJURIES

Various complications are possible after treatment of a PIP joint injury. Although joint stiffness and flexion contracture are most common, other complications include re-dislocation, posttraumatic arthritis, chronic swelling, or even permanent functional loss. Given the precise anatomy of the joint and its soft tissue stabilizers, even minor injury can afflict adhesion or misalignment among the delicate structures and lead to abnormal wear and stiffness. Nevertheless, underestimation of the severity of the injury by patients, health care providers, or coaches can delay treatment and increase the chances of complication.

There is no consensus for the best treatment avenue for PIP joint injuries. In addition, evidence suggests that posttreatment outcomes rarely return a full AOM.[37] However, studies indicate that outcomes are significantly improved when the injuries are tackled early (within 4 weeks of injury), regardless of treatment modality used.[39–42] To further diminish complications, evidence recommends early diagnosis and restoration through concentric reduction to facilitate early motion exercises, if feasible, for every injury.[9,37,43,44]

JOINT STIFFNESS OR FLEXION CONTRACTURE

Although many patients can tolerate around 15° to 20° of flexion contracture without any functional deficit, more severe contractures typically require corrective treatment.[45] Achieving a full AOM and stability of the joint, as well as harmonization of the complex structures surrounding the joint, is essential. PIP joint stiffness may be attributed to a combination of structures, including the bony parts, articular surface, joint capsule, collateral and retinacular ligaments, tendons or their sheaths, and the skin. Similarly, flexion contracture may be caused by a lack of extensor power at the PIP joint, decreased excursion of flexor tendons, capsular or ligamentous contractures, or bony blocks or exostoses resulting from malunited fractures.[46,47] Therefore, it is often extremely difficult to delineate the root cause of the contracture, especially in cases that also involve chronic stiffness.

Because joint stiffness and flexion contracture are the most common complications after PIPJ injury, it is important to understand the pathogenesis of the disease. Following acute injury of the PIP joint, the inflammatory processes of healing and hemarthrosis increase the joint's relative volume. In response, the PIP joint will accommodate up to 30° to 40° of flexion to maximize its volume. In conjunction with pulling forces from the flexor tendons, the finger is maintained in a flexed posture.[48,49] During the inflammatory period, scarring and fibrosis are initiated, causing adhesions along the tendons and underlying bony parts or the surrounding soft tissue. The adhesion-forming zone is not necessarily confined within the injury zone, and it may extend further beyond the affected area.[50] When the PIP joint remains in this position for an extended period of time, dense fibrotic scarring can occur. This process causes increased stiffness of the joint and difficulties with digit manipulation. To ensure the best outcomes, the surgeon should evaluate all potential causes and initiate treatment before the formation of dense fibrosis had begun.

Clinical Evaluation

Surgeons should focus their evaluation on defining the precipitating cause of stiffness and delineating the causative structure of stiffness. Details on injury mechanism, severity, duration of injury, prior treatment and rehabilitation, global function of hand, and occupation must be considered. Greater severity injuries will create more extensive scarring and adhesions.[44] Detailed history taking will guide the surgeon in determining a prognosis and facilitate the appropriate intervention technique. Because patient compliance plays a crucial role in the treatment process for PIP joint stiffness, it must be addressed in the evaluation stage.

Patients should be educated on the treatment protocol and possess an appropriate understanding of the treatment plan to ensure optimal healing.[51]

A stiff finger is characterized into one of the following groups[52]:

1. Skin/fascia-related problems
2. Muscle/tendon injuries or lesions
3. Capsule/joint ligaments contractures
4. Damage of articular bone

The affected finger is palpated, and the pliability, consistency, and mobility of skin are evaluated. If surgical intervention is deemed necessary, incisions should be planned, and any skin defect after contracture release should be estimated. In addition, local tissue rearrangement or skin flap should be planned, if indicated, to achieve tension free coverage.

The examiner must also evaluate the mobility of the joint. Any discrepancy between the active and passive AOM is measured. If the passive AOM is preserved but there is a limited active AOM, musculotendinous adhesion or injury exists. If both the passive and active AOMs are equally limited, there is a clear indication of joint involvement or bone block. However, examiners should be cautious because tendon involvement is often masked and may remain unknown with physical examination alone. Radiograph tests, such as radiographs or a computed tomographic scan, are suggested to illustrate the articular congruency and identify the bone block. In cases of chronic stiffness and contracture, intrinsic tightness must also be evaluated. Intrinsic tightness is confirmed if there is less PIP flexion when the metacarpophalangeal (MCP) joint is extended than when it is flexed. Furthermore, the physician should check for abnormal posture of the digit during posing and motion. Hyperextension of the distal interphalangeal (DIP) joint combined with a flexion stance at the PIP joint suggests a chronic central slip injury. A summary of the classification system for PIP joint stiffness, created by Jupiter and colleagues[53] and modified by Kaplan,[51] is presented in **Table 2**.

Prevention

Regardless of treatment type, it is generally difficult for one to regain a full ROM after stiffness or contracture has started to develop. Thus, prevention of joint stiffness or flexion contracture is often easier and may provide better outcomes than treatment. Stiffness and contracture of the PIP joint may be attributed to prolonged immobilization and low levels of patient participation owing to pain or edema.[51,54] To ebb the chance of fibrosis and stiffness, early and effective treatment

protocols are imperative. Appropriate fracture stabilization, maintenance of joint stability, and restoration of the soft tissue envelope permit early motion and can limit edema, thus lessening the chance of contracture.[37] Furthermore, the physician should initiate adequate pain control, edema control, and patient counseling measures simultaneously with treatment.

In addition, the patient should initiate tendon-gliding exercises during the first 4 weeks of injury to minimize tendon adhesion. Gaining 5 mm of tendon excursion and upwards to 30° to 40° in PIP joint motion are favorable prognostic signs.[49] Immobilization of the joint for longer than 3 weeks should be avoided.[45] Prolonged immobilization not only will facilitate stiffness of the PIP joint but also may escalate stiffening of the DIP joint and even nearby digits, which may not have been directly injured.[55] Similarly to most other injuries in which a short immobilization period is required, the hand can be safely splinted with the wrist positioned in 30° of extension, the MCP joints flexed at 70° to 90°, and the PIP joints fully extended. Safe positioning places the MCP and PIP collateral ligaments with maximum tautness and strengthens the volar plate, subsequently minimizing postimmobilization stiffness. Although this splinting technique may produce a slight degree of extension contracture at the PIP joint, correction of the extension contracture is considerably easier than flexion contracture.[56]

Nonoperative Treatment

Given that most patients can tolerate slight contractures without any functional deficit, treatment of PIP flexion contractures is not indicated until the degree of contracture is greater than 20°. However, some patients may seek treatment of a stiff finger or slight contractures to best suit their aesthetic preferences. Nonoperative treatments, such as serial casting or dynamic/static extension splinting, should be the primary treatment avenues in most cases.[44,45,53,57] Serial casting is preferred if the contracture is long standing or the degree of contracture is greater than 45°. On the other hand, splinting is suitable if examination reveals some joint mobility and a contracture of less than 45°. Previous research has reported that aggressive forces from a wire splint can produce pressure ulcers on the underlying skin when applied in cases of severe contracture (>45°).[58] Further studies report that the success rate of nonoperative treatment is highly dependent on the amount of time spent in the splint as well as patient compliance rates.[56,59,60]

Table 2
Stiff finger classification

	Motion Loss	Dorsal Disease	Palmar Disease	Possible Associated Conditions	Treatment
Type 1	Limited passive flexion Limited passive extension	Extensor adhesions Dorsal capsule-ligamentous contracture	A2 pulley insufficiency Palmar plate contracture Accessory collateral contracture Skin deficiency	Flexor tendon adhesions Flexor tendon disruption	Stage 1 • Extensor tenolysis • Dorsal capsulectomy • Flexor check Stage 2 • Flexor tenolysis, reconstruction • Palmar plate, checkrein release
Type 2	Limited passive flexion Limited active extension	Extensor adhesions Dorsal capsule-ligamentous contracture		Flexor tendon adhesions Flexor tendon disruption	Stage 1 • Extensor tenolysis • Dorsal capsulectomy • Flexor check Stage 2 • Flexor tenolysis, reconstruction
Type 3	Limited active flexion Limited passive extension		Flexor tendon adhesions Flexor tendon disruption A2 pulley insufficiency Palmar plate contracture Accessory collateral contracture Skin deficiency		Flexor tenolysis Flexor tendon reconstruction Pulley reconstruction Palmar plate, checkrein release ACL release Skin contracture release, resurfacing
Type 4	Limited active flexion Limited active extension	Extensor subluxation Excessive length of extensor tendon	Flexor tendon adhesions Flexor tendon disruption		Stage 1 • Extensor rebalancing, reconstruction Stage 2 • Flexor tendon tenolysis, reconstruction
Type 5	Limited passive extension		Palmar plate contracture Accessory collateral contracture Palmar fibromatosis Palmar skin contracture		Palmar plate, checkrein release ACL release Fasciectomy Skin contracture release, resurfacing
Type 6	Limited active flexion		Flexor tendon adhesions Flexor tendon disruption		Flexor tenolysis Flexor tendon reconstruction

(continued on next page)

	Motion Loss	Dorsal Disease	Palmar Disease	Possible Associated Conditions	Treatment
Table 2 (*continued*)					
Type 7	Limited passive flexion	Scar, burn contracture	Bone block		Skin contracture release, resurfacing Excision of bony block
Type 8	Limited active extension	Extensor disruption			Splinting Extensor tendon repair, reconstruction

From Kaplan FTD. The stiff finger. Hand Clin 2010;26(2):193; with permission.

Surgical Treatment

A surgical release operation may initiate an inflammatory cascade that promotes additional fibroses and adhesion. Therefore, surgery is only indicated after all nonoperative protocols have been attempted without evidence of improvement. Moreover, there is not a restricted time window in which surgery must be initiated. Some reports have shown that surgical intervention can aid a patient to achieve an AOM between 65° and 90°; however, slight flexion contractures (<25°) typically remain.[45] Nonetheless, others have reported unimpressive results or worsening outcomes.[13,61–63]

Open release of the PIP joint can be conducted using local, regional, or general anesthesia. However, a wide-awake local anesthesia technique is recommended because it permits the surgeon to directly observe the mobility of the PIP joint throughout the operation.[64] In cases involving multiple fingers or extensive scarring that require a more extensive tendon release to the hand and forearm, use of regional or general anesthesia is indicated.

When considering appropriate surgical techniques, the cause of the stiffness or contracture should first be classified as a bony abnormality or soft tissue imbalance. Bony abnormalities, such as bony blocking or ankylosis, should be corrected before addressing the soft tissue contracture.[65] We address three main techniques to release the soft tissue of the PIP joint that are commonly practiced today.

Percutaneous surgical release

In 1985, Stanley and colleagues[66] were the first to propose percutaneous surgical release for treating PIP joint flexion contracture. The investigators aimed to lessen the extent of surgery inflicted to the joint by using a limited incision to release the underlying ACL. A long-term study of 30 joints after a follow-up period averaging 34 months reported better outcomes among patients with osteoarthritis and postimmobilization stiffness, as opposed to those with inflammatory arthritis. Although approximately half of the study participants demonstrated improved outcomes and long-lasting results (average PIP joint flexion deformity angle improved from 78° to 34°; average AOM improved from 17° to 39°), outcomes in the other half remained unchanged or deteriorated.[67] Thus, the investigators concluded that percutaneous ACL release is properly indicated in stiff joints affected by capsuloligamentous disease that have not undergone previous surgery.[67] This operation is not always a suitable alternative for an open release but can be attempted before adoption of a more extensive technique.

The operation is performed using a Beaver knife insert through a dorsum 2-mm incision just lateral to the overlying head of the proximal phalanx. The blade is inserted between the head of the proximal phalanx and the collateral ligament and is swung back and forth to unleash the ACL entirely (**Fig. 5**). Blade direction is kept strictly in the sagittal plane to avoid inadvertent injury of the neurovascular bundles. The surgeon must use moderate force to manipulate the joint, break remaining adhesions, and split the flexor tendon sheath. Occasionally, surgeons may be able hear the sound of the intra-articular adhesions breaking. Aggressive force should be avoided, because it may jeopardize the volar plate or result in iatrogenic phalangeal fracture.

Open surgical release

Similar to percutaneous release, the goal of open surgical release is to eliminate any structures that restrict joint motion, yet maintain sufficient joint

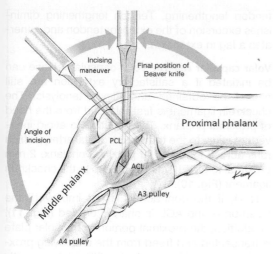

Fig. 5. Percutaneous surgical release technique to treat flexion contracture of the PIP joint. (*Courtesy* of C. Hokierti, MD, Bangkok, Thailand.)

stability. However, as previously mentioned, PIP joint stiffness or flexor contracture is usually caused by a combination of structures, and it is often impossible to delineate the prevailing causative structure in an individual finger through clinical evaluation alone. Previous literature has noted the benefits of a sequential release of involved structures; however, the order varies from author to author.[65,68,69] Most recommend progressively releasing from the proximal to distal ends and from extra-articular to intra-articular, checking for improvements after every structure released.[54,62,65,69–71] Sequential releases are recommended in the following order.

Flexor tenolysis This operation should be conducted under wide-awake local anesthesia, if feasible. In severe and long-standing contractures, the need for provisional soft tissue reconstruction using local tissue rearrangement or a flap should be considered and planned in advance (**Fig. 6**). To begin, underlying structures can be exposed via a midaxial or Bruner incision, yet the midaxial approach is most common. One study of 45 fingers found that patients with a midaxial incision exhibited a better AOM 1.5 years postoperatively when compared with those receiving a Bruner incision.[72] Nonetheless, the midaxial exposure is limited, and extending the incision beyond the proximal phalanx can be challenging. Given that adhesions or fibrosis is not necessarily confined within the digit and there is a possibility for extensive scarring, a Bruner incision may be more appropriate (**Fig. 7**).

After incision, the flexor tendons are released. Windows in the flexor tendon sheath are made

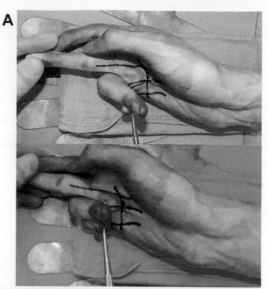

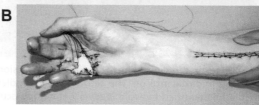

Fig. 6. This patient had a long-standing and severe flexor contracture of the right hand from Dupuytren disease. (*A*) The local tissue rearrangement incisions were designed. (*B*) At the end of the operation, the remaining incision was covered with a full-thickness skin graft from the forearm.

proximal to the A1 pulley, on the distal border of the A2 pulley, and proximal to the A4 pulley. The A2 and A4 pulleys are preserved to prevent bowstringing of the flexor tendons. The operator can use a traction force to break the flexor digitorum superficialis (FDS) and flexor digitorum profundus (FDP) from their adhesions. A Freer elevator is used to dissect the tendons from the pulley, surrounding tissue, and underlying bones (**Fig. 8**). The FDS should be adequately freed toward its insertion site. If resistance of the flexor tendons remains proximally, a counterincision in the distal forearm is needed (**Fig. 9**). The surgeon can then apply the traction force on the encountered tendon to facilitate adhesion lyses and tendon dissection.[69]

When tenolysis is adequately performed, manual traction on the tendon will reveal full extension of the PIP joint, but the patient may not be capable of full active PIP joint extension. Extension lag is frequently observed after PIP joint injury, because sustained stretching of the extensor tendon from the flexion contracture can cause

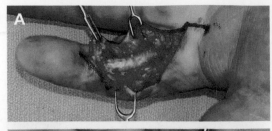

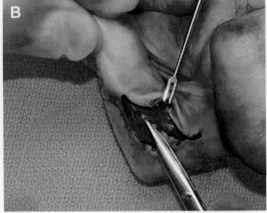

Fig. 7. Flexor tenolysis using (A) a Brunner incision and (B) a midaxial incision. The neurovascular bundles should be identified to avoid inadvertent neurovascular injury during the operation.

tendon lengthening. Tendon lengthening diminishes excursion of the extensor tendon and generates a lag in extension.[73,74]

Volar capsular release Volar capsular release can be initiated if a satisfactory extension arc still cannot be obtained after flexor tenolysis. The checkrein ligament is first released from the head of proximal phalanx. Take caution to avoid inadvertent injury to the transverse digital artery, which runs across the head of proximal phalanx, 2 mm proximal to the PIP joint and deep to the checkrein ligament (**Fig. 10**).

Next, if the contracture is not improved, the insertion of the ACL is sharply divided (**Fig. 11**). In addition, the proximal portion of the volar plate is transected and freed from the underlying proximal phalanx. Afterward, the PIP joint is gently manipulated until a functional AOM is obtained. Ultimately, if the flexor contracture still remains after release of the ACL and volar plate, the proper collateral ligaments may be progressively released until they are totally freed from their origin. The proper collateral ligaments should first be released from the volar origin, and then, if necessary, released from the dorsal origin. Using this tactic, stability of the PIP joint is maintained by the lateral retinacular fascia.[44,51,69] Once the final functional AOM is obtained, surgeons must then ascertain

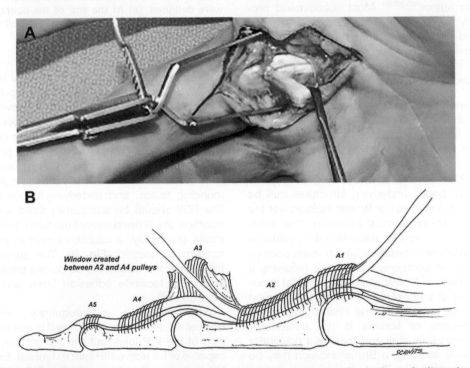

Fig. 8. (A) Traction force is applied to profundus and superficialis tendons individually to facilitate breaking of adhesion between both tendons. (B) A Freer elevator is used to dissect the peritendinous adhesion. ([B] From Kaplan FTD. The stiff finger. Hand Clin 2010;26(2):201; with permission.)

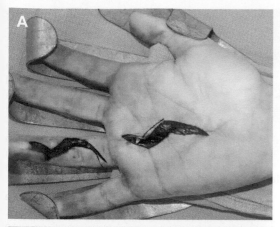

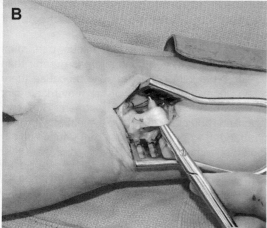

Fig. 9. (*A, B*) Incisions designed for flexor tenolysis.

normal circulation of the finger. If there is a possibility of circulation being compromised, the surgeon and patient should be accepting of a lesser motion arc because the viability of the digit is most important.

Existing literature suggests that it may be impossible to achieve a full AOM after open surgical release. Normally, the functional AOM for the PIP joint is between 36° and 86°, with an average

of 61°.[75] Open release typically shifts the AOM, such that 25° to 30° of extension is gained, yet there is a concomitant amount of flexion loss.[44,45] Nonetheless, an open release procedure should provide enough motion at the PIP joint for daily hand usage. Ghidella and colleagues[61] found that outcomes of open surgical release are most favorable in younger patients with a less severe diagnosis or a preoperative contracture of less than 45°. Conversely, adverse surgical outcomes are more commonly seen in patients who are older, who have had a large number of operative procedures, those with extensive extracapsular release, or those with severe joint deformity.[46,47,61]

Dynamic traction device application

In 1986, Schenck[76] proposed dynamic traction splinting and early passive movements as a viable treatment option for comminuted intra-articular fractures of the PIP joint. Dynamic traction splinting applies the ligamentotaxis principle, in which one gradually extends and distracts the PIP joint to overcome the deformation force. The benefits of this method have been generously demonstrated in the literature.[77–80] Avoiding the possibility of added injury from open release, application of a dynamic distraction device diminishes the extent of soft tissue dissection to prevent further fibrosis or stiffness. Moreover, this method transmits force directly to the phalangeal bone, avoiding the development of pressure sores that frequently accompany serial casting or splinting. Treatments using a distraction device have grown in popularity throughout the last decade, and a wide variety of designs have been developed. However, all distraction devices can be principally classified into 1 of 2 types: extension correction or distraction correction devices (**Fig. 12**).[81]

Past studies have demonstrated favorable outcomes using various distractor models. On average, patients gain 42° to 62° of motion, and the distraction method has been shown to improve the degree of contracture even in highly resistant

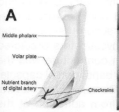
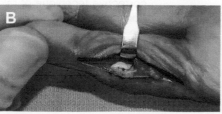
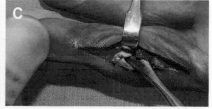

Fig. 10. Volar capsular release. (*A*) Relevant anatomy. (*B*) Incision of periosteal attachments of the volar plate. (*C*) Volar plate dissected. ([*A*] *From* Chung KC, Brown M. Capsulotomy for proximal interphalangeal contracture. In: Chung KC, editor. Operative techniques: hand and wrist surgery. 3rd edition. Philadelphia: Elsevier; 2018. p. 368; with permission.)

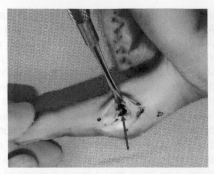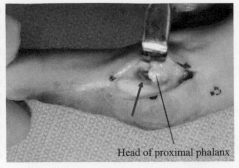

Head of proximal phalanx

Fig. 11. Arrows indicate where the true and accessory collateral ligaments are freed from the proximal phalanx.

cases.[82–84] In 2013, Houshian and colleagues[78,81] detailed the long-term outcomes of chronic post-traumatic PIP joint flexion contracture treated using a distraction device. During the distraction phase, the system was activated 1 mm each day. The distraction phase was terminated once a 5-mm joint opening or full extension of PIP joint was obtained; however, the device was kept in place for 1 week after successful distraction. Results showed that the average AOM had improved by 30° to 90° at an average of 54 months after device removal. Investigators emphasized the use of a distraction device to correct flexion contractures, as opposed to an extension device, because a distraction device can circumferentially lengthen the periarticular tissue, whereas an extension device only creates pronounced effects on the volar soft tissue. In addition, this study reported a combined complication rate of less than 15% for pin-tract infection, swelling, redness,

temporary flexion deformity of the DIP join, and pain, with all complications being completely resolved within a few weeks after the treatment period.

When using a distraction technique, care must be taken if the flexion contracture is greater than 80° or if the joint is hypermobile, because there is an increased chance of asymmetrical joint opening or subluxation after treatment. Serial radiographs and close follow-up evaluations are recommended to prevent further joint subluxation.[81] Patients with connective tissue diseases that affect the elasticity of the tissue, especially the neurovascular bundle, or delay healing require intensive monitoring during the distraction period or may be better suited for an alternate treatment method.

EXTENSION CONTRACTURE

Although less common than flexion contractures, extension contractures are another frequent complication following PIP joint injury. Kuczynski[85] proposed that extension contractures result from adhesion between deep surfaces of the extensor apparatus and the retinacular ligament with the underlying bone. In cases of long-standing contracture, the fibrosis and adhesion may also involve the collateral ligaments, causing a more profound stiffness of the joint. Around the same time, Egawa and colleagues[86] presented their corrective technique of releasing the lateral band from the central band and dorsal capsule over the PIP joint in an effort to accomplish a greater flexion arc. However, the investigators predicted that the cause of extension contracture was the adhesion among the central band, dorsal capsule, and the lateral band. Because the lateral band had shifted dorsally from adhesion of the dorsal capsule and central slip, its release may restore the volar alignment and improve the extension arc. Long-standing extension contracture may also result from intrinsic contracture.[87]

Fig. 12. (A) Extension correction device. (B) Distraction correction device. (Courtesy of C. Hokierti, MD, Bangkok, Thailand.)

A

B

Nonetheless, adhesions of the extensor apparatus are most commonly the cause of the contracture.[69] Illuminating the imperative cause of disease will aid the surgeon to determine an appropriate structural release sequence that avoids unnecessary surgical exposure and reduces opportunity for further inflammation or consequential fibrosis.

Prevention

The same measures described for overcoming flexion contracture can be applied to prevent extension contracture. Early mobilization after establishing concentric reduction with adequate joint stability is the most important preventive paradigm.

Nonoperative Treatment

There are several available modalities for nonoperative treatment of PIP joint extension contractures. Two methods, taping and interphalangeal slings, follow a similar concept. Both mold the finger posture to achieve a specific position and are gradually adjusted to provide a gentle prolonged stretch. Oppositely, a dynamic flexion splint applies passive force across a joint in one direction while permitting active motion in the opposite direction. All of the nonoperative treatment options facilitate plastic deformation, and, as a result of viscoplastic properties, tissue formation is permanently lengthened. Therefore, any type of static or dynamic splinting can correct the contracted joint.[60,88]

Despite the high prevalence of extensor contracture, reports on outcomes after nonoperative treatment are limited. Existing literature does indicate that nonoperative treatment can improve the arc of extension in cases where the cause of contracture was solely capsular or intrinsic muscle adhesion.[59,89] Similarly to treatment of flexion contracture, any surgical procedure may add some intent of injury and promote further scar and adhesion. Therefore, nonoperative treatment should be the first line of treatment considered for all contractures. For rare cases, such as a patient who presents with a contracture with a chronic ulcer on the dorsum of finger or bony ankylosis, the nonoperative phase can be skipped because open surgical correction is inevitable.

Surgical Treatment

Surgical treatment is indicated when nonoperative treatments are unable to improve the AOM. Given the risks of operative intervention, a nonoperative regiment should be continued if it continuously reveals positive gains in ROM.[69]

The literature contains only a few case reports to guide expectations, and results vary substantially. In one report, Mansat and Delprat[54] investigated outcomes after surgical correction of extension contracture. Among the 246 contracture releases of the PIP joint performed, of which 45% were extension contractures, the degree of flexion improved by an average of 28°, whereas the PIP ROM improved from 19°-34° preoperatively to 8°-62° postoperatively.[54] There are 2 options used for surgical correction of a PIP joint extension contracture.

Extensor tenolysis

Extensor tenolysis is performed under wide-awake local anesthesia with or without a tourniquet. If a tourniquet is used, it should be placed at the forearm for a limited time period (no longer than 2 hours) to diminish pain. The wide-awake approach permits the patient to maintain active control and move their hand throughout the operation. Active movement by the patient will provide an indication of the adequacy of surgical release and can be used to further break existing adhesion. Furthermore, the patient can participate throughout the progression of the surgery and observe the final results, which may encourage them to take a proactive role in the recovery process.

Egawa and colleagues[86] were the pioneers who first presented open surgical release for correction of a PIP joint extensor contracture. Their procedure involved extensor tenolysis and release of the lateral band from the central band. Inoue[90] reported that, on average, the patients who underwent this procedure gained 56° of flexion but lost 9° of extension.

Surgeons have the option between a dorsal or dorsolateral approach. These approaches are pointed at the extensor apparatus, which is most commonly the structure responsible for the contracture. A curvilinear incision is made over the PIP joint. This incision design permits proximal or distal incision extension, which may be necessary for accurate determination of normal tissue planes. Skin flaps are meticulously elevated from the underlying tendon by sharp dissection. Care should be taken to preserve the paratenon of the extensor tendon. Next, the extensor apparatus and lateral bands are circumferentially freed using a scalpel or Freer elevator. The extensor tendon should be freed entirely from the base of proximal phalanx to the dorsal capsule or central slip insertion. Caution must be taken to avoid iatrogenic avulsion of the central slip, terminal tendon, or triangular ligament. In the scenario that there is some contracture of the DIP joint, tenolysis can be extended distally to reach the terminal tendon insertion. Afterward, the extensor tendon and lateral band are completely released. Longitudinal parallel incisions are made between the central tendon and the lateral bands at the level of PIP joint (**Fig. 13**). These incisions will release the lateral band from the central tendon and can restore volar shift. The passive AOM should be

assessed. If full passive flexion is achieved, the tourniquet is deflated. The patient is asked to actively flex the affected finger while, simultaneously, the surgeon gently manipulates the PIP joint. Further extensor tenolysis is required if the patient cannot obtain a functional flexion arc. In this case, proximal extension of the incision may be necessary.

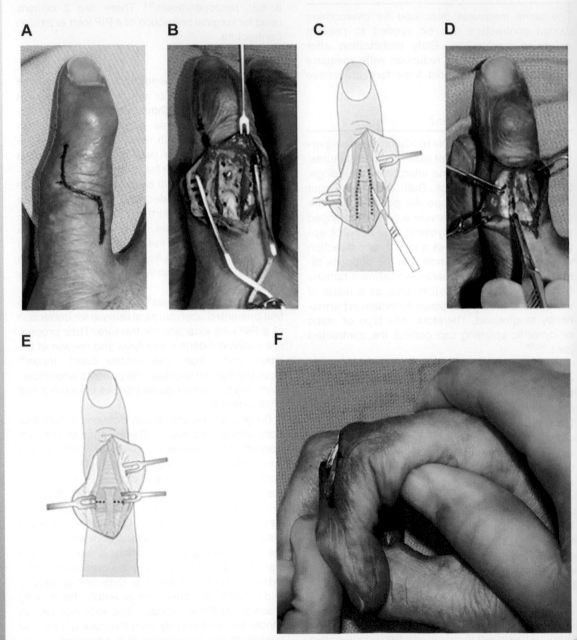

Fig. 13. Extensor tenolysis. (*A*) Extensor structures approached via a curvilinear dorsal incision. (*B, C*) Lateral bands are separated from the central tendon by making bilateral longitudinal incisions along the border of the central tendon. (*D, E*) Dorsal capsulotomy and collateral ligament excision are performed through the interval of the lateral band and central tendon. (*F*) The AOM is evaluated. ([*C, E*] *From* Yang G, McGlinn EP, Chung KC. Management of the stiff finger: evidence and outcomes. Clin Plast Surg 2014;41(3):509; with permission.)

A finger that is stiff in extension also has a chance of developing flexor tendon adhesion, indicating the need for flexor tenolysis. Thus, it is crucial to test the excursion of the flexor tendons. Excursion of the flexor tendons can be tested by asking the patient to actively flex the finger during the operation or by directly pulling the flexor tendons via a volar stab incision. Because it is impossible to determine the necessity of flexor tenolysis preoperatively, the patient should be informed of the possibility of subsidiary flexor tenolysis before the operation.

Dorsal capsulotomy

If all previously described treatment methods have been attempted without restoration of passive flexion, dorsal capsulotomy is indicated. The dorsal capsules are exposed through the interval between the lateral band and central slip. An incision is made on the dorsal capsule while gently forcing the PIP joint in flexion. A Freer elevator is used to free any intra-articular adhesion and fibrosis around the volar plate. If flexion is limited after dorsal capsulotomy, partial or total collateral ligament excision can be safely performed without consequent PIP joint instability[62] **(Fig. 14)**. The

success of the open release is justified when the patient can actively reproduce the same amount of function that was achieved at the operating scene.

RE-DISPLACEMENT AND RE-DISLOCATION

Occasionally, a chosen treatment option cannot maintain sufficient joint stability, leading to re-displacement or re-dislocation. Re-displacement of a seemingly stable reduction may also arise from poor initial positioning, too rapid mobilization into extension, or hardware failure.

The prevalence rate of re-displacement varies within the literature, because it is highly dependent on the severity of disease and the mode of treatment. For example, re-displacement has been reported in up to 31% of patients who underwent volar plate arthroplasty for PIP dorsal fracture dislocation.[25,42,78,91,92]

Prevention and Treatment

Surgeons must carefully evaluate the pathology of the injury and select the best treatment to provide adequate stability. Complication rates are markedly high in patients who undergo a procedure

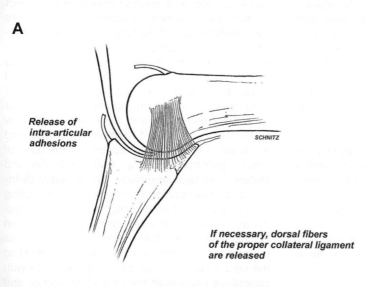

A

Release of intra-articular adhesions

SCHNITZ

If necessary, dorsal fibers of the proper collateral ligament are released

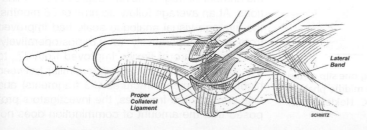

B

Proper Collateral Ligament

Lateral Band

SCHNITZ

Fig. 14. Dorsal capsulotomy. (*A*) Release of the dorsal capsule by making a transverse incision and using a Freer elevator to facilitate lysis of the intra-articular fibrosis. (*B*) Partial or total collateral ligament excision by insertion of a blade between the head of the proximal phalanx and the collateral ligament and swinging it back and forth. (*From* Kaplan FTD. The stiff finger. Hand Clin 2010;26(2):200; with permission.)

that does not appropriately match the pathology, and previous research reveals that the major cause of complications is attributed to inappropriate treatment.[25,42,92,93]

Preventing re-displacement is achieved through the appropriate initial treatment. Nonetheless, certain treatment types are associated with higher rates of re-displacement. For example, volar plate arthroplasty has a high reported rate of re-displacement because the head of the proximal phalanx can become embedded into the advanced volar plate.[25] In addition, the bony defect depth at the volar lip of middle phalanx may be wider than the thickness of the volar plate. Consequently, the volar plate provides insufficient support to produce a buttress effect.[8] To overcome this discrepancy, the bony defect can be augmented with a bone graft from the excised fragmented bone.[92] Alternatively, Wiley[94] described a technique using one slip of the FDS tendon and attaching it to the base of the middle phalanx at the volar lip defect (**Fig. 15**). Although large-scale studies on the outcomes of this procedure have not been performed, their small case series of 3 patients reported satisfactory results without re-displacement.[94]

Maintaining an appropriate postoperative follow-up protocol is essential. Serial radiography should be performed periodically. Mangelson and colleagues[45] recommend a follow-up visit every 7 to 10 days for 4 weeks with serial radiographic evaluation. The appropriate interval for an individual's follow-up schedule depends on disease severity and patient compliance. In the case that there is increased potential for displacement and treatment may not provide complete stability, the follow-up schedule should be revised for more frequent visits.

Treatment of a re-displaced joint usually requires a more aggressive revision or salvage operation. A revision operation should be chosen based on 3 criteria: reduction achieved, stability maintained, and an acceptable condition of remaining cartilage. If the surgeon cannot satisfy all 3 criteria with revision, a salvage operation such as arthrodesis or implant arthroplasty is

recommended.[45] The most commonly selected revision operation is a hemihamate autograft. The literature reports favorable outcomes for this operation in patients with involvement of more than 50% of the articular surface of the middle phalanx and in cases of chronic dorsal fracture dislocation of the PIP joint. In addition, the use of a hemihamate autograft operation has been shown to improve the AOM, reduce pain, and maintain stability of PIP joint.[95–97] In one example, Calfee and colleagues[95] followed 22 patients who underwent hemihamate autograft for an average of 4.5 years postoperatively. Investigators found that the postoperative AOM improved from 19° to 89°, and no patients reported significant postoperative pain.

MALUNION

Neglect of a PIP joint fracture dislocation or inadequate prior treatment can further result in malunion. Malposition of the bony structures can facilitate abnormal wear or interference to the AOM. Consequently, arthritis or ankylosis may develop. Malunions of periarticular fractures of the PIP joint are scantly reported. Similar to the treatment of re-displaced joints, surgeons can use a revision or a salvage operation to correct a malunion. Various revision operations are commonly practiced, including corrective osteotomy with ORIF, volar plate arthroplasty, and hemihamate autograft. Acceptable results following corrective osteotomy with ORIF are demonstrated in the literature.[98–102] For example, Del Pinal and colleagues[102] examined outcomes using their osteotomy technique and ORIF with miniscrew and/or cerclage wire in 11 patients who sustained a malunited intra-articular fracture of the base of middle phalanx. Using a modified Eaton and Malerich shotgun approach, the operator delineated cartilage-containing fragments by removing fibrous tissue and new bone. Next, articular fragments were disimpacted and elevated. Open wedge osteotomy of the volar lip fragment was performed to restore the volar buttress. They filled the void underneath the elevated fragments with cancellous bone graft from the distal radius, and fixation was performed, if necessary, based on the number of fragments and degree of comminutions. At an average follow-up time of 28 months, the average visual analogue scale had improved from 9.1 preoperatively to 0.8 postoperatively. The average arc of flexion improved from 77° to 84°. Because these results were similar between highly comminuted fractures (>3 fragments) and less comminuted fractures, the investigators proposed that the amount of comminution does not

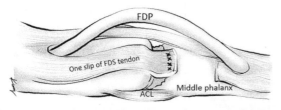

Fig. 15. Wiley's technique of attaching one slip of the superficial tendon to the base of the middle phalanx at the volar lip defect. (*Courtesy of* C. Hokierti, MD, Bangkok, Thailand.)

play a substantial role in predicting outcomes of osteotomy and internal fixation. Investigators also emphasized that the quality of the remaining cartilage was the most crucial factor to undergo osteotomy and ORIF.[102]

Despite reports of favorable outcomes after osteotomy and ORIF, many surgeons prefer to reconstruct the volar buttress of the middle phalanx with the volar plate or a hemihamate autograft. A malunion that has a high degree of comminution is technically demanding, and surgical restoration of the concentric reduction is fraught with potential risks, such as loss of fixation, avascular necrosis, or loss of joint mobility.[103] Thus, surgeons may be more comfortable with the volar plate arthroplasty or hemihamate autograft procedure.

O'Rourke and colleagues[104] published an 11-year review of 59 intra-articular fractures of the phalanges. Although 17% of joints showed radiological evidence of arthritis at the final follow-up visit, only one patient had persistent symptomatic pain. Nevertheless, if the PIP joint becomes arthritic, a salvage operation is indicated. Salvage procedures can provide the patient with a painless joint and improve hand function. Arthrodesis is indicated for patients with intense hand usage, insufficient bone stock, or lack of stability to support an implant. Otherwise, implant arthroplasty is typically selected to reduce pain and achieve functional motion. If arthrodesis is selected, the position of the fused PIP joint must accommodate the basic functions of the hand.

Prevention

Exemplary management of any PIP joint fracture can prevent malunion. Careful evaluation to determine the disease abnormality, selection of the best treatment option, and intensive postoperative follow-up care are fundamental to avoid subsequent complication. Early intervention is encouraged to decrease the need for a salvage operation and preclude reconstruction.

SWAN-NECK DEFORMITY

Hyperextension deformity of the PIP joint, regardless of subluxation, may develop secondary to an unhealed volar plate. Patients are unable to flex the PIP joint and afflict painful snapping of the lateral bands during forceful flexion. The deformity can lead to swan-neck deformity by the chronicity of tendon shifting. A treatment of swan-neck deformities should aim to relieve painful motion while maintaining joint stability. However, treating a chronic swan-neck deformity of the PIP joint can be a greater technical challenge owing to scar deformation. If the joint movement is supple and the PIP joint is well aligned with established stability, a swan-neck deformity can be treated using an extension block splint and buddy taping to initiate early motion exercises. Open surgical intervention is indicated if the following is a factor:

- The hyperextension deformity is persistent,
- The patient cannot tolerate splinting, or
- The underlying abnormality requires surgical correction (eg, malunion or re-displacement).

For open interventions, surgeons have the choice between volar plate reattachment or FDS tenodesis. Stiffness of the periarticular soft tissue may preclude the possibility of volar plate reattachment, in which case FDS tenodesis is the best option. Previous literature has demonstrated satisfactory operative outcomes with correction of the swan-neck deformity after FDS tenodesis.[105–107] In one example, Catalano and colleagues[106] reviewed their 15 years of experience treating patients with posttraumatic chronic hyperextension of the PIP joint using FDS tenodesis (**Fig. 16**). Out of 12 total patients, 10 returned with a good or excellent outcome, and the average ROM improved from 31°-92° preoperatively to

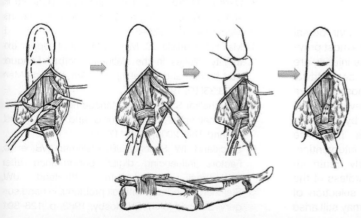

Fig. 16. The steps of flexor tenodesis. The ulnar slip of the FDS is identified at the cruciate pulley and transected. The end of the distal portion of the ulnar slip of the FDS is secured through the A2 pulley and sutured to itself. Note the slight degree of PIP flexion after FDS tenodesis. (*Adapted from* Wei DH, Terrono AL. Superficialis sling (flexor digitorum superficialis tenodesis) for swan neck reconstruction. J Hand Surg Am 2015;40(10):2071; with permission.)

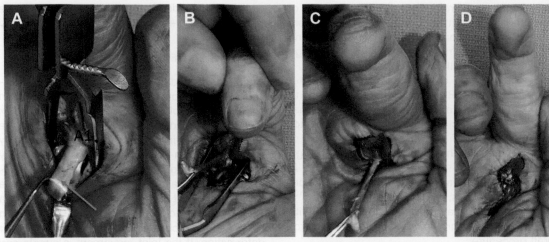

Fig. 17. Modified FDS tenodesis at the A1 pulley. (*A*) The FDS is identified just proximal to the A1 pulley. (*B*) Radial and ulnar slip of FDS is transected 1 cm proximal to the A1 pulley. (*C*) The distal portion of the transected FDS is sutured to the cut edge of the A1 pulley. (*D*) Tension is set to maintain the PIP joint in 20° of flexion.

12°-100° postoperatively. Nonetheless, several studies have reported that this technique will lead to inevitable flexion contracture.[108–110] Most surgeons advocate 20° to 30° of PIP joint flexion to facilitate an adequate functional AOM.[111] Considering the scar and adhesion of PIP joint that may arise by performing FDS tenodesis at the A2 pulley, the senior author has modified this operation by performing FDS tenodesis at the A1 pulley instead (**Fig. 17**).

Prevention

Owing to the nature of injury, preventing a volar plate injury is nearly impossible. Nonetheless, early detection is a key element to ensure adequate recovery. Chronic hyperextension deformity can lead to a fixed swan-neck deformity. Treatment protocols for the fixed deformity are more challenging and may require a more aggressive salvage operation.

SUMMARY

PIP joint injuries are common. In particular, dorsal fracture dislocations continue to be the most prevalent pattern of injury. However, these injuries are frequently overlooked because they seem trivial in nature. Given the high rate of postoperative complications for PIP joint injuries, every injured finger should be carefully evaluated by a trained physician. All pathologic findings must be addressed before pursuing a specific intervention. Current evidence supports that early treatment can improve surgical outcomes regardless of the treatment method chosen. Despite selection of the proper treatment, complications may still arise

because of the delicate anatomic structure of the PIP joint. The most prevalent complications, stiffness and flexion contracture, are more easily prevented than treated. To lessen the chance and severity of any complication, the chosen treatment should provide concentric alignment and facilitate early ROM exercises.

ACKNOWLEDGMENTS

The authors thank Drs Nasa Fujihara and Chananya Hokierti for their generous figure contributions.

REFERENCES

1. Leibovic SJ, Bowers WH. Anatomy of the proximal interphalangeal joint. Hand Clin 1994;10(2): 169–78.
2. Court-Brown CM, Wood AM, Aitken S. The epidemiology of acute sports-related fractures in adults. Injury 2008;39(12):1365–72.
3. Degroot H 3rd, Mass DP. Hand injury patterns in softball players using a 16 inch ball. Am J Sports Med 1988;16(3):260–5.
4. Mall NA, Carlisle JC, Matava MJ, et al. Upper extremity injuries in the National Football League: part I: hand and digital injuries. Am J Sports Med 2008;36(10):1938–44.
5. Chinchalkar SJ, Gan BS. Management of proximal interphalangeal joint fractures and dislocations. J Hand Ther 2003;16(2):117–28.
6. Strickland JW, Steichen JB, Kleinman WB, et al. Factors influencing digital performance after phalangeal fracture. In: Strickland JW, Steichen JB, editors. Difficult problems in hand surgery. St Louis (MO): CV Mosby; 1982. p. 126–39.

7. Hess F, Furnstahl P, Gallo LM, et al. 3D analysis of the proximal interphalangeal joint kinematics during flexion. Comput Math Methods Med 2013; 2013:138063.

8. Bowers WH, Wolf JW Jr, Nehil JL, et al. The proximal interphalangeal joint volar plate. I. An anatomical and biomechanical study. J Hand Surg Am 1980;5(1):79–88.

9. Blazar PE, Steinberg DR. Fractures of the proximal interphalangeal joint. J Am Acad Orthop Surg 2000;8(6):383–90.

10. Dias JJ. Intraarticular injuries of the distal and proximal interphalangeal joints. In: Berger RA, Weiss AC, editors. Hand Surgery. Volume 1. First editon. Philadelphia: Lippincott Williams & Wilkins; 2004. p. 153–74.

11. Kiefhaber TR, Stern PJ, Grood ES. Lateral stability of the proximal interphalangeal joint. J Hand Surgery 1986;11(5):661–9.

12. Minamikawa Y, Horii E, Amadio PC, et al. Stability and constraint of the proximal interphalangeal joint. J Hand Surgery 1993;18(2):198–204.

13. Page SM, Stern PJ. Complications and range of motion following plate fixation of metacarpal and phalangeal fractures. J Hand Surgery 1998;23(5): 827–32.

14. Schenck RR. Classification of fractures and dislocations of the proximal interphalangeal joint. Hand Clinics 1994;10(2):179–85.

15. Day CS, Stern PJ. Fractures of the metacarpals and phalanges. In: Wolfe SW, Hotchkiss RN, Pederson WC, et al, editors. Green's operative hand surgery. 6th edition. Philadelphia: Churchill Livingstone; 2011. p. 239–90.

16. London PS. Sprains and fractures involving the interphalangeal joints. The Hand 1971;3:155–8.

17. Rhee RY, Reading G, Wray RC. A biomechanical study of the collateral ligaments of the proximal interphalangeal joint. J Hand Surgery 1992;17(1): 157–63.

18. Eaton RG, Sunde D, Pang D, et al. Evaluation of "neocollateral" ligament formation by magnetic resonance imaging after total excision of the proximal interphalangeal collateral ligaments. J Hand Surgery 1998;23(2):322–7.

19. Greg Merrell JFS. Dislocations and ligament injuries in the digit. In: Wolfe SW, Hotchkiss RN, Pederson WC, et al, editors. Green's operative hand surgery. Philadelphia: Churchill Livingstone; 2011. p. 293–4.

20. Ford DJ, el-Hadidi S, Lunn PG, et al. Fractures of the phalanges: results of internal fixation using 1.5mm and 2mm A. O. screws. J Hand Surg Br 1987;12(1):28–33.

21. Weiss AP, Hastings H 2nd. Distal unicondylar fractures of the proximal phalanx. J Hand Surg 1993; 18(4):594–9.

22. Fahmy NR, Harvey RA. The "S" Quattro in the management of fractures in the hand. J Hand Surg Br 1992;17(3):321–31.

23. Sammut D, Evans D. The bone tie. A new device for interfragmentary fixation. J Hand Surg Br 1999; 24(1):64–9.

24. Jupiter JB, Belsky MD. Fractures and dislocations of the hand. In: Browner BD, Jupiter JB, Levine AM, Trafton PC, editors. Skeletal trauma. Philadelphia: W B Saunders; 1992. p. 959–63.

25. Hastings H 2nd, Carroll CT. Treatment of closed articular fractures of the metacarpophalangeal and proximal interphalangeal joints. Hand Clin 1988;4(3):503–27.

26. Kiefhaber TR, Stern PJ. Fracture dislocations of the proximal interphalangeal joint. The J Hand Surg 1998;23(3):368–80.

27. Morgan JP, Gordon DA, Klug MS, et al. Dynamic digital traction for unstable comminuted intra-articular fracture-dislocations of the proximal interphalangeal joint. J Hand Surg 1995;20(4):565–73.

28. Agee JM. Unstable fracture dislocations of the proximal interphalangeal joint. Treatment with the force couple splint. Clin Orthop Relat Res 1987;(214):101–12.

29. Stern PJ, Roman RJ, Kiefhaber TR, et al. Pilon fractures of the proximal interphalangeal joint. J Hand Surg 1991;16(5):844–50.

30. Calfee RP, Sommerkamp TG. Fracture-dislocation about the finger joints. J Hand Surg 2009;34(6): 1140–7.

31. Lee LS, Lee HM, Hou YT, et al. Surgical outcome of volar plate arthroplasty of the proximal interphalangeal joint using the Mitek micro GII suture anchor. J Trauma 2008;65(1):116–22.

32. Viegas SF. Extension block pinning for proximal interphalangeal joint fracture dislocations: preliminary report of a new technique. J Hand Surg 1992;17(5):896–901.

33. Newington DP, Davis TR, Barton NJ. The treatment of dorsal fracture-dislocation of the proximal interphalangeal joint by closed reduction and Kirschner wire fixation: a 16-year follow up. J Hand Surg Br 2001;26(6):537–40.

34. Phair IC, Quinton DN, Allen MJ. The conservative management of volar avulsion fractures of the P.I.P. joint. J Hand Surg Br 1989;14(2):168–70.

35. Williams RM, Hastings H 2nd, Kiefhaber TR. PIP fracture/dislocation treatment technique: use of a hemi-hamate resurfacing arthroplasty. Tech Hand Up Extrem Surg 2002;6(4):185–92.

36. Freiberg A. Management of proximal interphalangeal joint injuries. Can J Plast Surg 2007;15(4): 199–203.

37. Bindra R, Colantoni Woodside J. Treatment of proximal interphalangeal joint fracture-dislocations. JBJS Rev 2015;3(12).

38. Salter RB. The physiologic basis of continuous passive motion for articular cartilage healing and regeneration. Hand Clin 1994;10(2):211–9.

39. Tekkis PP, Kessaris N, Enchill-Yawson M, et al. Palmar dislocation of the proximal interphalangeal joint–an injury not to be missed. J Accid Emerg Med 1999;16(6):431–2.

40. Grant I, Berger AC, Tham SK. Internal fixation of unstable fracture dislocations of the proximal interphalangeal joint. J Hand Surg Br 2005; 30(5):492–8.

41. Dionysian E, Eaton RG. The long-term outcome of volar plate arthroplasty of the proximal interphalangeal joint. J Hand Surg 2000;25(3):429–37.

42. Eaton RG, Malerich MM. Volar plate arthroplasty of the proximal interphalangeal joint: a review of ten years' experience. J Hand Surg 1980;5(3):260–8.

43. Khouri JS, Bloom JM, Hammert WC. Current trends in the management of proximal interphalangeal joint injuries of the hand. Plast Reconstr Surg 2013;132(5):1192–204.

44. Hogan CJ, Nunley JA. Posttraumatic proximal interphalangeal joint flexion contractures. J Am Acad Orthop Surg 2006;14(9):524–33.

45. Mangelson JJ, Stern P, Abzug JM, et al. Complications following dislocations of the proximal interphalangeal joint. J Bone Joint Surg Am 2013; 95(14):1326–32.

46. Curtis RM. Capsulectomy of the interphalangeal joints of the fingers. J Bone Joint Surg Am 1954; 36-A(6):1219–32.

47. Curtis RM. Management of the stiff proximal interphalangeal joint. J Hand Surg Eur Vol 1969;1(1):32–7.

48. Allieu Y, Ould Ouali A, Gomis R, et al. Simple arthrolysis for flexor rigidity of the proximal interphalangeal joint. Ann Chir Main 1983;2(4):330–5.

49. Freeland AE, Hardy MA, Singletary S. Rehabilitation for proximal phalangeal fractures. J Hand Ther 2003;16(2):129–42.

50. Schneider LH. Tenolysis and capsulectomy after hand fractures. Clin Orthop Relat Res 1996;(327): 72–8.

51. Kaplan FT. The stiff finger. Hand Clin 2010;26(2): 191–204.

52. Yang G, McGlinn EP, Chung KC. Management of the stiff finger: evidence and outcomes. Clin Plast Surg 2014;41(3):501–12.

53. Jupiter JB, Goldfarb CA, Nagy L, et al. Posttraumatic reconstruction in the hand. J Bone Joint Surg Am 2007;89(2):428–35.

54. Mansat M, Delprat J. Contractures of the proximal interphalangeal joint. Hand Clin 1992;8(4):777–86.

55. Merritt WH. Written on behalf of the stiff finger. J Hand Ther 1998;11(2):74–9.

56. Glasgow C, Fleming J, Tooth LR, et al. The long-term relationship between duration of treatment and contracture resolution using dynamic orthotic devices for the stiff proximal interphalangeal joint: a prospective cohort study. J Hand Ther 2012; 25(1):38–46 [quiz: 47].

57. Harrison DH. The stiff proximal interphalangeal joint. Hand 1977;9(2):102–8.

58. Fess EE. Splints: mechanics versus convention. J Hand Ther 1995;8(2):124–30.

59. Hunter E, Laverty J, Pollock R, et al. Nonoperative treatment of fixed flexion deformity of the proximal interphalangeal joint. J Hand Surg Br 1999;24(3): 281–3.

60. Prosser R. Splinting in the management of proximal interphalangeal joint flexion contracture. J Hand Ther 1996;9(4):378–86.

61. Ghidella SD, Segalman KA, Murphey MS. Long-term results of surgical management of proximal interphalangeal joint contracture. J Hand Surg 2002;27(5):799–805.

62. Diao E, Eaton RG. Total collateral ligament excision for contractures of the proximal interphalangeal joint. J Hand Surg 1993;18(3):395–402.

63. Pittet-Cuenod B, della Santa D, Chamay A. Total anterior tenoarthrolysis to treat inveterate flexion contraction of the fingers: a series of 16 patients. Ann Plast Surg 1991;26(4):358–64.

64. Lalonde DH, Kozin S. Tendon disorders of the hand. Plast Reconstr Surg 2011;128(1):1e–14e.

65. Dukas AG, Wolf JM. Management of complications of periarticular fractures of the distal interphalangeal, proximal interphalangeal, metacarpophalangeal, and carpometacarpal joints. Hand Clin 2015;31(2):179–92.

66. Stanley JK, Jones WA, Lynch MC. Percutaneous accessory collateral ligament release in the treatment of proximal interphalangeal joint flexion contracture. J Hand Surg Br 1986;11(3):360–3.

67. Cerovac S, Stanley J. Outcome review on the percutaneous release of the proximal interphalangeal joint accessory collateral ligaments. Orthop Rev 2009;1(2):e19.

68. Levaro F, Henry M, Masson M. Management of the stiff proximal interphalangeal joint. J Am Soc Surg Hand 2003;3(2):78–87.

69. Watt AJ, Chang J. Functional reconstruction of the hand: the stiff joint. Clin Plast Surg 2011; 38(4):577–89.

70. Abbiati G, Delaria G, Saporiti E, et al. The treatment of chronic flexion contractures of the proximal interphalangeal joint. J Hand Surg Br 1995; 20(3):385–9.

71. Gould JS, Nicholson BG. Capsulectomy of the metacarpophalangeal and proximal interphalangeal joints. J Hand Surg 1979;4(5):482–6.

72. Brüser P, Poss T, Larkin G. Results of proximal interphalangeal joint release for flexion contractures: midlateral versus palmar incision. J Hand Surg 1999;24(2):288–94.

73. Vahey JW, Wegner DA, Hastings H 3rd. Effect of proximal phalangeal fracture deformity on extensor tendon function. J Hand Surg Am 1998;23(4):673–81.

74. Beekman RA, Abbot AE, Taylor NL, et al. Extensor mechanism slide for the treatment of proximal interphalangeal joint extension lag: an anatomic study. J Hand Surg 2004;29(6):1063–8.

75. Hume MC, Gellman H, McKellop H, et al. Functional range of motion of the joints of the hand. J Hand Surg Am 1990;15(2):240–3.

76. Schenck RR. Dynamic traction and early passive movement for fractures of the proximal interphalangeal joint. J Hand Surg 1986;11(6):850–8.

77. Houshian S, Gynning B, Schroder HA. Chronic flexion contracture of proximal interphalangeal joint treated with the compass hinge external fixator. A consecutive series of 27 cases. J Hand Surg Br 2002;27(4):356–8.

78. Houshian S, Jing SS, Kazemian GH, et al. Distraction for proximal interphalangeal joint contractures: long-term results. J Hand Surg 2013; 38(10):1951–6.

79. Kasabian A, McCarthy J, Karp N. Use of a multiplanar distracter for the correction of a proximal interphalangeal joint contracture. Ann Plast Surg 1998; 40(4):378–81.

80. Bain GI, Mehta JA, Heptinstall RJ, et al. Dynamic external fixation for injuries of the proximal interphalangeal joint. J Bone Joint Surg Br 1998;80(6):1014–9.

81. Houshian S, Jing SS, Chikkamuniyappa C, et al. Management of posttraumatic proximal interphalangeal joint contracture. J Hand Surg 2013;38(8):1651–8.

82. Hastings H 2nd, Ernst JM. Dynamic external fixation for fractures of the proximal interphalangeal joint. Hand Clin 1993;9(4):659–74.

83. Inanami H, Ninomiya S, Okutsu I, et al. Dynamic external finger fixator for fracture dislocation of the proximal interphalangeal joint. J Hand Surg 1993;18(1):160–4.

84. Patel MR, Joshi BB. Distraction method for chronic dorsal fracture dislocation of the proximal interphalangeal joint. Hand Clin 1994;10(2):327–37.

85. Kuczynski K. The proximal interphalangeal joint. Anatomy and causes of stiffness in the fingers. J Bone Joint Surg Br 1968;50(3):656–63.

86. Egawa T, Doi T, Iwasaki N. Lateral band release for post-traumatic extension contracture of the PIP joint. Seikeigeka (Orthop Surg) 1968;19:1076–8.

87. Shin AY, Amadio PC. The stiff finger. In: Wolfe SW, Hotchkiss RN, Pederson WC, et al, editors. Green's operative hand surgery, vol. 1. Philadelphia: Churchill Livingstone; 2011. p. 370–2.

88. Bonutti PM, Windau JE, Ables BA, et al. Static progressive stretch to reestablish elbow range of motion. Clin Orthop Relat Res 1994;(303):128–34.

89. Weeks PM, Wray RC Jr, Kuxhaus M. The results of non-operative management of stiff joints in the hand. Plast Reconstr Surg 1978;61(1):58–63.

90. Inoue G. Lateral band release for post-traumatic extension contracture of the proximal interphalangeal joint. Arch Orthop Trauma Surg 1991;110(6):298–300.

91. Chalmer J, Blakeway M, Adams Z, et al. Conservative interventions for treating hyperextension injuries of the proximal interphalangeal joints of the fingers. Cochrane Database Syst Rev 2013;(2): CD009030.

92. Deitch MA, Kiefhaber TR, Comisar BR, et al. Dorsal fracture dislocations of the proximal interphalangeal joint: surgical complications and long-term results. J Hand Surg 1999;24(5):914–23.

93. Hamilton SC, Stern PJ, Fassler PR, et al. Mini-screw fixation for the treatment of proximal interphalangeal joint dorsal fracture-dislocations. J Hand Surg 2006;31(8):1349–54.

94. Wiley AM. Instability of the proximal interphalangeal joint following dislocation and fracture dislocation: surgical repair. Hand 1970;2(2):185–91.

95. Calfee RP, Kiefhaber TR, Sommerkamp TG, et al. Hemi-hamate arthroplasty provides functional reconstruction of acute and chronic proximal interphalangeal fracture-dislocations. J Hand Surg 2009;34(7):1232–41.

96. Williams RM, Kiefhaber TR, Sommerkamp TG, et al. Treatment of unstable dorsal proximal interphalangeal fracture/dislocations using a hemi-hamate autograft. J Hand Surg 2003; 28(5):856–65.

97. Yang DS, Lee SK, Kim KJ, et al. Modified hemihamate arthroplasty technique for treatment of acute proximal interphalangeal joint fracture-dislocations. Ann Plast Surg 2014;72(4):411–6.

98. Ishida O, Ikuta Y. Results of treatment of chronic dorsal fracture-dislocations of the proximal interphalangeal joints of the fingers. J Hand Surg Br 1998;23(6):798–801.

99. Wolfe SW, Katz LD. Intra-articular impaction fractures of the phalanges. J Hand Surg 1995;20(2):327–33.

100. McCue FC, Honner R, Johnson MC, et al. Athletic injuries of the proximal interphalangeal joint requiring surgical treatment. J Bone Joint Surg Am 1970;52(5):937–56.

101. Zemel NP, Stark HH, Ashworth CR, et al. Chronic fracture dislocation of the proximal interphalangeal joint-treatment by osteotomy and bone graft. J Hand Surg 1981;6(5):447–55.

102. Del Pinal F, Garcia-Bernal FJ, Delgado J, et al. Results of osteotomy, open reduction, and internal fixation for late-presenting malunited intra-articular fractures of the base of the middle phalanx. J Hand Surg 2005;30(5):1039.e1-14.

103. Harness NG, Chen A, Jupiter JB. Extra-articular osteotomy for malunited unicondylar fractures of the proximal phalanx. J Hand Surg 2005;30(3):566–72.

104. O'Rourke SK, Gaur S, Barton NJ. Long-term outcome of articular fractures of the phalanges: an eleven year follow up. J Hand Surg Br 1989; 14(2):183–93.

105. Brulard C, Sauvage A, Mares O, et al. Treatment of rheumatoid swan neck deformity by tenodesis of proximal interphalangeal joint with a half flexor digitorum superficialis tendon. About 23 fingers at 61 months follow-up. Chir Main 2012;31(3):118–27 [in French].

106. Catalano LW 3rd, Skarparis AC, Glickel SZ, et al. Treatment of chronic, traumatic hyperextension deformities of the proximal interphalangeal joint with flexor digitorum superficialis tenodesis. J Hand Surg 2003;28(3):448–52.

107. Lane CS. Reconstruction of the unstable proximal interphalangeal joint: the double superficialis tenodesis. J Hand Surg 1978;3(4):368–9.

108. Boyer MI, Gelberman RH. Operative correction of swan-neck and boutonniere deformities in the rheumatoid hand. J Am Acad Orthop Surg 1999; 7(2):92–100.

109. Horner G, Terrono AL. Soft tissue procedures for the rheumatoid swan neck finger deformity. Tech Hand Up Extrem Surg 2000;4(1):22–9.

110. Froelich JM, Rizzo M. Reconstruction of swan neck deformities after proximal interphalangeal joint arthroplasty. Hand (N Y) 2014; 9(1):93–8.

111. Wei DH, Terrono AL. Superficialis sling (flexor digitorum superficialis tenodesis) for swan neck reconstruction. J Hand Surg 2015;40(10): 2068–74.

Therapy Concepts for the Proximal Interphalangeal Joint

Nathan P. Douglass, MD, Amy L. Ladd, MD*

KEYWORDS

- Therapy • Proximal interphalangeal joint • Stiffness • Modalities • Orthoses

KEY POINTS

- Injuries to the proximal interphalangeal joint follow 3 phases of healing—inflammatory, fibroblastic, and remodeling.
- Blocking, static, and dynamic orthoses have multiple applications, including protecting injured structures and preventing and treating finger stiffness.
- Hand therapists use modalities, including edema wraps, cryotherapy, scar massage, ultrasound, electrical stimulation, and contrast baths.
- Modalities have multiple purposes, including edema control, pain reduction, desensitization, and neuromuscular reeducation.

INTRODUCTION

The anatomy of the hand is complex, with little room for edema and low tolerances for scar formation. A disruption in the delicate balance in 1 structure often leads to dysfunction in other structures in the same finger. For example, a mallet injury of the distal interphalangeal joint (DIPJ) may lead to hyperextension at the proximal interphalangeal joint (PIPJ).[1] Adjacent fingers may also become affected, such as the quadriga effect from flexor digitorum profundus scarring or overtightening.[2] Comprehension of the nature of the specific PIPJ disorder is, therefore, necessary when designing a hand therapy program. The program requires not only focus on PIPJ motion but also positioning and motion of adjacent joints and fingers. Furthermore, the program changes depending on the timing of the injury and the phases of healing of soft tissues and bone.

Although improving motion in the hand and fingers is crucial in the improvement of patient function, additional hand therapy techniques focus on edema, atrophy prevention, neuromuscular reeducation, and desensitization. The efficacy of a hand therapy program hinges on communication between physician and therapist, the relationship between the therapist and patient, and the active participation of the patient.

PHASES OF HEALING

Inflammatory Phase

The inflammatory phase, as its name suggests, is characterized by increased blood flow and increased inflammatory mediators, such as tumor necrosis factor α and transforming growth factor β.[3–5] Neutrophils and macrophages egress from vasodilated blood vessels and begin the process of phagocytosis and wound healing with

Funding Sources: None related to this topic.
Conflicts of Interest: None related to this topic.
Department of Orthopedic Surgery, Robert A. Chase Hand & Upper Limb Center, Stanford University, 450 Broadway Street, Pavilion C, Redwood City, CA 94063, USA
* Corresponding author.
E-mail address: alad@stanford.edu

Hand Clin 34 (2018) 289–299
https://doi.org/10.1016/j.hcl.2018.01.001
0749-0712/18/© 2018 Elsevier Inc. All rights reserved.

production of collagen III.[4] The process lasts from approximately several days to 1 week, with variation depending on the degree of injury, patient age, and patient health status.[4]

Treatment during the inflammatory phase focuses on pain control, immobilization, and edema control.[6] Range-of-motion activities are generally begun as soon as possible but are often limited by the immobilization modality or patient pain tolerance during the inflammatory phase. The simplest method for edema control is elevation of the extremity and is recommended in nearly all injuries and postoperative conditions. Prefabricated pillows and shoulder slings, which place the hand at heart level, are used routinely. Other modalities used during the inflammatory phase include cryotherapy and retrograde massage.[5]

Fibroblastic Phase

The fibroblastic phase begins after the acute inflammatory phases wanes during the first week and lasts approximately 3 weeks.[6] The period is characterized by increased fibroblast activity and deposition of disorganized collagen.[6] The resulting tissues repaired with cross-linked collagen may have less elasticity than the native tissue, and cross-links may occur across tissue planes leading to stiffness.[7] In earlier stages, this stiffness is often characterized by a soft endpoint but may become a hard endpoint with maturation.[3] Edema, hyperemia, and pain may further limit motion during the earlier phases.

Thus, therapy during the fibroblastic period continues to focus on edema control with increasing emphasis on active and passive motion exercises to reduce the risks of joint contractures and soft tissue adhesions.[8] Depending on the injury sustained or surgery performed, patients may use orthoses for protecting injured structures and remove the orthoses for therapy exercises. Dynamic or blocking orthoses are commonly used. Motion exercises focus on tendon gliding or joint immobilization. Scar massage is initiated after incisions are well healed.[9]

Remodeling Phase

The remodeling phase is characterized by continued collagen synthesis and maturation of collagen cross-linkages.[6] Contractures with a soft endpoint may progress to firm endpoints and permanent contracture if not treated promptly and appropriately. Increasing emphasis is placed on regaining or maintaining range of motion. Care should be taken with passive flexion of the PIPJ because aggressive tension can lead to attenuation of the central slip and extensor lag.[10]

Stiffness and anxiety related to the injury can lead to further disuse resulting in a cascade of further edema, muscle atrophy, and contracture. In some patients this cascade may lead to complex regional pain syndrome (CRPS) or variants thereof. Modalities, including contrast baths, heated ultrasound, paraffin baths, and initiation or continuation of active range-of-motion exercises, are beneficial. In patients with a history of CRPS or those with signs concerning for its onset, mirror therapy may be beneficial.[11–13]

Joint contractures in some patients develop from chronic disorders. Examples include chronic inflammation (eg, rheumatoid arthritis) or neurologic (stroke) or chronic musculotendinous abnormalities (eg, chronic boutonniere deformity). A carefully designed therapy program with orthoses can still be beneficial in long-standing contractures despite remodeling.[10,14]

MOTION EXERCISES

In the early phases of healing, hand therapy exercises focus on the prevention of tendon adhesions. The normal smooth gliding of tendons is maintained by the lubricating synovial fluid within the tendon sheath. Disruptions to this environment may occur with direct tendon trauma, with opening of the tendon sheath incision for surgical exposure, or from surrounding inflammatory processes. Passive and active motion are begun as soon as the nature of the surgery or injury allows.

Contributors to increased tendon gliding resistance include postoperative edema, annular pulleys, extensor tightening, and joint stiffness.[15] Cao and Tang[16] showed that resistance was greatest in the first 4 days after surgery and correlated with edema. Resistance significantly decreased after 6 cycles of passive motion. The investigators recommended starting motion exercises on postoperative days 4 to 7, depending on the severity of edema. Starting the therapy session with passive motion exercises and then proceeding to active motion exercises lessens gliding resistance and improves subsequent tendon excursion with the active exercises.[16]

Active joint motion exercises produce up to 79% more tendon excursion than passive motion exercises.[17] Active motion exercises should, therefore, be used whenever possible when trying to prevent tendon adhesions.

Differential tendon gliding exercises mobilize 1 tendon with minimized motion to adjacent tendons sharing the same sheath or compartment to prevent tendon to tendon adhesions. For example, the PIPJ may be held in extension to immobilize the flexor superficialis tendon while isolated motion through the DIPJ promotes flexor profundus tendon motion. As little as 3 mm of motion may be needed to help prevent such adhesions and can be amplified with use of synergistic finger and wrist motion.[18] Multiple tendon gliding exercises have been described.[19] A simple program follows the fingers through multiple positions: hand flat, hook fist, composite fist, intrinsic plus, and fingertips to palm (**Fig. 1**).

Communication between physician, therapist, and patient is essential for early initiation of motion exercises while taking care to protect vulnerable structures, such as skin incisions, tendon repairs, and fractures.

ORTHOSES

Orthoses have been made from a long list of materials for thousands of years and for a multitude of purposes.[20] A comprehensive review of orthoses types and uses is beyond the scope of this article. The most common functions of orthoses for PIPJ disorders are to aid in pain control while soft tissues heal, protect injured or repaired structures, stabilize joints or fractures, and prevent or correct deformity.

After surgery, immobilization with orthoses is often used during the inflammatory period to aid in soft tissue rest and wound healing. Immobilization orthoses stop all motion at selected joints. Although the position of the PIPJ and metacarpophalangeal joint (MCPJ) may vary from extension (eg, Dupuytren disease) to flexion (eg, flexor tendon repair), hands that are immobilized for longer than 1 week to 2 weeks are generally placed in the safe position (**Fig. 2**). The wrist is placed in 30° of extension, the MCPJ at 70° to 90°, and the PIPJ and DIPJ in full extension. The safe position places collateral ligaments on maximal tension, helping to prevent joint contracture.

Buddy Taping

One of the simplest forms of orthosis is buddy taping or straps (**Fig. 3**). The injured digit is linked to an adjacent digit through the use of a nonrigid material connecting both proximal phalanges. The uninjured digit encourages motion of the injured digit while reducing radioulnar stresses to the PIPJ. Buddy taping is often indicated in stable injuries to the PIPJ, such as simple dislocations,[21] and injuries to the metacarpals.[22] In 1 study, buddy taping showed better outcomes than blocking splints in the treatment of simple PIPJ dislocations.[23] Buddy taping can have drawbacks, such as low patient compliance and skin injuries.[24]

Blocking Splints

Blocking splints are a type of restriction orthosis that limit the range of motion via an external force. They are typically used to prevent joint motion in 1 direction while allowing passive or acting motion in the opposite direction. Dorsal blocking splints are often used in the treatment of unstable dorsal PIPJ dislocations (**Fig. 4**). The splints prevent the joint from extending to an unstable position, while allowing early active flexion. In other cases, a dorsal blocking splint may protect a repaired flexor tendon from extension, while allowing passive or active flexion.

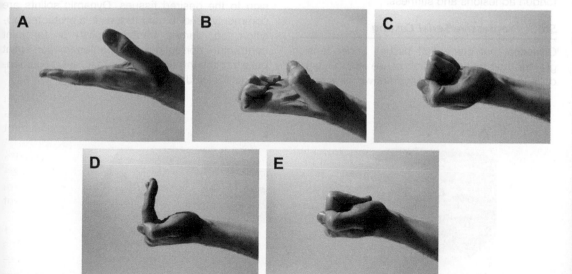

Fig. 1. Differential tendon gliding exercises involve actively placing the hand in a cycle of positions, including (*A*) hand flat, (*B*) hook fist, (*C*) composite fist, (*D*) intrinsic plus, and (*E*) fingertips to palm.

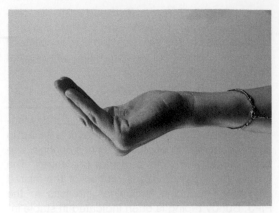

Fig. 2. The safe position places the wrist at 30° extension, MCPJ at 70° of flexion, and the interphalangeal joints in full extension.

Immobilization of 1 joint augments flexion and extension forces across the adjacent non-immobilized joints. Blocking splints with the MCPJ flexed can help promote isolated active PIPJ extension.[3]

Relative motion (RM) orthoses maintain the injured finger(s) in 15° to 30° of MCPJ extension (Fig. 5) or flexion (Fig. 6) relative to the other uninjured fingers, depending on the injury being treated.[25,26] RM extension splints reduce tension on the extensor apparatus and are commonly used for extensor tendon injuries.[26] RM flexion splints promote PIPJ extension and are commonly used for Dupuytren disease and boutonniere deformities.[26] Both the RM flexion and extension splints allow immediate controlled active motion of the MCPJ, PIPJ, and DIPJ and help prevent tendon adhesions and stiffness.

Static Progressive/Serial Casting

Orthoses that place soft tissues under tension greater than resting tension cause lengthening of collagen fibers, in a process known as creep.[27]

As soft tissues lengthen, joints obtain greater range of motion.

Static progressive splinting or serial casting (Fig. 7) are similar methods often used to treat contractures. Their efficacy depends on the force of joint distraction and the time duration of stretching. The viscoelastic properties of ligaments and other soft tissues allow these tissues to stretch over time with a steady force applied. Excessive force may cause microtrauma in soft tissues, leading to additional inflammation, pain, and scarring. Flowers[28] proposed a decision hierarchy for the amount of force that should be applied to stiff joints but the optimal force remains unknown. Therapists should err on the side of low tissue tension because inexperienced therapists tend to place too much force on tissues because additional motion can be gained with a longer duration of therapy.[29]

Flowers and LaStayo[30] developed the term, total end range time (TERT), to describe the accumulated time in which a joint is placed under tension with an orthosis. In their study of 20 PIPJ contractures casted twice over a period of 9 days, they demonstrated that improvements in motion were proportional to TERT. Subsequent studies[31–33] have also demonstrated improved motion with longer durations of splinting. Serial casting in rheumatoid arthritis and juvenile idiopathic arthritis can also be beneficial for chronic atraumatic PIPJ contractures.[14]

Dynamic Splinting

Dynamic orthoses are composed of a static base with an elastic material that imparts constant tension to the desired tissues. Dynamic splints are commonly used to hold tissues in a protected position (eg, James traction splint) or for joint contracture corrections. The James traction splint pulls traction through the fingernail, using ligamentotaxis for PIPJ fractures.[34]

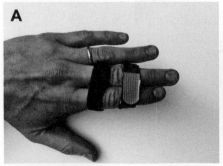
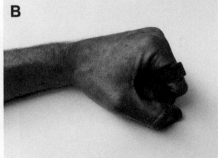

Fig. 3. (A) Dorsal and (B) lateral views of buddy straps, which allow controlled motion at the MCPJ and interphalangeal joints.

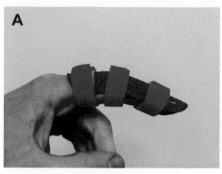
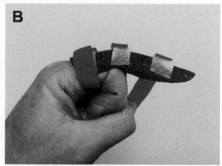

Fig. 4. (A) The dorsal blocking splint limits extension at the PIPJ while allowing for (B) active flexion within the splint.

Patients may find it difficult to wear dynamic splints for greater than 12 hours per day.[35] Flexion deficits respond quicker to dynamic splinting than extension deficits.[33] Contracture resolution is correlated with the number of weeks of treatment, with continued improvements in extension contracture up to 17 weeks.[33]

Better outcomes can be expected in patients who seek treatment earlier, those with less pretreatment stiffness, and those with flexion rather than extension deficits.[36]

WOUND MANAGEMENT

Primarily closed wounds or incisions progress through the same phases of healing as deeper tissues. During the remodeling phase, scar mobilization with various forms of massage can help reduce adhesions among the soft tissue layers, including tendons, and improve suppleness and softness to the skin. The force used should be gentle. If the force used is too great, it may cause further inflammation. Massage is typically performed with the assistance of a thick lubricating cream (vitamin E lotion, cocoa butter, and so forth) and a slow, deep circular motion performed several times daily prior to range-of-motion exercises.

Scar pads are typically made of silicone and assist in protecting sensitive scars from abrasion. Micropore or paper tape can also be used. Vibration is routinely used on incisional scars to reduce sensitivity (**Fig. 8**). Abundant sunscreen should be applied to immature scars to protect from

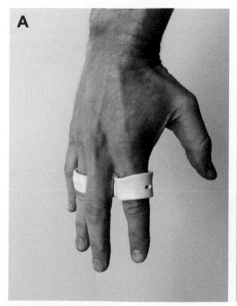
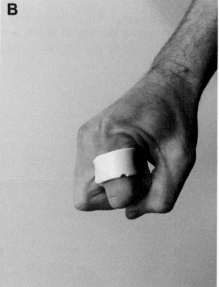

Fig. 5. The RM extension splint maintains the injured finger in approximately 30° of extension compared with the other digits throughout the range of (A) extension and (B) flexion.

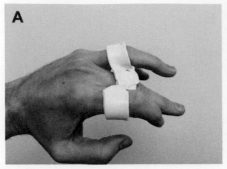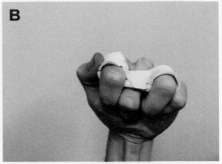

Fig. 6. The RM flexion splint maintains the injured finger in approximately 30° of flexion compared with the other digits throughout the range of (*A*) extension and (*B*) flexion.

sunburn, irritation, and darkening. Immature scars are pink or red, thick, itchy, or sensitive. Keloid scars involve hypertrophy of skin tissues beyond the initial zone of injury, are less amenable to therapy, and have a high recurrence rate.[7] Skin scar tissue that is limiting motion can be gently stretched to the point of scar blanching.[37] Pressure garment therapy, silicone sheets, and silicone sprays may help in preventing scar hypertrophy.[38]

Open or granulating wound management focuses on débridement of necrotic tissue while maintaining the fragile granulation tissue of the wound bed to allow continued healing. Techniques for gentle wound débridement include using soap and water, pulsed lavage, frequent dressing changes, and whirlpool therapy. Thicker eschars can be débrided surgically or enzymatically.

EDEMA CONTROL

After an injury or surgery, the inflammatory cascade causes increased leakage of proteinaceous material from capillary beds into the interstitial space resulting in swelling. Acutely, swelling reduces the pliability of the skin, restricting motion. Chronically, the deposition of proteins and collagen can result in scarring and stiffness. In addition to stiffness, finger edema may cause altered sensitivity and discomfort.

Increases in the severity and area of edema contribute to a proportional increase in the gliding resistance of tendons in cadaveric studies.[39] Reduction in postoperative edema may contribute substantially to improvements in tendon gliding and reduction in tendon adhesions.

Methods for edema control include elevation, edema wraps, elastic gloves, string wrapping, and retrograde massage. All methods cause increased interstitial pressure and promote lymphatic and venous drainage. String wrapping is performed by wrapping a rope or cordlike material progressively around the digit from distal to proximal, left in place for 5 minutes and then removed for immediate initiation of motion exercises.[40] Utilization of multiple techniques is likely superior to using 1 technique alone.[40]

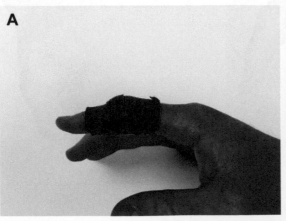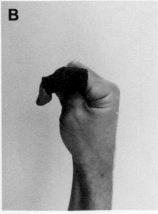

Fig. 7. Thermoplastic PIPJ splints stretch the PIPJ into extension while allowing free (*A*) extension and (*B*) flexion at the MCPJ and DIPJ.

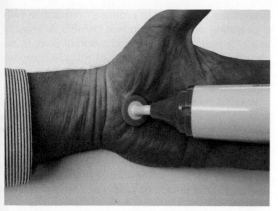

Fig. 8. Scar massage techniques include the use of vibrating devices for both softening of scar tissue and desensitization.

DESENSITIZATION

Patients with PIPJ injuries often experience some degree of swelling and stiffness. Even with minor finger edema, patients often complain of altered sensation. More significant injuries may include elements of direct nerve injury or alterations in nerve signaling with hypothesia or hyperesthesia. At an extreme, this can manifest as CRPS, a potentially devastating and disabling condition often characterized by exaggerated pain from nonpainful stimuli.

Desensitization techniques gradually reintroduce normal stimuli in a form of sensory reeducation. A typical program begins with a soft texture, such as moleskin, rubbed over the affected area several times daily until numbness occurs (**Fig. 9**). The process repeats with gradually rougher or noxious stimuli. The gate theory of pain developed in 1965[41] proposed the use of nonpainful stimuli to suppress signals of painful stimuli in the spinal cord, although more recent research has shown the mechanisms of pain and nerve signaling to be more complex.[42]

Graduated tactile stimulation is assisted by the use of various modalities including paraffin baths (**Fig. 10**), fluidotherapy, contrast baths, and putties. Extremes of temperature should be avoided during the desensitization process. A graduated desensitization program in 1 study showed statistically significant improvements ($P \leq .001$) after 6 weeks with reduced discomfort at rest and with use or touch, a decreased size of the sensitive skin area and a higher occupational performance in daily occupations.[43]

MODALITIES

Modalities is a collective term referring to a variety of techniques or devices used by therapists to assist in pain modulation, edema control, desensitization, range of motion, strengthening, neuromuscular reeducation, and tissue healing.

Cryotherapy

Cold therapy, or cryotherapy, is the application of a cold material to the site of concern to induce vasoconstriction, decrease the metabolic rate, and potentially provide an analgesic effect.[44] Delivery devices of cold therapy include cold or ice packs, contrast baths, cold water immersion, wraps, and coolant sprays. In animal models, cryotherapy has been shown to decrease leukocyte-mediated capillary leak, leading to reductions in edema.[45] Cryotherapy is especially beneficial in the acute postinjury period and once active motion has been initiated. Caution should be advised in patients with sensory nerve injuries or impairments.

Heat Therapy

Heat therapy can be delivered through paraffin baths, thermal ultrasound, heating pads and wraps, and warm soaks. Therapeutic temperatures range from 36°C to 45°C.[44,46] In contrast to

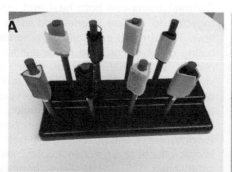
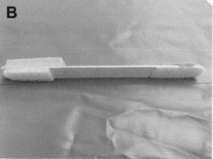

Fig. 9. (*A*) A hand therapist's toolbox of textiles with varying degrees of roughness used for desensitization. (*B*) Patients are given a modified tongue depressor with 4 textures for use at home.

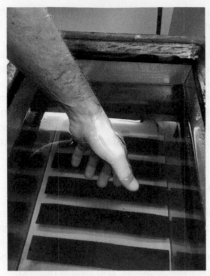

Fig. 10. Paraffin baths are widely used for heat therapy and tactile desensitization.

cold therapy, heat therapy increases blood flow through vasodilation, helping to remove inflammatory agents and pain mediators and reduce edema and pain. It also increases collagen extensibility and may help decrease muscle spasms.[45] Heat therapy may be most beneficial once a patient's therapy protocol allows for active motion. Caution is advised in the presence of moderate to severe edema due to the possibility of exacerbating the swelling.

Ultrasound

Ultrasound has a wide range of applications and can be generally categorized as either thermal (also known as continuous ultrasound) or nonthermal (also known as low-intensity or pulsed ultrasound). Thermal ultrasound is generally used as a form of heat therapy given its heating effect on deeper tissues. Nonthermal ultrasound has a wide range of clinical applications from improvement in fracture healing,[47] joint pain from osteoarthritis,[48] and tendon healing in acute injuries.[49,50] It has questionable effects on chronic tendinopathies.[51–53] The evidence for ultrasound is limited by the wide range of clinical applications, variations in protocols, and low-level evidence studies.

Electrical Modalities

Electrical modalities are generally used for either pain modulation or neuromuscular reeducation.

Neuromuscular electrical stimulation (NMES) is performed by passing an electrical impulse from through electrodes placed on the skin over targeted muscles. Individual muscle bellies or muscle groups are stimulated to produce contraction with a pulsating alternating current. NMES is broadly used for motor relearning, reduction of pain, muscle strengthening, prevention of muscle atrophy, prophylaxis of deep venous thrombosis, and improvement of tissue oxygenation.[54]

In hand therapy, NMES is useful to slow disuse atrophy, neuromuscular reeducation after tendon transfer, facilitate tendon gliding after tendon repair or tenolysis, and reduce edema through motion activities, which promote venous and lymphatic drainage. NMES may be particularly useful in patients hesitant to attempt active motion.

Transcutaneous electrical stimulation (TENS) units connect to electrodes placed on the skin and transmit either low-frequency high-intensity or high-frequency low-intensity pulsed currents.[44] The electrical stimulation is thought to modulate nerve pathways and reduce pain. A Cochrane review showed weak evidence to support the use of TENS for acute pain.[55]

Fluidotherapy

Fluidotherapy is a dry heat modality consisting of finely divided solids suspended in an air stream, combining heat therapy and tactile stimulation. It is an effective agent in raising the temperature of deep tissues in a dry environment.[56,57] In 1 study, fluidotherapy was shown to decrease the distal sensory latency of the superficial radial sensory nerve action potential.[58]

Paraffin Therapy

Paraffin baths (see **Fig. 10**) are 1:7 mixtures of mineral oil and paraffin wax heated to 53°C. Although widely used as a heat and tactile modality, there is a paucity of evidence on its effects. A Cochrane review showed short-term benefit of paraffin baths in combination with exercises for arthritic fingers.[59]

Contrast Baths

Contrast baths use both heat and cold therapy together to reduce edema and increase blood flow. The affected extremity is immersed in alternating baths of cold and hot water for predetermined amounts of time. The alternating vasodilation and vasoconstriction is thought to help promote circulation and lymphatic drainage to reduce swelling. Although widely used, its impact on edema control and functional benefit is controversial and no relationship between physiologic effects and functional outcomes has been established.[44,60] Potential contraindications include insensate hands, open wounds, heat or cold intolerance, and peripheral vascular disease.

Continuous Passive Motion

Continuous passive motion devices cycle joints passively through a predetermined arc of motion. Theoretically, the convenience and defined parameters of motion enable patients to participate in greater and more effective daily passive motion exercises; however, there is a lack of evidence to recommend continuous passive motion after hand injuries or surgery.[27,61,62]

THE HAND THERAPIST, PHYSICIAN, AND PATIENT RELATIONSHIPS

Hand therapy programs are often recommended after injuries to PIPJ due to the frequency of finger edema and stiffness. Communication between the hand therapist, surgeon, and patient is critical for ensuring the protection of injured/repaired structures while allowing early mobilization for optimal outcomes. Explicit limitations on motion or activity should be made clear to the patient and therapist. Providing the therapist with an operative note may clarify the extent and specifics of the injury to better guide rehabilitation.

Participation in hand therapy and home exercise programs is crucial for many types of PIPJ disorders. Poor compliance with hand therapy after Dupuytren release for severe PIPJ contracture results in worse outcomes.[63] Patients with higher costs of hand therapy visits attend therapy less and have worse outcomes after flexor tendon repair.[64] The optimal amount of therapy varies by injury pattern and patient. One study showed no clear relationship between the amount of hourly motion exercises and final active or passive range of motion after flexor tendon repair.[65]

SUMMARY

The principles of hand therapy for PIPJ disorders include protecting injured structures, minimizing patient discomfort, and optimizing patient recovery. Orthoses are commonly used in the earlier phases of healing for soft tissue rest, protection, and comfort. Experienced hand therapists use a range of modalities for edema control, pain reduction, desensitization, and neuromuscular reeducation. Guided motion exercises and home exercise programs help prevent adhesions and stiffness. The utilization of hand therapy programs results in better patient outcomes for many types of PIPJ injuries.

REFERENCES

1. Posner MA, Green SM. Diagnosis and treatment of finger deformities following injuries to the extensor tendon mechanism. Hand Clin 2013;29:269–81.

2. Schreuders T. The quadriga phenomenon: a review and clinical relevance. J Hand Surg Eur 2012;37: 513–22.

3. Cooper C. Fundamentals: hand therapy concepts and treatment techniques. In: Cooper C, editor. Fundamentals of hand therapy. 2nd edition. St Louis (MO): Mosby; 2014. p. 1–14.

4. Thomopoulos S, Parks WC, Rifkin DB, et al. Mechanisms of tendon injury and repair. J Orthop Res 2015;33:832–9.

5. Comer GC, Clark SJ, Yao J. Hand therapy modalities for proximal interphalangeal joint stiffness. J Hand Surg Am 2015;40:2293–6.

6. McGee CW. Preventing and treating stiffness. In: Cooper C, editor. Fundamentals of hand therapy. 2nd edition. St Louis (MO): Mosby; 2014. p. 524–41.

7. Dorf E, Blue C, Smith BP, et al. Therapy after injury to the hand. J Am Acad Orthop Surg 2010;18:464–73.

8. Pitts DG, Willoughby J, Morgan RK. Clinical reasoning and problem solving to prevent pitfalls in hand injuries. In: Cooper C, editor. Fundamentals of hand therapy. 2nd edition. St Louis (MO): Mosby; 2014. p. 87–102.

9. Comer GC, Gordon C, Yao J. Hand therapy modalities following extensor mechanism surgery. J Hand Surg Am 2015;40:2081–4.

10. Houshian S, Jing SS, Chikkamuniyappa C, et al. Management of posttraumatic proximal interphalangeal joint contracture. J Hand Surg Am 2013;38: 1651–8.

11. Smart KM, Wand BM, O'Connell NE. Physiotherapy for pain and disability in adults with complex regional pain syndrome (CRPS) types I and II. Cochrane Database Syst Rev 2016;(2):CD010853.

12. Ezendam D, Bongers RM, Jannink MJA. Systematic review of the effectiveness of mirror therapy in upper extremity function. Disabil Rehabil 2009; 31:2135–49.

13. Moseley LG, Gallace A, Spence C. Is mirror therapy all it is cracked up to be? Current evidence and future directions. Pain 2008;138:7–10.

14. Ugurlu U, Ozdogan H. Effects of serial casting in the treatment of flexion contractures of proximal interphalangeal joints in patients with rheumatoid arthritis and juvenile idiopathic arthritis: a retrospective study. J Hand Ther 2016;29:41–50.

15. Wu YF, Tang JB. Tendon healing, edema, and resistance to flexor tendon gliding. Hand Clin 2013;29: 167–78.

16. Cao Y, Tang JB. Resistance to motion of flexor tendons and digital edema: an in vivo study in a chicken model. J Hand Surg Am 2006;31:1645–51.

17. Korstanje J, Schreuders T, van der Sijde J, et al. Ultrasonographic assessment of long finger tendon excursion in zone V during passive and active tendon gliding exercises. J Hand Surg Am 2010; 35:559–65.

18. Horii E, Lin GT, Cooney WP, et al. Comparative flexor tendon excursion after passive mobilization: an in vitro study. J Hand Surg Am 1992;17:559–66.

19. Wehbe MA. Tendon gliding exercises. Am J Occup Ther 1987;41:164–7.

20. Fess EE. A history of splinting: to understand the present, view the past. J Hand Ther 2002;15: 97–132.

21. Birman MV, Rossenwasser MP. Proximal interphalangeal joint fracture dislocations in professional baseball players. Hand Clin 2012;28:417–20.

22. van Aaken J, Fusetti C, Luchina S, et al. Fifth metacarpal neck fractures treated with soft wrap/buddy taping compared to reduction and casting: results of a prospective, multicenter, randomized trial. Arch Orthop Trauma Surg 2016; 136:135–42.

23. Paschos NK, Abuhemoud K, Gantsos A, et al. Management of proximal interphalangeal joint hyperextension injuries: a randomized controlled trial. J Hand Surg Am 2014;39:449–54.

24. Won SH, Lee SHSY, Chung CY, et al. Buddy taping: is it a safe method for treatment of finger and toe injuries? Clin Orthop Surg 2014;6:26–31.

25. Howell JW, Merritt WH, Robinson SJ. Immediate controlled active motion following zone 4-7 extensor tendon repair. J Hand Ther 2005;18:182–9.

26. Hirth MJ, Howell JW, O'Brien L. Relative motion orthoses in the management of various hand conditions: a scoping review. J Hand Ther 2016;29:405–32.

27. Glasgow C, Tooth LR, Fleming J. Mobilizing the stiff hand: combining theory and evidence to improve clinical outcomes. J Hand Ther 2010;23:392–401.

28. Flowers KR. A proposed decision hierarchy for splinting the stiff joint, with an emphasis on force application parameters. J Hand Ther 2002;15:158–62.

29. Pitts DG, Fess EE. Orthoses. In: Cooper C, editor. Fundamentals of hand therapy. 2nd edition. St Louis (MO): Mosby; 2014. p. 103–14.

30. Flowers KR, LaStayo P. Effect of total end range time on improving passive range of motion. J Hand Ther 1994;7:150–7.

31. Prosser R. Splinting in the management of proximal interphalangeal joint flexion contracture. J Hand Ther 1996;9:378–86.

32. Glasgow C, Wilton J, Tooth L. Optimal daily total end range time for contracture: resolution in hand splinting. J Hand Ther 2003;16:207–18.

33. Glasgow C, Fleming J, Tooth LR, et al. The long-term relationship between duration of treatment and contracture resolution using dynamic orthotic devices for the stiff proximal interphalangeal joint: a prospective cohort study. J Hand Ther 2012;25: 38–47.

34. Goldman SB, Amaker RJ, Espinosa RA. James traction splinting for PIP fractures. J Hand Ther 2008;21: 209–15.

35. Glasgow C, Fleming J, Tooth LR, et al. Randomized controlled trial of daily total end range time (TERT) for Capener splinting of the stiff proximal interphalangeal joint. Am J Occup Ther 2012;66:243–8.

36. Glasgow C, Tooth LR, Fleming J, et al. Dynamic splinting for the stiff hand after trauma: predictors of contracture resolution. J Hand Ther 2011;24: 195–206.

37. Moore ML, Dewey WS, Richard RL. Rehabilitation of the burned hand. Hand Clin 2009;25:529–41.

38. Steinstraesser L, Flak E, Witte B, et al. Pressure garment therapy alone and in combination with silicone for the prevention of hypertrophic scarring. Plast Reconstr Surg 2011;128:306–13.

39. Cao Y, Tang JB. Investigation of resistance of digital subcutaneous edema to gliding of the flexor tendon: an in vitro study. J Hand Surg Am 2005;30:1248–54.

40. Flowers KR. String wrapping versus massage for reducing digital volume. Phys Ther 1988;68:57–9.

41. Melzack R, Wall PD. Pain mechanisms: a new theory. Science 1965;150:971–8.

42. Mendell LM. Constructing and deconstructing the gate theory of pain. Pain 2014;155:210–6.

43. Goransson I, Cederlund R. A study of the effect of desensitization on hyperaesthesia in the hand and upper extremity after injury or surgery. Hand Ther 2011;16:12–8.

44. Hartzell TL, Rubinstein R, Herman M. Therapeutic modalities - an updated review for the hand surgeon. J Hand Surg Am 2012;37:597–621.

45. Deal DN, Tipton J, Rosencrance E, et al. Ice reduces edema. A study of microvascular permeability in rats. J Bone Joint Surg Am 2002;84–A:1573–8.

46. Artzberger SM. Edema reduction techniques. A biologic rationale for selection. In: Cooper C, editor. Fundamentals of hand therapy. 2nd edition. St Louis (MO): Mosby; 2014. p. 35–50.

47. Rutten S, van den Bekerom MPJ, Sierevelt IN, et al. Enhancement of bone-healing by low-intensity pulsed ultrasound. JBJS Rev 2016;4:1.

48. Jia L, Wang Y, Chen J, et al. Efficacy of focused low-intensity pulsed ultrasound therapy for the management of knee osteoarthritis: a randomized, double blind, placebo-controlled trial. Sci Rep 2016;6:35453.

49. Yeung CK, Guo X, Ng YF. Pulsed ultrasound treatment accelerates the repair of Achilles tendon rupture in rats. J Orthop Res 2006;24:193–201.

50. Ng CO, Ng GY, See EK, et al. Therapeutic ultrasound improves strength of achilles tendon repair in rats. Ultrasound Med Biol 2003;29:1501–6.

51. Larsson MEH, Kall I, Nilsson-Helander K. Treatment of patellar tendinopathy - a systematic review of randomized controlled trials. Knee Surg Sports Traumatol Arthrosc 2012;20:1632–46.

52. D'Vaz AP, Ostor AJK, Speed CA, et al. Pulsed low-intensity ultrasound therapy for chronic lateral

epicondylitis: a randomized controlled trial. Rheumatology 2006;45:566–70.

53. Khanna A, Nelmes R, Gougoulias N, et al. The effects of LIPUS on soft-tissue healing: a review of literature. Br Med Bull 2009;89:169–82.

54. Sheffler LR, Chae J. Neuromuscular electrical stimulation in neurorehabilitation. Muscle Nerve 2007;35:562–90.

55. Johnson MI, Paley CA, Howe TE, et al. Transcutaneous electrical nerve stimulation for acute pain. Cochrane Database Syst Rev 2015;(6):CD006142.

56. Borrell RM, Parker R, Henley EJ, et al. Comparison of in vivo temperatures produced by hydrotherapy, paraffin wax treatment, and fluidotherapy. Phys Ther 1980;60:1273–6.

57. Vardiman JP, Jefferies L, Touchberry C, et al. Intramuscular heating through fluidotherapy and heat shock protein response. J Athl Train 2013;48:353–61.

58. Kelly R, Beehn C, Hansford A, et al. Effect of fluidotherapy on superficial radial nerve conduction and skin temperature. J Orthop Sports Phys Ther 2005;35:16–23.

59. Welch V, Brosseau L, Casimiro L, et al. Thermotherapy for treating rheumatoid arthritis. Cochrane Database Syst Rev 2002;(2):CD002826.

60. Breger Stanton DE, Lazaro R, MacDermid JC. A systematic review of the effectiveness of contrast baths. J Hand Ther 2009;22:57–70.

61. Handoll H, Madhok R, Howe T. Rehabilitation for distal radial fractures in adults. Cochrane Database Syst Rev 2002;(2):CD003324.

62. Massy-Westropp N, Johnston R, Hill C. Postoperative therapy for metacarpophalangeal arthroplasty. Cochrane Database Syst Rev 2008;(1):CD003522.

63. Misra A, Jain A, Ghazanfar R, et al. Predicting the outcome of surgery for the proximal interphalangeal joint in Dupuytren's disease. J Hand Surg Am 2007;32:240–5.

64. Toker S, Oak N, Williams A, et al. Adherence to therapy after flexor tendon surgery at a level 1 trauma center. Hand 2014;9:175–8.

65. Dobbe JGG, van Trommel NE, Ritt MJPF. Patient compliance with a rehabilitation program after flexor tendon repair in zone II of the hand. J Hand Ther 2002;15:16–21.

Moving?

Make sure your subscription moves with you!

To notify us of your new address, find your **Clinics Account Number** (located on your mailing label above your name), and contact customer service at:

Email: journalscustomerservice-usa@elsevier.com

800-654-2452 (subscribers in the U.S. & Canada)
314-447-8871 (subscribers outside of the U.S. & Canada)

Fax number: 314-447-8029

Elsevier Health Sciences Division
Subscription Customer Service
3251 Riverport Lane
Maryland Heights, MO 63043

*To ensure uninterrupted delivery of your subscription, please notify us at least 4 weeks in advance of move.

Moving?

Make sure your subscription moves with you!

To notify us of your new address, find your Clinics Account Number (located on your mailing label above your name), and contact customer service at:

Email: journalscustomerservice-usa@elsevier.com

800-654-2452 (subscribers in the U.S. & Canada)
314-447-8871 (subscribers outside of the U.S. & Canada)

Fax number: 314-447-8029

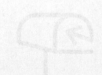

Elsevier Health Sciences Division
Subscription Customer Service
3251 Riverport Lane
Maryland Heights, MO 63043

ELSEVIER

Printed and bound by CPI Group (UK) Ltd, Croydon, CR0 4YY

03/10/2024

01040298-0012